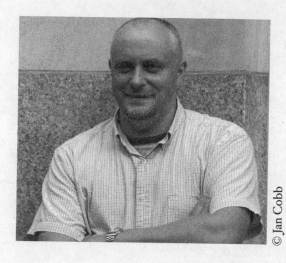

© Ian Cobb

About the Author

IAN JACKMAN has written and cowritten numerous books, including the *New York Times* bestseller *Stickin'* by James Carville. Jackman worked at a major New York publishing house, and he was also the managing director of the Modern Library.

EAT THIS!

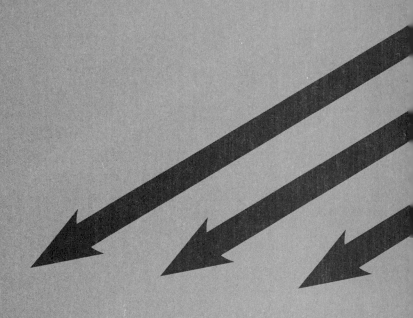

HARPER

NEW YORK • LONDON • TORONTO • SYDNEY

EAT THIS!

1,001 Things to Eat Before You Diet

Ian Jackman

HARPER

Be careful out there. I don't have any food allergies or sensitivities, so I can eat what I like. If you do have allergies, and you're interested in something mentioned in this book, make sure you check out the ingredients first.

HarperCollins books may be purchased for educational, business, or sales promotional use. For information please write: Special Markets Department, Harper-Collins Publishers, 10 East 53rd Street, New York, NY 10022.

FIRST EDITION

Designed by Jamie Kerner-Scott

Library of Congress Cataloging-in-Publication Data is available upon request.

ISBN: 978-0-06-088590-8
ISBN-10: 0-06-088590-4

07 08 09 10 11 DIX/RRD 10 9 8 7 6 5 4 3 2 1

For Kara, Sam, and Lindsay

CONTENTS

EAT THIS!

INTRODUCTION

When one considers the millions of permutations of foods and wines to test,
it is easy to see that life is too short for the formulation of dogma. Each
eater can but establish a few general principles that are true only for him.

—A. J. Liebling, *Between Meals* (1962)

Good food is one of life's great pleasures. A lobster roll from a seaside store in Maine—big chunks of meat touched with mayonnaise, topped with paprika, and piled into a toasted hot dog roll. A North Carolina pulled-pork sandwich with peppery slaw cut with vinegar. A breakfast burrito packed with chorizo and eggs smothered in cheese and green chile in a Santa Fe restaurant. Summer's best sweet corn and tomatoes you serve with your grilled chicken. A perfect sweet white nectarine. Simple, memorable, delicious.

In an age of elevated food and diet anxiety, we still deserve to enjoy what we eat. As A. J. Liebling points out, there's so much food (and drink)—surely even more than was readily available in his day. Still, it's easy to get stuck in a rut of bland familiarity. As far as what we eat is concerned, like the rest of the industrialized world, America has moved from being a nation of food producers to being a nation of eaters. In 1900, half the workforce toiled on farms. Today, while more than twelve million Americans work in restaurants, and four in ten people will do so at some point in their lifetimes, there are less than one million full-time farmers and farmworkers.

We're much farther removed from the original sources of our nutrition than at any other time in history. This is not literally the case, for as the population increases and shifts around the country, subdivisions encroach toward and onto what was once farmland. The separation is apparent, however, in how we shop for our food. Has there ever been a greater disconnect between what we eat and the food supply whence it comes? For most of our produce, we rely upon supermarkets and what they decide to stock. Before refrigeration and mass transportation, the food we bought was grown and raised nearby. Now we have to be reminded to "shop local," to buy from our neighboring farms. And when we eat out across this enormous country, we often eat the same stuff from the same restaurant chains.

So much of what we eat is banal and bland, even when it's not particularly healthy. A modest amount of exploring, away from the processed and everyday and toward the fresh and unusual, yields whole new avenues of food choice. This is what this book tries to do, to respectfully point out realms of food experience you might enjoy. Researching this book, I discovered many different foods I didn't know I liked; much of them I didn't know even existed. I'm ready to keep turning my thoughts afield: to new towns, new regions, new eating experiences—and I hope that this book will inspire you to do the same.

The best place to start looking for new food to eat is right where you are. Think, what grows locally? In many towns, farmers bring the produce to the people, at green markets that are springing up to satisfy our increased interest in fresh food. Seek and you will probably find a cornucopia—the never-ending horn of plenty of mythology overflowing with food and drink. It may well look something like what Prudence Wickham grows in the first chapter.

So what are the *Eat This* criteria? One key word is *local*. (Think global, eat local, as someone smart once said.) Our focus is on locally bought food and neighborhood restaurants. I'm not interested in fancy restaurants, such as the one I went to where the waiter smugly made a point of correcting my pronunciation of a word on the menu. Even if he was technically correct, I felt belittled. The food itself is more important than the cool factor of the restaurant or any particular chef. I'm certainly not qualified to anoint the *best* of anything. (Who is?) It's very easy to get in deep water making claims about the best barbecue, for instance. The 1001 things are picked out in bold type in the text. At the end of each chapter I have picked out a couple of places and dishes that I particularly like and are worthy of a visit.

Nor is *authenticity* a particularly vital consideration. It's invariably a tiresome argument, but like all but the most zealous of libertarians, I'm prone to draw the line here, but also over there. (I won't abide carrots in my Irish stew, but I feel that my proprietary attitude is allowed because my mother's Irish.) The key factor is, the food just has to be *good*.

What I seek is a mouthwatering cross section that everyone, including me, can seek to experience. After living my first twenty-eight years in the United Kingdom, I moved to the United States in 1992. I've been constantly amazed and excited by the food I've found in my new home country. All the time, I'm discovering a New World of eating. Throughout the book, I've relied on the help of local experts (and my friends) to point the way for me. I've tried much of the food discussed in this book, but what I haven't comes recommended by other people in parts of the country I've yet to visit. This book has turned into my personal reference guide and eating to-do list. Not much beats happening upon a place on the way from one town to another, tasting something you've never tried, and loving it. I can't wait for the new eating delights that await me. I hope you can join me for some of them.

As for the subtitle, I've never found that "dieting," as such, works for me. The thought of being "on a diet" is debilitating, but I do try to watch what I eat, which isn't the same thing as being on a diet. Within the bounds of generally healthy and sensible eating there is a lot of latitude, which is where this book resides for me.

A word about the organization of this book. The most efficient way to categorize the food mentioned here was to think of how we eat it. Unless we grow the stuff ourselves or forage for it in woods and hedgerows, we get sustenance in one of two ways. Either we go shopping for ingredients that we prepare ourselves or we pay someone else to make the food for us in a restaurant or a similar commercial enterprise. So, in part one, we look at the fruits and vegetables, the meat and fish, the sauces and preserves we prepare at home or eat as they come. Along the way, we might digress to discuss a little of the history of one food, or how another is grown or raised. (I find a little bit of context makes for a tasty condiment.) Then, in part two, there are the individual dishes and meals we buy complete. So the sausage is in the first section, the hot dog in the second. Part one and part two: ingredients and meals; eat in and eat out.

Please note that within this general rubric, we're not sticking to any hard-and-fast rules. Many people, this shopper included, are undisciplined food marketers. Out we go to buy some fruit, and a couple of pounds of sausage find their way into the basket. And we're quite likely to stop at the ice cream stand on the way back home. Some terminological inexactitude and category laxity are allowed, where it's convenient. So, for example, there are restaurants mentioned in part one. For our purposes, the tomato is a fruit and sweet corn, a vegetable. And what to do with candy and ice cream, which are produced for us? They don't constitute a meal, at least not usually, so they go in part one, where the sauces and preserves reside for the same reason. Pastrami sandwiches stay in the deli section and not the sandwich section. To smooth over any inconsistencies and to facilitate navigation, there are two indexes, one by food and one by region, and there is contact information for the establishments mentioned.

Two other notes: The shopping information is added to show you what you can find online or over the phone. In most cases, I haven't ordered from these sources, though in many I certainly intend to. So I'm not endorsing one over another, nor am I vouching for the quality of the products they sell.

Stores and restaurants open and close and change locations. Restaurants are notoriously difficult to keep open. Cabana Carioca, my favorite eatery in Midtown Manhattan, for one, closed down during the period I was writing this book. Many of the places we feature in this book have been open for decades, but it's inevitable that one or two will succumb to redevelopment or some other form of attrition over time. We apologize in advance should this prove to be the case. Also, if I mention a price for something, there is, of course, no guarantee that it will be the same tomorrow or whenever you happen to be passing by. And menus change too. As I know to my cost, it's always best to call ahead before you set out for somewhere . . . Of course, we've also tried to ensure that the contact information we've included is up-to-date, but e-mail addresses and phone numbers are subject to change as well.

Toward the end of my eating research, I sat late one night, pleasantly full of wonderful fresh seafood, in a restaurant in the West Village in New York City with an old friend and two professional chefs from the West Coast, one of whom was my friend's husband. The chefs had been in New York a couple of days and had eaten at numerous restaurants old and new, well known and otherwise, the length and breadth of the city. As the two compared notes, I listened with fascination. The chefs used the precise language of the experienced and highly-trained expert—how fresh or vital this or that ingredient was, or how a particular piece of charcuterie was slightly rancid, or how a wine had a woodsy or mushroomy aroma. What they returned to, though, when they talked about the food, was whether it was prepared with *love* or with *soul*. "There's no love there," one would say of a particular restaurant, "there's no soul."

Thinking back, my best *Eat This* experiences have been about food that was made and presented with this love and soul I heard being described. In some cases, I believe you can actually taste it in the food. Come share the pleasure. As I found researching this book, people enjoy talking about good food and like nothing better than passing on recommendations. So make your own food lists. Take a friend and stop at that old neighborhood restaurant you've driven by a hundred times. Spend a little more at the farm stand for locally produced fruit and vegetables. Eat something you've never tried before.

Thinking about all this food has spiked my appetite, so let's eat.

Part I

EATING IN

1

FRUIT (MOSTLY)

We had an abundance of mangoes, papaias and bananas here, but the pride of the islands, the most delicious fruit known to men, cherimoya, was not in season. It has a soft pulp, like a pawpaw, and is eaten with a spoon.
—Mark Twain's Letters from Hawaii (1866)

Route 25 winds through the farmland and vineyards of the North Fork of Long Island. By the side of the road in the village of Cutchogue sits the Wickham family farm stand, where the main attraction is the wonderful local fruit. If you stop there once during the high summer season, it's almost impossible to drive straight past ever again. As you approach, you'll start thinking about the extraordinary white and yellow peaches or the tiny Suffolk red grapes. You'll wonder what that morning's sweet corn is like. Then your mind will wander to one of the many varieties of tomato; then to the blueberries, blackberries, and raspberries. By the time you're contemplating what's in the cheese locker today and you remember the homemade doughnuts, you've turned off the road and into the dusty parking lot.

The current custodians of the family business are Prudence Wickham and her husband, Dan Heston, along with Prudence's uncle Tom Wickham. Other family members share ownership, but these three live and work here. They're part of a very long line of Wickhams who have been farming this land since 1680. When Prudence talks about the land grab the family suffered after the Revolutionary War, she sounds like she's still miffed about it on her ancestors' behalf. More recent incursions from pillaging property developers have been fended off. The family has sold development rights to their land, mostly to the state and county, and it's good to think that the monstrous and ugly houses long a feature of the South Fork, and which are now cropping up to the north, won't be built on this bit of eastern Long Island at least.

This is the kind of place where you can feel close to the source of what you're eating. Directly behind the structure that houses the retail operation are the pick-your-own apple and peach trees. Buy some of the family's produce and talk to Prudence Wickham for a couple of minutes. She grew all the crops here, so she can tell you everything you could possibly ever think to ask about them, including their lineage and the history of the land they grow on. The location of the farmhouse has changed more than once. It's now situated down a lane that begins behind the stand and through the fruit trees. "You want to have a buffer between you and the rest of the community," says Prudence. "Everybody wants to live next to a farm, until they live next to a farm."

Cutchogue is situated on a narrow sliver of rich farmland between the abundant waters of Peconic Bay and Long Island Sound. Says Prudence, "It used to be that anyone who was farming out here was also working the water. When my great-grandfather was farming he did as much with the water as he did with the land. He did the farming in the summer; in the winter he was mostly working the bay and had one of the largest fleets of boats out here doing commercial fishing. That has changed because farming has specialized more and the knowledge required to put these crops out has increased. Farmers have been forced to make the decision: Are you going to go fishing or are you going to stick with the land?" The Wickhams decided to stay ashore, although nothing is far from the water in this part of the world—there's water on three sides of the farmland. The Wickhams own about 292 acres, but some of that is salt marsh, where food crops won't grow. After the Second World War there was an initiative to make the country self-sufficient in food. The Army Corps of Engineers helped design a system of dikes that drains when the tide is low and blocks the water when the tide is high. Priorities have changed since the forties. "Imagine messing around with the wetlands today," Prudence says. "Drying them up so you could farm. It's a whole different culture, and people's expectations are different. We're careful with them."

The location does have its benefits: water retains heat better than soil, so among other things, the buds of fruit trees and bushes don't freeze during cold snaps in the spring. The other factor is the sun—fruit needs a lot of sunlight to ripen, and Cutchogue officially gets more hours of sunshine than any other town in New York State; more than the sometimes fog-bound Hamptons, a few miles south. So the Wickhams are able to grow fruit you wouldn't expect to find this far north, like nectarines and apricots.

When the Long Island Railroad started running between the city of Brooklyn and Greenport in 1844, no one was growing nectarines in Cutchogue. Farming was concentrated on vegetables like Brussels sprouts, potatoes, broccoli, and cauliflower. The farm also produced seeds, and at one time the Wickhams were the world's largest suppliers of cauliflower, broccoli, and Brussels sprouts seeds. The railroad changed the farmers' focus from local markets to the big one in New York City. Today, if you take the first left from the farm stand, you'll find yourself on Depot Road, so called because there used to be a train stop there, with a storehouse to hold potatoes for shipment to New York. Prudence's father, Jack, remembers the building being in use when he was a teenager.

For years the business was strictly wholesale. Then the farm started producing peaches and plums. Initially the fruit was sold from the back of a truck, then from a skid that was pulled down to the roadside every morning and back up to the farmhouse at night. After the Second World War, Prudence's grandfather John Wickham was sent to Argentina by the World Bank to help local farmers with their potato crops. In Argentina, John ate a nectarine and had some kind of eureka moment. He figured out that the place in Argentina that grew the nectarine he was eating was about the same distance from the equator as his farm in Cutchogue. He thought there was no reason why he couldn't grow this fabulous fruit himself. With all the nearby farms producing potatoes and vegetables, he was on the lookout for a new niche, and this was the perfect solution. John came home, and the first trees went in. The farm stand was built to sell this first crop of nectarines.

Two-thirds of what Prudence produces today is for the retail market. Retail is a completely different game from the wholesale business. It's a specialty market catering to people looking for items they can't find in the grocery store. These are discerning customers who are prepared to pay a premium for the freshest high-quality produce. Wholesale, the farmer has to worry about appearance and uniformity first and second, and taste somewhere down the line. He also needs produce resilient enough to stand transportation. "It's gotta be able to bounce," as Prudence puts it.

Take the average supermarket tomatoes. While they are tasteless, pale, and woody, they manage by some miracle to be all the same shape and size. (If this is what customers want, when did we get to be so dumb?) Prudence's tomatoes have blemishes; they're of different sizes and odd shapes, but inside they're almost crimson in color, and they taste fantastic. Bite into a vine-ripened tomato, sprinkled with sea salt, and eat it with crusty bread and some nutty **Manchego cheese** out of the Wickhams' cold cellar. Summer eating doesn't get any better. (The Wickhams provide everything you need for lunch—baguettes are shipped in from a bakery in Brooklyn. I ate mine with the obligatory tomato and Spanish **Valdeon cheese,** a salty cow/goat's milk semi-hard cheese wrapped in sycamore leaves.)

While Prudence and I are talking, Tom Wickham stops by and I ask him about the ripening of tomatoes. The Wickhams let their tomatoes ripen on the vine, and they pick them and bring them straight to the stand. Larger operations will pick their fruit when it's green and truck it long distances to where it needs to be. The process of ripening fruit can be artificially prompted by exposing it to ethylene gas. If you pump ethylene into the trailer containing the tomatoes and drive three days, your tomatoes will arrive a uniform reddish color. But they're not actually ripe—they've just been fooled by the gas into coloring up. This is why supermarket tomatoes often feel like baseballs.

Much of the reason Prudence sells directly to the public is that she can't afford to accept what wholesalers will give her. While a wholesaler might pay 50 to 52 cents a pound for apples—a price that has been constant for a couple of years—she can't afford to sell them for less than $1.20, which means she has to bypass the middleman and sell directly to the public. The Wickhams' costs are high. Everything has to be trucked out to the eastern end of Long Island. Gas is like gold, labor is expensive, and basic agriculture costs more, too. If you want to spread lime, it'll cost about thirty-five dollars a ton in Cutchogue, three times what it might cost at the eastern shore of Maryland, say, where the land is very similar.

It has long been a Wickham expectation that family members establish a career away from the farm, or get a college degree, before they decide whether they want to work the land full-time. Prudence's father trained as an engineer and moved to Maryland; her aunt has a doctorate in education. Prudence herself earned a master's degree and spent twelve years as a clinical nurse specialist at the Johns Hopkins Hospital in Baltimore, working with terminally ill children. Prudence's father remains very involved in the farm and he flies up to New York to help out on the weekends. Prudence's husband, Dan, was a professional arborist who lived a couple of miles down the road from the Wickhams in Maryland. He'd never seen the Cutchogue farm before he and Prudence got married. Prudence says that as an arborist, Dan was used to working with huge trees, so switching to more diminutive fruit trees was a piece of cake. "You people are sweating about pruning *these?*" Dan said upon seeing the farm for the first time.

It's obvious that Prudence has attacked her second career with gusto. She's very proud of the farm and the varied bounty it produces. Prudence points out that most farm stands specialize in one to six crops, but the Wickhams sell twenty-nine. The stand is open as soon as the asparagus and rhubarb are ready, in April, and it operates until the apples run out, which is around Christmas Eve. Ask her to choose what she likes to eat best and Prudence finds it very difficult to favor one fruit or vegetable over any other. She enjoys the sweet and tart Mutsu apple. And while she likes the strong flavor of a great yellow peach, when a sweet white peach like a Raritan Rose comes in, Prudence prefers that. Of the Raritan Rose, she says, "When they are really going, they're just to die for."

The peaches were magnificent this particular year. The abundant sunshine we enjoyed made for fine fruit, although dry weather meant higher costs for the farmer. The trees that John Wickham planted aren't on the irrigation grid that serves much of the farm. Water has to be piped in to stop the peach trees from dropping their fruit before it has a chance to ripen. North Fork land, however, benefits from a high water table. "Dig down anywhere here four to thirteen feet and you'll hit freshwater springs," says Prudence. "It's beautiful water—fast flowing and constant." It allows the Wickhams to irrigate at a thousand gallons a minute from one pump all summer long.

On a hot, still day inside the wooden farm stand, as you feel the weight of the ears of corn, it's easy to think that things haven't changed much around here in a long time. But the farm is a dynamic as well as a living enterprise. This long summer would turn to fall as surely as every other. Toward the end of the season there was a little more time for the Wickhams to explore some of the new ideas they're constantly investigating as they look to improve or expand their business. The farm already does a lot more than grow food. The family operates a bed-and-breakfast in a lovely old house on the road down to neighboring New Suffolk. Prudence is focusing on the tours the farm runs, which are educational as well as entertaining, with subjects like the environment, women and farming, and the process of pollination. These sessions are designed to go beyond the traditional

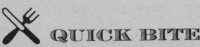

QUICK BITE

Everyone knows that Georgia is the Peach State, although it ranks third in the country in peach production after California and South Carolina (the Palmetto State). Georgia works hard to keep peaches front and center: the peach is the state fruit. In 1924, two Georgia counties in the center of the state were merged to form Peach County. About forty varieties of Georgia peaches are available from around the middle of May through August. The original Georgia peach is the **Elberta** variety, developed in the state by Sam Rumph, who named it for his wife.

farm hayride in an effort to bring people closer to the realities of the farm and farming.

Prudence is also thinking of expanding the apple cider business, first into sparkling cider and maybe into hard cider one day. The decision to start making an alcoholic product will need careful consideration because it would introduce an adults-only element into what is now a G-rated universe. But if she doesn't make hard cider, she may have to get out of the cider business altogether. New regulations require the pasteurization or UV treatment of all types of cider, and Prudence will need as much revenue as possible to make the whole enterprise viable.

Land is at such a premium out here that the farming is extremely intensive, with farmers employing all the progressive techniques they can. The result is a higher dollar volume from farming in Suffolk County than in any other county in New York. (Much of this bounty is due to the county's vineyards, in whose development John Wickham also played a role.) The need to eke as much out of the small parcel of land as possible entails some compromises. Prudence says she has to use pesticides, for worms in the apples and peaches, for example. She also has to use some fungicides because the moist environment can encourage fungi to grow.

Prudence has learned everything she knows from her family and by working on this land. There's no substitute for getting to know one place intimately, and for the ability to try something out in the field. Tom Wickham has a doctorate in agricultural engineering from Cornell, and one generation has passed down both its book learning and its experience to the next. It's all very well reading about a process in a book, but unless you know the nuances of your own land you can get in trouble. Take apple thinning, for example. There are two ways of doing it: you can pick off a percentage of the apples by hand or you can spray a hormone that causes some of the apples to drop. But different species react differently. Spray indiscriminately, and one type of tree may drop all its fruit. It's only through trial and error that you know what will work for you.

The Wickhams are always striving to learn. "When we take vacations we stop at other farms to see what's going on," Prudence says. "We're often amazed at the difference in attitude. People are much more lax. Out here we've got to be right up to date. We need to know the latest techniques. Even if you're not using them, you have to know why you're not using them."

Naively, I asked Prudence if she gets to slow down after the holidays. No chance. By the end of January, she has to be seeding tomatoes for the hothouses so they have a chance to ripen by the first week in May. She has to plant other crops, repair buildings, and plan and research for the next year. If you're trying a new tomato, for example, what's the best way to grow it? Planning reaches far beyond the next season. If Prudence decides to put in a new peach or apple tree, she's not going to see any return for seven years.

Prudence and Tom made a presentation of their fruit during the inaugural Hamptons Wine and Food Festival, at the Hayground School in Bridgehampton. Everything Prudence passed around during her lecture was grown on the Wickhams' farm, and much of it had been on the vine or the tree the day before. Guided through a smorgasbord of soft fruit, apples, berries, and melons by an expert like Prudence, you can begin to identify and appreciate subtle variations in flavor.

Prudence begins her fruit talk by establishing the difference between *flavor* and *sweetness*. Whether they realize it or not, most people favor one over the other, and the majority prefer a sweeter fruit to one with a more intense flavor. Think about a white peach (which is very sweet) and a yellow peach (which has a more intense peach flavor). Which do you like better?

WICKHAM'S FRUIT FARM FRUIT

MELONS

Amy. An orangey-gold melon hailing originally from the Canary Islands. Amy has firm flesh and a high water content. Amy's seeds are very expensive (about a dollar each).

Angel. Not as sweet as Amy, but has a stronger flavor.

Gold Star. A muskmelon, one of the cantaloupes. It has a strong odor, is very juicy, and is hard to find.

GRAPES

Suffolk Red. Specific to East End Long Island. They're very small but they burst with an intense flavor. "Don't be fooled by the size of these grapes," says Prudence. "They're hard to sell because they're small, but they're good—so sweet."

TOMATOES

Striped Stuffer. So called because (a) they have stripes, and (b) they're hollow and are specifically designed to be stuffed with something like chicken salad. This is a modern rather than an heirloom variety.

Green Zebra. An heirloom variety. Surprisingly sweet, says Prudence, and indeed it is. Prudence tells us that people say tomatoes used to be prepared so they tasted much sweeter. "The reason for that is that our grandparents used to sugar them before they added salt and pepper."

QUICK BITE

What is an heirloom tomato? It's a variety whose seeds are open-pollinated, which means they're not hybrids. Any seed, not just that of the tomato, can be heirloom. Nancy Rommelmann in her fascinating book, *Everything You Pretend to Know About Food*, says, "Heirloom fruits and vegetables are grown from seeds that have been handed down for at least three generations, and sometimes hundreds of years (not century-old seeds, of course, which would not germinate, but seeds from the plants of seeds your grandmother sowed)."

Black Krim. This strong-flavored heirloom variety has green shoulders (the area around the stalk), a pinkish bottom, and a body that can be the color of chocolate. Many heirlooms have the same green shoulders. Their refusal to grow the same size or shape, and their possession of variegated skin, are some of the features of the heirloom tomato.

Kellog. Another heirloom variety.

Tangerine Gold. This is a modern tomato, more uniform and superficially more attractive than an heirloom.

Sun Gold. Cherry tomatoes. Over the summer I buy at least one pint pot of these bright yellow orbs every time I go to the farm stand. Before I reach home, my purchase is four or five tomatoes short every time. They look great; they taste even better, juicily sweet/tart.

Celebrity. These are very hard to grow because they sunburn easily. They used to be the standard American red tomato but have been superseded by easier-grown varieties.

Prudens. The paler the tomato, the lower the acidity. Pink tomatoes like Prudens are less acidic than red ones. The paler the fruit, the more delicate the flavor, too.

PRUDENCE'S TIPS

"When you're buying melons, look for even webbing [the raised pattern on the skin], good size and color. Do you know what a good size or color is for a particular melon? Me neither, so go ask someone. Sniffing it, shaking it, thumping it—they won't work."

◆ "Never put tomatoes in the fridge—they lose their flavor quickly."

◆ "What do you do about fruit flies getting in the house [when you bring in produce]? Just before you come in, tap the [produce] container and the flies will get airborne momentarily. Before they have a chance to alight, put the container in a bag and get inside. Put the bag in the fridge for half an hour. Remove the fruit and throw out the bag and the fruit container, and you should be fine. Just remember to eat the fruit quickly."

◆ "We have beehives on the farm for pollination. If you want the bees to stay at home, block one of the two entrances [of the hive]—they will not go out the same entrance they came in."

APPLES

Ginger Gold. This is a new variety. It will take thirty years to find out if it works in the market.

Gravenstein. You see this only on farm stands because it didn't work in the wholesale market. It has a complex flavor but is an "unattractive" fruit.

Burgundy. A tart apple that's good for baking.

Sansa. This is still new, meaning that the variety was released in the late eighties. Sweet.

Zestar! Created by the University of Minnesota and released in 2003. Note: its name is Zestar!, not Zestar? or Zestar; but Zestar!

Empire. Also a product of academia, this graduated from Cornell University in 1966.

Jonagold and **Mutsu,** which weren't in season this day, are the farm's most popular apples. I love the Mutsu (which is more commonly known in stores as Crispin), which originated in Japan as a variant of the Golden Delicious. The sweet Jonagold is a cross between the Golden Delicious and Jonathan.

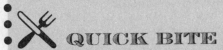

QUICK BITE

Cornell's New York State Agriculture Experiment Station, in Geneva, New York, has produced Empire, **Cortland**, Jonagold, Jonamac, and **Macoun** apple varieties that now make up about a fifth of the New York State apple crop. Geneva doesn't breed just apples. Very tasty **Castleton** plums, a European variety of plum, also hails from Cornell, among other fruit and veg.

Call ahead and see what's available at the farm stand. The Wickhams will ship gift boxes of apples anywhere in the USA: 1-631-734-6441 / www.wickhamsfruitfarm.com. Or go visit a farm in your area.

On a fabulous clear day in mid-September, the Milk Pail Farm in Water Mill, on eastern Long Island, offered a good variety of apples to pick. The locality had received upwards of eight inches of rain a couple of days before, and ponds of water stood around. The Milk Pail was previously a dairy and potato farm that has turned to apple growing in the last twenty-five years. You can cart home half a bushel (about twenty pounds) of apples you pick yourself for twenty-three dollars. This day, the farm offered **Royal Gala, Honeycrisp,** Cortland, **McIntosh, Jonamac,** and Empire, some of the earlier types of apple. Super-tart Honeycrisp is my favorite of these.

Honeycrisp, a cross between Macoun and Honeygold varieties developed at the University of Minnesota in 1991, is a rising star among apples. Although somewhat difficult to grow, the apple has an exceptional taste that makes it highly sought after. The Honeycrisp was the subject of a column in the *New York Times* where it was described as the "iPod of apples" because of the buzz surrounding it.

The Honeycrisp . . . really is kind of amazing: firm, wonderfully flavorful, tart and sweet at the same time. It's no wonder that they often sell for twice as much as other apples and that growers sound like used-car dealers when they talk about them.
—Peter Applebome, New York Times *(October 15, 2006)*

The Milk Pail pick-your-own operation opens around Labor Day and runs past Halloween and into November, if the weather cooperates. We visited toward the middle of October and found **Idared, Golden Delicious, Red Delicious,** Jonagold, **Fuji, Cameo,** Mutsu, Empire, and **Stayman.** Straight off the tree, these apples were great. Here, even the often bland and tasteless Golden Delicious actually lived up to its name.

MILK PAIL APPLE VARIETIES

The Milk Pail orchard grows twenty-six varieties of apples. In order of their maturing on the Milk Pail's trees (from Paulared to Pink Lady), they are:

Paulared	Jonamac
Empress	Royal Gala
Ginger Gold	Honeycrisp
Sansa	Macoun
Zestar!	Cortland
McIntosh	Empire

Mutsu	Winesap
Jonagold	Braeburn
Russet	Cameo
Red Delicious	Fuji
Golden Delicious	Granny Smith
Lady Apples	Gold Rush
Idared	Pink Lady

The Halsey family at the Milk Pail has been farming in this part of the world for 350 years—those working now are the eleventh and twelfth generations of Halseys on Mecox Bay. The family runs two other operations: The Country Store and Amy Flowers. The former on Route 27 (the Montauk Highway), selling apples, cider and donuts, maple syrup, cheese, jams, and honey. The store is near the turning for the orchard and its neighboring pumpkin patch. Amy Flowers is open May to August in nearby Water Mill.

Check the Web site www.milk-pail.com for apple availability. The Country Store is open all winter and will ship by UPS to anywhere in the country. Contact: 1-631-537-2565.

PLUMS

The northeastern plum season as a whole runs from May through October, but within that time some individual plums are in season for only a month and a half; some cherries, for just two weeks. So you may be restricted to what is ripe when you visit a farm stand. There are essentially two kinds of plums commercially grown in this country: Japanese and European. Japanese plums generally come first, peaking in August, while European plums are found later in the summer. In our Wickham tasting session, we tried **Methley** and **Shiro** plums, both Japanese plums. To me, the plum is an underappreciated fruit, especially when the skin is tart and the flesh is flush with sweetness—unbeatable.

European plums have darker (purple to black) skins and yellow flesh. They might be called "prune" plums, for that is the dried fate of many of these fruits. I like the big, sweet **Empress** plum, a European, prune-type freestone plum.

BERRIES

Elliot blueberries. If you grow blueberries you have to net them against birds. The Wickhams' net covers an acre. In the whole world of food, there's nothing better for you than blueberries.

Caroline raspberries. This small and very sweet variety is Dan's favorite. **Titan** is larger.

Black Satin blackberries. Zing!

QUICK BITE

At the Central Market in Lancaster, Pennsylvania, I bought some jam made from **wineberries.** I wasn't familiar with the wineberry—the gentleman at the stand told me he picks them himself along the side of the road and in the woods. A little research shows that the wineberry was introduced into this country by fruit breeders and produces a raspberry-like fruit. (The jam tasted like raspberry jam.) The plant has done so well and is so vigorous it is deemed a pest to native flora.

This is what is generally available, and when, at the Wickham's Farm Market.

May asparagus, rhubarb, tomatoes, cucumbers, greens

June asparagus, rhubarb, tomatoes, cucumbers, strawberries, greens

July tomatoes, cucumbers, cherries, raspberries, peaches, apricots, nectarines, blueberries, sweet corn, greens

August tomatoes, peaches, nectarines, blackberries, blueberries, raspberries, melons, apples, sweet corn, greens

September tomatoes, peaches, raspberries, melons, grapes, apples, pears, cider, greens

October apples, pears, grapes, cider, greens

November apples, pears, cider

December apples, cider

Unless you live in Cutchogue or New Suffolk, New York, this list is going to look different for the fresh produce in your area, but only slightly so in much of the country. North Carolina, for example, is quite similar. See the state agriculture department site: www.ncagr.com/markets/chart.htm (where there are links to farmers markets).

Like many pick-your-own enterprises, Anderson Orchard in Mooresville, Indiana, shows apple and other fruit availability on its Web site. I can see that my favorite Honeycrisp apple is available here from late August to late September. Find who near you sells what, and when.

And check out this U.S. Department of Agriculture (USDA) chart for the availability (and safe handling) of many popular fruits and vegetables: www.fas.usda.gov/htp/Hort_Circular/2005/09-05/Handling%20Charts.pdf. Many vegetables, like broccoli, carrots, cauliflower, and celery, grow at their peak in California all year round.

The most useful comprehensive Web site is **www.pickyour own.org,** which has state-by-state listings of U-Pick farms and provides availability information and picking tips for a wide range of fruits and vegetables.

PEACHES

Says Prudence, "A freestone peach is one whose flesh comes away from the stone. The other kind is the cling peach. Early peaches are always cling peaches; late are always freestone. It's not a varietal difference; it's just the way the peach *is*."

Among the yellow flesh peaches are: **Loring; Topaz,** a buttery freestone; **Jim Dandee,** a relatively new peach introduced in 1980; and **Ernie's Choice,** an even younger variety, this one coming out of New Jersey in 1991. We tried **Sunfre,** a nectarine, and a couple of white-flesh peaches, **Red Rose,** and the **Raritan Rose,** Prudence's favorite.

At the Food Festival, Prudence's audience was bombarded with small wedges of fruit, and I gave up trying to describe the flavor of each because I quickly ran out of adjectives. I sat back and enjoyed the fresh summery flavors. It's true to say that everything tasted wonderful.

Freshness can be guaranteed when you buy direct from the farm. Not only can you pick up the fruit and look it over, you can probably see exactly

QUICK BITE

On a July pizza expedition into Brooklyn I picked up a couple of pints of right-in-season New Jersey blueberries at a supermarket to nosh on for the journey home. I stood on a subway platform and broke into the plastic pack, bit into a blueberry, and said out loud, "Wow." Absolutely fresh-to-bursting, each berry was firm and smooth and alive with sweet/tart juice.

where it grew. Try the best varieties that grow near you and eat them when they have been picked that day or thereabouts and they will taste fantastic, too. You can supply your own adjectives.

In Portland, Oregon, Caprial and John Prence celebrate the finest local produce, both at their restaurant, Caprial's Bistro, and on their television show, *Caprial and John's Kitchen*. "I would say the best thing about the Northwest is our range of fresh produce," says Caprial. "The list is so long: salmon, oysters, ling-cod, berries, apples, pears, peaches, hazelnuts, cheese (both cow and goat), wild mushrooms, lamb, pork, many, many veggies . . ."

Needless to say, what you looked for would depend upon the season. "In the spring it's morel mushrooms and spring salmon," says Caprial. "In the summer it's more mushrooms, berries like **Marion,** strawberries, raspberries, **loganberries,** and blackberries. Also peaches and more salmon. In the fall there are apples, pears, oysters, more mushrooms, and hazelnuts. And, anytime, our great wines. I'd send you downtown to our farmers market that is growing each year, and we also have a market in almost every neighborhood. "Our restaurant, Caprial's Bistro, works with all these great products, so does Higgins [Restaurant and Bar] and Wildwood [Restaurant and Bar] and many other great restaurants in the city. A tour of wine country would also be great, with lots of farm stands on the way."

GOOSEBERRIES

Until I spotted a tiny, six-ounce pack of Oregon **gooseberries** at a Whole Foods in West Hollywood, I hadn't seen any of these small hairy fruits in years. The gooseberry was one of my favorite childhood fruits (together with the raspberry). My dad's aunt and uncle, who lived on our road, had a couple of very fecund gooseberry bushes in their garden, and every now and then I'd go over and eat them in reverse order of size, from the

QUICK BITE

The mild springs and moderate summers of Oregon's Willamette Valley are perfect for berry growing. A loganberry is a cross between a blackberry and a red raspberry. The Marionberry was born and bred in Oregon, and named for the state's Marion County. A Marionberry is the result of the union of **Chehalem** and **olallieberry** varieties of blackberries, and they are harvested around the second week in July through the second week in August. There's a whole world of berries out there: dig in!

The Oregon Raspberry and Blackberry Commission (www .oregon-berries.com) will sell you berry products online and has a comprehensive listing of stores selling Marionberries (at www .marionberries.com). Trader Joe's, Whole Foods, and Wild Oats are good national bets.

Washington State is another big berry producer. Author Susan Volland likes a **strawberry shake** made from the Klicker family's strawberries, served at the Dairy Queen in Walla Walla, Washington, but only in June and July. Make a meal of it with the renowned **Walla Walla sweet onion rings**.

ripest (and sweetest) to the smallest and, frankly, unripest and potentially stomachache-inducing. There was no price sticker on the pack of Whole Foods gooseberries. I asked, and they turned out to be $6.99, but I was on vacation, so I indulged. The berries were unbelievably tart. Had they been on the bush back home, they'd have been among the last I'd have picked.

There's a good reason why I hadn't run across commercial gooseberries in the United States. Gooseberry shrubs and other members of the *Ribes* genus, like red currants and black currants, are banned in some parts of the country because they host an essential stage in the life cycle of white pine blister rust, which can devastate valuable forests. No other type of plant will do; the fungal spores of the rust must visit a berry bush to spread, and while the *Ribes* hosts are unaffected, the pine trees are ruined. So no *Ribes* genus berry bushes, no white pine blister rust.

This inadvertent disease carrying means that in many states certain *Ribes* are prohibited by law. In Ohio, for example, the European black currant is a "public nuisance," and it's unlawful to "possess, transport, plant, propagate, sell, or offer for sale, plants, roots, scions, seeds or cuttings of these plants . . ." (And, come to think of it, I never see red currants.) It's not a consistent ban: in some places gooseberries are reprieved; in others they're banned.

In any case, my Oregon gooseberries must have been American gooseberries, not the European variety I knew. Over here, the fruit is smaller and rounder, while the British version can grow to the size of a small plum, provided some small boy doesn't grab them before they're ripe. Gooseberries wilt under intense sunlight, so they'll take in Oregon and northern California, where the season runs mid-May to August. Most of the fruit gets processed rather than sold out of stores to nostalgia cases like myself. Scientists are working on a rustproof gooseberry variety, so maybe I'll see more around sometime in the future.

🛒 See if there's a Whole Foods near you: www.wholefoodsmarket .com.

KIRSTEN DIXON'S ALASKA

Two hundred miles northwest of Anchorage, along the Iditarod Trail in Alaska, is the Winterlake Lodge. It is possible to reach the lodge by trail, but only under your own steam, or with a team of dogs in winter. The most practical way to get there is to take a fifty-minute flight by small plane from Lake Hood, which is next to the Anchorage International Airport. In the summer, floatplanes are able to land on Winter Lake, which adjoins the lodge; in winter, ski planes touch down on the lake's frozen surface.

Kirsten Dixon owns the lodge with her husband, Carl. Winterlake Lodge is open to guests year-round. Kirsten is a highly accomplished chef who cooks in a location that presents some particular challenges, especially when it comes to shopping. There's no road, as such, so most of her food has to be delivered by air. Kirsten contracts with a number of purveyors and suppliers in Anchorage who specialize in getting provisions to places that aren't accessible by road. Air taxis ply their trade from Lake Hood, where the cheapest small plane to hire for home delivery is a Cessna 206, a single-engine prop plane. It costs $550 to transport a thousand pounds of supplies in one of these out to the lodge.

It pays for Kirsten to be extremely well organized and to plan ahead, because she can't pop round the corner for a stick of butter or a couple of onions if she runs out. She says it used to be a challenge to think about how much flour she'd need for the next three months, but now it's second nature. Another problem most of us don't face is having our greens freeze in the plane on the way home, which can happen to Kirsten in winter.

In addition to the food that's flown in, local farmers have standing orders with Kirsten to supply the lodges with organic produce. Kirsten also has a garden of nearly an acre, where she grows her own herbs in the summer months.

Visitors come to Winterlake Lodge and stay a day or two. They pay an all-inclusive price, covering accommodation and meals along with outdoor activities like dog mushing, snowmobiling, and skiing in the winter, and sport fishing, hunting, and hiking in the summer. Near the lodge is a succession of evocatively named points to observe and explore: Trimble Glacier and the Rainy Pass; the Happy River and Canyon Creek; the Upper Skwentna River and Red Creek. Kirsten always has something cooking on or in the stove, a tray of chocolate cookies to be served with locally picked blueberries, perhaps. She has kitchens here and at Redoubt Bay Lodge, which is closed in the winter, and at headquarters back in Anchorage. There are monthly cooking classes at Winterlake, with themes like "the winter kitchen" or "wild Alaska berries."

As with Prudence Wickham's, Kirsten Dixon's life revolves around food. The women might live in radically different environments but each has an intimate knowledge of the land where she lives and works. Prudence lives a short truck or train ride from one of the largest markets—and perhaps the single richest one—in the world, but her farming costs are high and her land is limited in size. It's expensive and difficult to get to Kirsten Dixon's kitchen, but she lives right in the middle of the greatest wild abundance in the country. Both women have recognized the great opportunities in their particular situations and worked around the obstacles.

There are a lot of culinary influences at work in Alaska. In Anchorage, there are people from Korea, Japan, the Philippines, and the South Sea Islands, all of whom bring something to the table. There is a Scandinavian presence, and historically the dominant influence has been from Russia. Alaska was a part of the Russian Empire until the United States purchased it in 1867 for $7.2 million. Kirsten says she finds a direct reminder of the state's Russian heritage when she comes across a **hot fruit soup** in some Arctic community.

Many Americans have found their way up to Alaska from the Lower 48. There are relics of California, like the sourdough bread that came north with prospectors at the time of the Gold Rush. Kirsten is from the

Bay Area herself. She first came to Alaska as a nurse with the public health service. Many first-generation Alaskans go there as teachers or government workers, or to work in the oil business, and end up staying on. These are people who find that the different lifestyle in Alaska resonates with them. Kirsten Dixon's third book is about what might be called alternative communities in the state, such as the group of Russian Orthodox monks who have retreated to Kodiak Island and whose great hobby is roasting coffee.

Kirsten says that many Alaskans are in tune with the food culture of their region. The *Anchorage Daily News*'s T. C. Mitchell talks about the farmers markets that have sprung up in the past few years, as they have all over the country "because people are starting to understand where their food comes from, and they like to interact with the farmers." For Kirsten, this involves taking more responsibility for gathering her own food. Someone in Alaska is more likely to go out and fish and stock up the freezer than in most parts of the country. Many Alaskans live without refrigeration, so they have to do their own canning and preserving, old practices that resonate throughout Alaskan cooking and food preparation. As Kirsten says, "It really is the last frontier out here."

CONTRIBUTION
Dana Cree

Dana Cree is a Seattle-based pastry chef and author of the terrific dessert-filled blog, Phatduck, and she now writes for Tasting-Menu (www.tastingmenu.com)—check it out.

"I grew up and still live in Seattle, so my entire life has been eating in this area. My great-grandma was a cattle rancher in eastern Washington, during the days when you still drove the cattle through the mountains to pasture each year. Her daughter—my grandma—was the cook of the house. Eventually she became the first college-educated person in our family, when she earned a degree in home economics. My youth was filled with old-fashioned cooking from the Pacific Northwest. Here are my regional specialties."

HUCKLEBERRIES

"First is a regional flavor that haunts my childhood memories— **wild huckleberries.** These dark cousins of the blueberry have an intense flavor all their own, and great staining power. They grow wild throughout eastern Washington State.

"Back then, we would take a camping trip and pick them for the week before Labor Day. Cooked into pancakes over the campfire, they were breakfast every morning. Then when we got home, jam was made, and the **huckleberry pies** began to come. The pie is best with a hint of lemon, cinnamon, and a binding starch to thicken the immense amount of juice the berries release. A reserve of berries was always frozen to ensure the Thanksgiving table would have a pie or two, but about half of them would end up on top of vanilla ice cream before the big day. My family on the East Coast searches [the huckleberry] out on visits—I think they like the name.

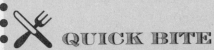

QUICK BITE

Andy Van Laar of Andy's Valley Service, on Highway 141 in Trout Lake, Washington, told me that he harvests huckleberries beginning around August 1 through Labor Day, both for a couple of local restaurants and for freezing to sell to his customers through the winter.

"As an adult I have put [huckleberries] on my own dessert menu in ice creams, cobblers, a shortcake, and my favorite, a **huckleberry cheesecake** topped with white chocolate. A regional specialty for these tart berries is a **huckleberry buckle.** The only source our restaurant has for them is a forager who will pick them while mushroom hunting. Other than that, there is a gas station in Trout Lake that sells them by the gallon."

HAZELNUTS

"Hazelnuts, or filberts, are also a large regional specialty. They come from Oregon mostly. I have recently been introduced to very nice hazelnuts from a farm called Holmquist [Hazelnut] Orchards. These hazelnuts [the **DuChilly hazelnut**] have a very delicate edible skin rather than the fibrous paper that usually envelopes the nut."

 Visit the Holmquist Hazelnut Orchards, in Lynden, Oregon, or buy all manner of hazelnut products—whole hazelnuts, flavored hazelnuts, hazelnut oil and flour—by phone or online: 1-800-720-0895 / www.holmquisthazelnuts.com.

NUTS

I have had a mixed time with peanuts in this country. On a visit to Yankee Stadium some years ago (Frank Tanana was pitching), I broke a tooth on a dry roasted peanut. Foolishly, I was chowing down on them whole, and one of my molars, weakened presumably by its long acquaintance with British dentistry, broke in two. I'll nibble a salted peanut every now and then, but my current nut of choice is the **almond.** On a trip through Georgia I picked up some **boiled peanuts** and enjoyed this regional delicacy immensely.

When people told me about boiled peanuts, they were more precise about where such peanuts are found than about any other dish. Kathleen Purvis, food editor of the *Charlotte Observer,* said, "As the daughter of Georgians who was raised in eastern North Carolina, I was an anomaly in my love of boiled peanuts. They're very region-specific: Virginians and North Carolinians hate them; South Carolina, Georgia, and North Florida natives love them."

John Kessler of the *Atlanta Journal-Constitution* told me, "The swampy land to the south of Georgia runs into Florida and Alabama, where it's peanut country: **fried peanuts,** boiled peanuts, green peanuts." (Green peanuts are fresh peanuts straight out of the field, which are said to make the best boiled peanuts, as opposed to raw peanuts that are green peanuts that have been dried.) Jacksonville native Katelyn Doyle was even more specific:

> **QUICK BITE**
>
> To represent the comely cashew nut, Linda Carucci, curator of COPIA, the American Center for Wine, Food, and the Arts, in Napa, California, nominates the "unusual and scrumptious" **Cashew Pakoras** at Namaste, an Indian restaurant in Concord, California.

boiled peanuts aren't big in her town, "but they're huge north of Palatka," a small town to the south.

As I write, I have in front of me a jar of North Carolina **salt peanuts** from Blue Smoke, the New York City barbecue restaurant. "Specially prepared for Blue Smoke by the First Methodist Men's Club of Mount Olive, North Carolina," it says on the label. Order them as an appetizer at the restaurant and carry home the leftovers (should there be any) in the jar. I love these supercrunchy peanuts.

Roberta Lawson Duyff is a St. Louis–based nutrition expert and author of *365 Days of Healthy Eating from the American Dietetic Association* and *The American Dietetic Association Complete Food and Nutrition Guide*. The city of St. Louis, Roberta is keen to make clear, is a modern and sophisticated food city. She points out that St. Louis University is one of the very few places in the country where it's possible to get a chef's degree and a dietetics certification. In the city there's a commitment to great-tasting food and to great nutrition. As elsewhere, the local markets showcase produce specific to the area. In the Clayton Market, for example, there are superb **lavender honeys** to be had. Missouri is also a center for the **American Eastern black walnut,** whose high tannin content lends it a different taste from that of other walnuts.

The Hammons company in Stockton, Missouri, processes walnuts, and provides recipes (black walnut sheet cake and brownies; **Missouri Pumpkin Black Walnut Pie,** etc.) on its Web site (www .black-walnuts.com).

Joe Bonwich of the *St. Louis Post-Dispatch* reports that the University of Missouri is engaged in repopulating the Missouri River Valley with **chestnuts,** the last trees having died out here forty or fifty years ago. There is a test farm producing four thousand to five thousand pounds of nuts a year. The last few years, the university's Center for Agroforestry has hosted a chestnut roast in New Franklin, Missouri, with samples of local chestnuts, pecans, and black walnuts available.

Both Joe Bonwich and Roberta Duyff single out the local peaches. A lovely indigenous peach crop is to be found in the hills above the Mississippi and along the Missouri River immediately to the north of St. Louis. Southeastern Missouri is in the boot-heel part of the state, and in the city of Campbell, Missouri, a peach fair has been held every August since 1944.

Between the Civil War and Prohibition, the Missouri Valley was one of the largest wine-producing regions in the country. The industry was killed off by Prohibition but has made a comeback in recent years, and good wine is being made in the region again. Roberta Duyff told a fascinating story about hardy Missouri stock being shipped to France when some of the great French vineyards were ravaged by phylloxera in the nineteenth century. There are numerous Missouri wineries once more, many using the Norton grape, which was made the Missouri state grape in 2003. Some Missouri wine is sickly sweet, says Joe, but some is very good.

CHERRIES

A great northwestern contribution to the national fruit treasury is the **Rainier cherry**. It's native to Washington State and is yellow with a rosy pink design on the skin. Rainier cherries are notable for their size. They are huge. And when they're ready, they simply burst with juice. There is a strictly limited season for these cherries, so buy some if you happen to come across them. Many are picked and sent to Japan, Korea, and Singapore. In New York they can fetch twenty dollars a pound. (I recently put some Rainier cherries on a supermarket checkout belt and the kindly cashier, concerned for my financial well-being, tried to talk me into buying regular cherries instead. And these Rainiers were $7.99 a pound, not $20.)

Visit the Olmstead Orchards in Grandview, in the Yakima Valley, east of Seattle. Here they know how to treat cherries right, so go to the orchard and pick yourself some gorgeous fruit. Having been warned about the shortness of the season, I went to the Olmstead Web site one July 3 to order some cherries and found the season's crop had already sold out.

You can put your name down to be notified when the next year's crop of cherries is available. Go to www.olmsteadorchards.com.

Ninety percent of U.S. **tart cherry** production comes from about two million trees in a five-county region in the state of Michigan. Traverse City hosts the National Cherry Festival each July. The Cherry Republic Company in Glen Arbor, Michigan, is one of the largest producers. Jason Homa from Cherry Republic told me about the tart cherry. The first trees were planted in the nineteenth century, when settlers began large-scale logging in the area. Europeans brought fruit trees with them and found the cherries did very well. The trees like the sandy soil with its good drainage. In an area hard by Lake Michigan there is a microclimate that moderates temperature swings in spring and summer. It also stays cold later in the year, which keeps the trees from blossoming too early. By the time they do blossom, the risk of frost has passed.

The Montmorency tart cherries are all ready at the same time and get moldy very fast once they're ripe. The cherries are mailed out on just one day each year, and what isn't purchased the Cherry Republic is left with to use at once, so by necessity much of the crop is processed. The tartness of the cherries allows them to be used in many products you wouldn't expect to be made of fruit. Cherry Republic sells cherries 160 different ways: jars of cherries and cherry syrup; cherry-themed baked goods and dessert toppings; cherry olive tapenade and cherry salsa; chocolate-covered cherries and cherry chocolate chili; cherry barbecue sauce and cherry mustard. Cherries are also put into nonfood products like body lotion, bath salts, and lip balm. Producers are working to develop the Balaton variety of cherry, which is heartier and with a more forgiving growing season.

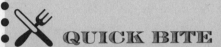

QUICK BITE

The brief cherry season is one of the fresh produce markers on the calendar each year. My friend Bud makes a fine tart **Cherry Pie** when the New Jersey cherries are ready. It's a lip-smacking pie calling out for ice cream accompaniment. Chef Eric Villegas makes a **Michigan Tart Cherry Sorbetto** at his Restaurant Villegas, in Okemos, Michigan.

Cherry Republic (motto: "Life, Liberty, Beaches, and Pie"): 1-800-206-6949 / www.cherryrepublic.com.

DATES

Every Christmas growing up I'd dig into all of the packs of dates from exotic climes we'd have around for the festive season. The fruit was so firmly shoehorned into its little coffin it was hard work to lever out the first date with the twiggy plastic forkette that came with the box. I imagine we got our dates from one of the major producers among the nations of North Africa: Algeria or Morocco; perhaps Egypt. Dates have been grown in the Persian Gulf since 4000 BCE, and today the world leaders in date production are Egypt, Saudi Arabia, and Iran.

Meanwhile, 7,500 miles west of Cairo and 100 miles east of Los Angeles lie the Coachella Valley and the city of Palm Springs. They grow dates here, too, mostly around the town of Indio. California's date growers gave the Middle East a four-thousand-year head start—the first growers here came at the start of the twentieth century—and this is a much smaller scale of operation. In California's date country the land is under heavy pressure from developers because this is a beautiful part of the world to retire to.

Sean Dougherty of the Hadley date orchard explained to me that dates need very specific conditions in which to thrive, namely, hot and dry summers, fairly cool evenings, good soil, and a plentiful water supply—pretty much what brings the retirees here, too. Date production is labor intensive, with workers having to make six preparatory visits per year to each tree. Partly for this reason, date farming hasn't broken out and grown in the area as much as that for grapes or almonds.

Many of the dates are of the **Medjool** and **Deglet Noor** varieties. I love to eat them straight out of the tub as a sweet snack, but in California, the **date shake** is the preferred vehicle. The shakes come in various flavors like vanilla or banana. Drink/eat one at the Riverside County Fair and Date Festival, held each February in Indio.

Sweet Energy of Colchester, Vermont, will ship Medjool and Deglet Noor dates, Turkish figs, ginger, apricots, and other lovely treats. Contact: 1-800-979-3380 / www.sweetenergy.com.

I've found dates featured to great effect in a couple of wonderful dishes. At Lupa, in New York City, you must try the **Apician Spiced Dates with Mascarpone**. *Apician* can refer to Marcus Gavius Apicius, a Roman chef who, two thousand years ahead of his time, wrote a cookbook. On the other hand, *Apician* can simply mean "fancy," in an epicurean sense. This date recipe is not in Apicius's book, but it is in *Cooking for Mr. Latte*, by the

New York Times's Amanda Hesser. Eat the dish and read the recipe and you'll see that the spiciness is provided by peppercorns, allspice, cloves, and honey, while orange and cinnamon add depth to the rich, complex sauce. At Lupa, the dates plump up wonderfully, with spicy and slightly tart flavors cutting the sweetness of the date with a touch of creamy cheese beneath. Fantastic.

Chef Janos Wilder presents an **Oaxacan Avocado, Date, and Tangerine Salad** with romaine, anise-citrus vinaigrette, pepitas, and queso fresco at his J Bar, in Tucson. It's a lovely, fresh appetizer salad with a lot of zing. (Pepitas are pumpkinseeds, by the way.) The dates are the chewiest ingredient in the salad, so they stick around your mouth, washed by the sweet tangerine juice and vinaigrette mingled with the crunchy seeds and the smooth avocado. There's such a lot going on here, you'll find quite different sensations to savor the second time you try the dish.

In terms of growing food, the most abundant state in the nation is California. The variety of fine produce available is stunning. I recall my first visit to a fresh market in California, a large fresh-food emporium in San Jose. My friends and I were picking up a picnic lunch, and our cart swelled with glorious fruits and cheeses. This was the first time I'd seen a **pluot,** the artificially engineered plum/apricot hybrid. Its boldly colored flesh is super sweet, and I remember well being knocked out by the things.

ORANGES

About half of all the nation's fruit acreage is concentrated in the state of California. While Florida outstrips California in total orange production (in 2006–2007, by about 135 million boxes to 33 million boxes; 33 million boxes of oranges is about 1.25 million tons of fruit), if you're eating a **navel orange,** it's likely to be from California. The most popular eating orange, and the Florida staple, is the **Valencia** orange. Navels start to come in around the middle of November and last into the late spring (in Florida through the end of January). Valencias are commonest March to June.

Around the holidays, I love to pick up little crates of **clementines.** Clementines, usually from Spain, are a cross between an orange and a man-

QUICK BITE

The pluot is one of the creations of the California company Zaiger Genetics, founded by biologist Floyd Zaiger, which has also made the aprium (a cross between an apricot and a plum); the nectaplum; the nectarcot; the peacotum (peach/apricot/plum); and the plumcot.

I picked up a few **Honeydew nectarines** at Schmidt's Market in Southampton, New York, this summer. It is a smallish, pale green fruit with a matte finish. The flesh was a uniform light lime green, too, and there seemed to be a whiff of melon about the taste, which was full of flavor and slightly less sweet than that of a regular nectarine. They're well worth tracking down. Despite the name, there's no honeydew in the Honeydew nectarine; it is the result of crossbreeding among nectarine varieties only. The fruit is a trademark of the Ito Company of Reedley, California, and it loves the heat of the San Joaquin Valley. Ito also developed the Mango™ Nectarine (not related to a mango) and the UFO white peach (not related to any alien life-form.) Check out www.itopack.com for all their exclusive fruits.

Before we get too sniffy about artificial hybrids, most of what we eat, vegetable and animal, has been bred to our specifications. Take the carrot. It is not naturally orange, but was made that way hundreds of years ago by loyal Dutch farmers who decided that their national color was more patriotic than the vegetable's regular purple, white, or yellow.

darin. As with all citrus fruit, pick one up. If it feels like a piece of cotton wool, there's not going to be a lot of juice in it. Mountains of oranges, tangerines, and clementines say Christmas to me.

Citrus lends itself well to shipping. Check out the produce at Melissa's, of Los Angeles, including **blood oranges, Cara Cara oranges,** lemon-impersonating **Bergamot oranges,** and **Tarocco oranges,** red fruit originally grown in Italy but now produced in California: 1-800-588-0151 / www.melissas.com.

The Showcase of Citrus, in Clermont, Florida, just ten minutes from Disney World, has a pick-your-own operation (closed May–October). It will ship boxes (bushels, half bushels, and quarter bushels) of mixed types of oranges, grapefruit, Honey-bells, tangerines, and **kumquats**: 1-352-394-4377 / www.showcaseofcitrus.com.

The fecundity of California's eighty thousand farms is demonstrated by the claims so many California towns make to being the "world capital" of one particular food crop or another. My attention was drawn to this fact by a fun article in the *Los Angeles Times* by Andy Meisler. Here are Gridley, World Kiwi Capital; Castroville, World Artichoke Capital; Corona, World Lemon Capital; and Yuba City, World Prune Capital, all towns demonstrating their civic pride and marketing chops. Pull off the road and wind down your window for a different taste of California, says Meisler, only don't roll down your window near Gilroy, he points out, it being the World Capital of Garlic.

World Avocado Capital is Fallbrook, California, where Rudolf Hass developed the avocado that bears his name. I love an avocado split in half, with its stone removed, eaten with balsamic vinegar poured in the hole up to the brim. I'll have the other half, too, if it's going begging. In Southern California there are sundry more imaginative ways to eat an avocado. Maria Hunt from the *San Diego Tribune* — San Diego is about an hour from Fallbrook — suggests an **avocado shake,** a Vietnamese specialty made from avocado, condensed milk, and crushed ice; and **avocado toast,** ripe avocado spread like butter over a piece of toast with a sprinkle of salt on top. The name of the avocado, incidentally, comes from the Nahuatl language of the Aztecs and the word *ahuacatl,* or "testicle."

DURIAN DURIAN

The flesh is whitish or coffee-colored with a creamy texture and a distinctive putrefying smell that becomes nauseating when the fruit is overripe.
— Larousse Gastronomique (*1988 edition*)

Among the charitable, printable comparisons: overripe cheese. Rotting fish. Unwashed socks. A city dump on a hot summer's day. Historians report that Sir Stamford Raffles, who established Singapore as a British trading post in 1819, held his nose and ran in the other direction if he caught even a whiff of the dreaded fruit. Another former British governor likened the stench to carrion in custard.
— *Philip Shenon,* New York Times (*July 18, 1994*)

On the one hand, the **durian** is reviled and abhorred for the odor that causes it to be banned on the Singapore subway system. On the other, it is the "King of Fruits," beloved by devotees in its native Southeast Asia and around the world. (Durian is the king, and the tropical Asian fruit the mangosteen is the queen.) My friend Paula promised me there'd be durians at the Chinese supermarket we were visiting in Flushing, Queens. (Markets like this are your best bet for finding a durian.) Paula, who is from China, is in the anti-durian camp; her mother loves them. We found the durians, giant, frozen, and hostile-looking. They're spiky buggers—I picked one up, and the sharp barbs drew blood from my thumb. One got Bob, Paula's husband, too. Bob said you have to respect a fruit that fights back. The durian was brownish and of a misshaped globular form, and in the basket it went.

At the checkout, the frozen durian weighed in at 5.2 pounds. At $1.29 a pound that equaled $6.71. I didn't know then whether it was a bargain or not. A label on it read Mornthong, which indicated it was from Thailand, I believe, one of the main supplier nations. A durian can grow to the size of a man's head, and weigh a good deal more than 5.2 pounds. We drove the durian home, and I left it in the kitchen overnight. I closed the door in case it got any ideas.

I looked at my durian the next morning, and as far as I could see it hadn't moved in the night. Because of the vicious spikes, it's difficult to

QUICK BITE

At the Gold City Supermarket there was a fabulous array of Asian produce, seafood, meat, and dry goods. The very first item I saw as I walked in was a pile of giant geoducks, among other assorted seafood, some of which were deceased, some not. At the fruit stand were Korean melons; longan, the lycheelike fruit from southern China; Korean pears; (pond) lily root; lotus root; and so on.

Check out the recipe for Lotus Root Soup in *My Grandmother's Chinese Kitchen* by Eileen Yin-Fei Lo. The soup is a Lunar New Year specialty—the words for "lotus root" are very similar to "achieve more," which is a very worthy New Year's resolution. And Eileen says, "It is also believed that the holes in the lotus root indicate that one should think things through." Even more sensible advice.

squeeze the thing to check for ripeness (which is our instinct with any fruit). I pressed down softly on one side, using half a pack of playing cards that were on the kitchen table, and there was some give. Leaning in, I detected a faint whiff of tropical-fruit smell. What was it like? Lychee, perhaps?

Later that day, when everyone else was out of the apartment, I cut into the durian with a large carving knife. The faint odor was multiplied instantly. Again I wavered, unsure of what I was experiencing—was it an aroma exotic and enticing or a plain rank smell? The fruit is divided into lobes, with large (edible if roasted) seeds and yellow, custardy flesh. I spooned out some of the flesh and liked it well enough. Neither by the smell nor the taste was I knocked out, however. I decided I would have to get a fresh durian in order to decide. Perhaps I could pick up some of the durian ice cream or wafers I'd seen at the supermarket. When I walked out of the kitchen and back in, the smell was a good deal stronger than I had realized when I was first in there. Later, when the durian was gone and most of the aroma had wafted out the window, all was well. I had survived my first encounter with the King of Fruit.

CHERIMOYA

Mark Twain's report on the **cherimoya** was made for the benefit of the readers of the *Sacramento Daily Union*, while he was staying in Waiohinu, on the island of Hawaii. At the time, no one reading this dispatch back home could have challenged Twain's lofty claims for the superior taste of cherimoya because the fruit wasn't introduced to California until 1871. The cherimoya has hardly become a household name in the intervening years. This twenty-first-century shopper had never heard of it before he saw a few on display in his local gourmet food store. I would have ignored the pale green, softball-size fruit had I not been on the lookout for novelties to eat. If I needed reminding, the cherimoya proved it's always worth trying something you've never eaten before.

With any fruit, there's a knack to knowing when it's ripe. The two I purchased developed a blackish tinge at the extremities overnight and were softly yielding to the touch. Good enough for me. The first fruit I ate by myself. I cut it in half, removed the hard black seeds, and began spooning out the substantial flesh. The off-white meat was similar in consistency to that of a pear, only softer and creamier. It was heavily and pleasantly scented and presented a definitely exotic taste, somewhat like a lychee or perhaps a muted passion fruit. Later my wife, Kara, said she detected a hint of coconut, but neither of us is well versed in tropical fruit to be able to properly locate the flavor.

AFRICAN HORNED CUCUMBER

Shopping for cherimoya one day, I bought a fruit I'd never seen before, identified as a "kiwano," a bright orange-and-yellow oblong with blunt spikes protruding from the surface, like a puffer fish in a disco suit. The acrylic body of the fruit gave no hint as to what it held inside. Back home, I waited a couple of days until I felt the fruit was soft to the touch and then cut into it. The pale green interior held serried ranks of seeds with a gelatinous covering. I had to dig hard with a spoon to get at the insides. The flesh looked like that of a cucumber and tasted something like it only with more acid and a faint hint of green apple taste.

It seems this fruit has identity issues—it's variously known as a kiwano (a name trademarked in New Zealand), **African horned cucumber,** African horned melon, English tomato, hedged gourd, horned melon, jelly melon, melano, and *métulon*. As it is native to the Kalahari Desert, and is heavily seeded inside, the *African horned cucumber* is, as far as I'm concerned, the best fit for what is in fact a member of the gourd family. From Africa, the fruit was introduced to Australia and is now grown in the United States and sold partly for its look as an ornamental fruit, which is a polite way of saying that on taste alone it's a tough sell.

The cherimoyas I had bought were from Chile, but I wanted to find out if they were grown in the United States, too, thus qualifying them for inclusion in this book. Sure enough, I found that there are cherimoya growers in California and indeed a California Cherimoya Association. I read a little online so I could ask a couple of semi-intelligent questions of the official cherimoya contact. The cherimoya is of the *Annona* genus, the same family as the custard apple (which is sometimes called the bullock's heart) and the guanabana (aka the soursop or graviola). A couple of times I read that *cherimoya* is just another name for a custard apple, so this was the first of my questions for George Emerich of the cherimoya association.

Mr. Emerich set me straight—the custard apple and the cherimoya are of the same genus but they aren't the same fruit. He told me you can find American-grown cherimoyas in some stores between November or December and May, but more reliably from Web sites like www.calimoya.com or www.cherimoya.com, both of which will ship you four- or five-pound boxes of the fruit. Calimoya.com is the info-packed Web site of Jay Ruskey, who has grown cherimoyas on his Condor Ridge Ranch in the hills around Santa Barbara since 1992 and currently has twenty-two acres of cherimoya under cultivation.

Condor Ridge Ranch sells cherimoyas, avocados, and other fruits: 1-805-685-4189 / www.calimoya.com.

Also try 1-866-464-3420 / www.cherimoya.com.

George Emerich added, "Cherimoyas are indigenous to the high altitudes (about seven thousand feet) in the South American Andes of Ecuador and Peru, where it is frost-free, the days are warm, and the nights are cool. They grow quite well along the coast of Southern California, up to about twenty-five miles inland. They don't thrive in the lowland tropics, such as Florida, as they are not very tolerant of hot nights." Frost is also a killer—many of California's cherimoya trees were wiped out this way in 1937. Another challenge to growing cherimoyas is the fact that they have to be pollinated by hand, which is a very labor intensive exercise. There are no natural pollinators in California. In fact, the male and female parts of the plant don't mature at the same time, and scientists aren't sure which beastie performs this essential service for the cherimoya in the Andean wild.

Having learned a little about it, I find the cherimoya amusingly finicky by nature as well as being endearingly odd to behold. The outside of my Chilean fruit had slightly raised, fish-scale-shaped details. George Emerich had recommended a Purdue University Web site that reproduces the superbly informative book *Fruits of Warm Climes*, by Julia Morton. In Peru, apparently, cherimoyas are named "according to degree of surface irregularity, as *lisa,* almost smooth; *impresa,* with 'fingerprint' depressions; *umbonada,* with rounded protrusions; *papilonado,* or *tetilado,* with fleshy, nipplelike protrusions"; and the unappetizing-sounding *tuberculada,* "with conical protrusions having wartlike tips."

Together with details on every aspect of growing cherimoyas, Julia

Morton includes numerous delightfully esoteric notes. In Bolivia, for example, consumers shake the fruit and if they hear the seeds rattle, they know it's ripe, while Italians look for the skin to begin to turn yellow and for the sweet scent of the fruit to be noticeable before they'll take one home. So next time I'm looking to buy, I'll know just when my cherimoya is getting to be ripe, and I hope you will, too.

As with all the finest fresh produce, a good cherimoya has the fine virtue of simplicity. In this case, you can't go wrong if you just cut it in half and eat it with a spoon. As George Emerich advises, "The subtle flavor may be ruined by any attempt to augment it."

FRUIT (MOSTLY) SUMMARY

RUN, DON'T WALK, FOR . . .

- **Farm-fresh fruit in season.** There's nothing like stopping at a farm stand and picking up fruit that has been ripening and soaking up the sun out in the field that very day. My favorites: peaches, tomatoes, apples—though, in truth, it's all good.

- Match your **tomato** with a lusty **cheese** and balance it on some **French bread.** Sprinkle with **Fleur de Sel,** open a cheap fruity red wine, and eat outside for the best summer lunch going.

- **Blueberries.** Gobble 'em up straight out of the container (though run them under the tap first). Not just flavorful, blueberries are packed with antioxidants: so good, and so good for you, too.

- **Raspberries.** Picked yourself, if possible.

- **Apician spiced dates with mascarpone** at Lupa in New York City. Any date is great: these dates are sublime.

IF YOU'VE NEVER TRIED . . .

- **Cherimoya.** Light, sweet, and sophisticated and very easy to prepare. Definitely worth looking for.

- **Rainier cherries.** Expensive, perhaps. Extraordinary, definitely.

- **The durian.** The King of Fruit. Or a nauseating stinker—take your pick.

2

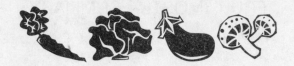

VEGETABLES

I found the hoe by the well-house and an old splint basket at the woodshed door, and also found my way down to the field where there was a great square patch of rough, weedy potato-tops and tall ragweed. One corner was already dug, and I chose a fat-looking hill where the tops were well withered. There is all the pleasure that one can have in gold digging in finding one's hopes satisfied in the riches of a good hill of potatoes.
—Sarah Orne Jewett, *The Country of the Pointed Firs* (1896)

If you think you're having a tough day, spare a thought for the fate of the trenched celery of Lancaster County. Having been grown from seed in one field beginning in April, the plants are ripped up and transplanted into another field in June and July. Some of the mature stalks, having been shielded from the harsh summer sun, are harvested from October on. These are the lucky ones. Over a few days in November, just as the season starts to turn to winter, the rest of the celery plants are cut away from their roots and buried in shallow trenches. Here the celery, deprived of nutrients from the soil, turns on itself for food, sustaining the fresh growth of a succulent new heart. Later, through February, the celery is disinterred from the cold ground, stripped down of its outer ribs, sold off and eaten.

Merv Shenk runs Hodecker's celery farm with his wife, Angie, near

Manheim, in Pennsylvania's Lancaster County. This is what is popularly known as Pennsylvania Dutch country, home to large communities of Amish and Mennonite people. I stand out in a wet celery field with Merv one August morning as the rows of transplanted celery stalks stretch out ahead of us. They stretch out, but not too far, because of the hundred and two acres on his farm, Merv has planted only ten acres of celery, which doesn't look like much when you see it in the field. But as Merv tells you about everything it takes to grow his special celery, you understand why he doesn't plant more. That and the fact that his family also runs a bed-and-breakfast business at their two-hundred-year-old Stone Haus Farm. Merv and Angie have a full house of guests this weekend, together with their three children, their chickens, cats, goat, and sheep, and fields of corn and soybeans to boot.

QUICK BITE

It was a treat for this English history buff to see a Lancaster County road sign pointing one way to York and another to Lancaster. English schoolboys and girls hear about the Wars of the Roses in the fifteenth century between the two dynasties with competing claims to the throne: the House of York (whose heraldic device was a white rose) and the House of Lancaster (a red rose). In Pennsylvania, I've seen the "Wars of the Roses" used to refer to the dessert cook-off at the Kitchen Kettle Village Rhubarb Festival (the cooks of York versus the cooks of Lancaster). In England, the rivalry is heatedly rejoined whenever Yorkshire and Lancashire giants Leeds and Manchester United play football against each other.

Merv has taken a gaggle of guests across the road that runs in front of his farmhouse to the celery patch. He's happy because it rained a quarter inch last night, after five weeks with almost no rain at all, and his celery needs the rain. More rain is promised today, which also makes Merv happy, happier than his vacationing guests, for whom every ride at Hershey Park up the road is going to be a water ride today.

In this field Merv is growing **blanched,** or bleached, **celery.** The celery is bleached by being shielded from the sun, which is the opposite of what you might expect from the name. The celery's not bleached *by* the sun, it's bleached because it doesn't see the sun at all. When exposed to sunlight, the chlorophyll in the plant turns it green, and the overwhelming majority of celery plants we see in the stores have the familiar green outer stalks. The Shenks keep their celery out of the sun either by wrapping each plant in a plastic sheet a few weeks before harvest or by burying it in the cold ground. This last is **trenched celery,** which Merv believes has the best and most delicate taste of all celery. The white-yellow stalks in the heart grow without the stringy tendons found in green celery, and they snap length-wise. The flavor is far removed from that of regular celery. This is a truly exclusive and unusual food—only a handful of farms in Lancaster, Lebanon, and York counties grow bleached celery.

The crop starts in a small patch of land behind the farmhouse and close to the well for ease of irrigation. Planting is in mid-April. Merv can hold the seeds for the entire planting in his hands, as eight ounces of celery seeds yield about three hundred thousand plants. The field holds twenty-two thousand plants an acre, and Merv might plant enough seed that he has fifty or a hundred thousand young plants over, which he can sell off before transplanting his own crop. First the seedbeds are packed down with a roller and covered to hold in moisture. At some point after the middle of June, the plants are uprooted and replanted using a special tractor-pulled planter. Four people—the Shenks get their extended family involved—sit on the back of the contraption and feed the plants into the machine. It takes about three hours to fill one acre.

When they're mature, the plants are covered by bleaching plastic held in place by wire. Thus is the sun kept off the stalks. (In the past, a clay tile sleeve would be used for this task.) From September, these celery plants can be harvested. The Shenks sell most of their celery to customers who come to the farm or from a stall in Lancaster's Central Market. In November, the shallow trenches are dug, the most laborious and back-breaking part of the whole operation, and the severed celery plants are buried in paper, straw, and plastic. This is the hardest work of the year. Referring to trenching, and smiling as he does so, Merv says that Mr. Hodecker used to say that to grow celery like this, you need a strong back and a weak mind.

When it comes to trenching, timing is important. You want the celery growing out in the field till the last possible minute, but if you leave it too late the plants might freeze where they stand. On the other hand, bury the celery before a warm spell of weather in November or December, and it might rot in the ground.

Merv believes that trenching celery emerged as a way to preserve the crop over the winter, in much the same way that people would store potatoes and other root vegetables in a cold cellar. The celery doesn't just survive like this, it thrives, growing its succulent new heart. The buried plant likes a cold winter to follow its wet summer, and as long as the temperature doesn't fall below 20 or 22°F for more than a couple of days, it will do fine. Buried like this, the celery will keep through February. The busiest selling season for the Shenks is between Thanksgiving and Christmas. Amish families will buy a big batch of celery for a wedding feast, which is held in the bride's home, and also in November or December, after the harvest is complete. Some customers will make a special trip after a frost, knowing the celery is especially good after a cold snap.

QUICK BITE

The 1918 edition of Fannie Farmer's *Boston Cooking–School Cook Book* mentions naturally white Kalamazoo celery. (She includes a recipe for **battered, fried celery** that might not suit modern tastes.) Celery was grown in the sandy soil of Kalamazoo from the mid-nineteenth century. The conditions turned out to be ideal—celery loves these "muck" soils more than the loamy ground of Pennsylvania. Kalamazoo celery became renowned nationally, in part because it was deemed to have medicinal qualities. In 1939, there were a thousand acres of celery planted, and Kalamazoo was Celery City. But blight, competition, and land development made inroads into production. The winds of change were strong: Kalamazoo became the site of the first pedestrian shopping mall in the United States, opened in 1959, and Kalamazoo is Celery City no more.

Most American celery now comes from California, where it's cut green and shipped the same day, and from Florida, where it grows from January to May, until the sun gets too intense for the plants.

The current site is the fourth location of Hodecker's celery farm. Merv Shenk learned the business from a farmer named Jay Hodecker, and when he passed away, Merv rented the celery farm in East Petersburg from Hodecker's estate for ten years. The Hodecker name was well established locally, so the Shenks kept it going. The family eventually settled in the same house Merv grew up in, working land that had been worked by his parents. Merv's forebears are Swiss Germans who moved to the area about two hundred years ago. There are enough Shenks to fill a page in the phone book, says Merv, and as we drove around we saw a street, a farm stand, and a church bearing the name.

You drive by countless fields planted with corn as you traverse Lancaster County. Merv showed us his cornfield, tattered leaves bearing the marks of a June hailstorm. This corn will be turned into cattle feed. Shenk also grows soybeans that will go to feed dairy cows or chickens, and the farm grows winter wheat from October through early July. Corn is relatively easy to grow compared with celery—harvesting takes about a half day. For that, a farmer might clear a hundred dollars an acre. While the return on celery is measured in the thousands of dollars per acre, it's about a hundred times more work.

If you always shop at a supermarket, it's possible to forget that all fresh food is seasonal. Supermarkets can ship produce in from a place where it is seasonal, home or abroad. There is nothing wrong with this, but following the cyclical tastes of the seasons can be enormously rewarding. The timing of what is good, and when, differs slightly every few miles you travel down the road. Anne Quinn Corr is an instructor in the Nutrition Department at the University of Pennsylvania and author of *The Seasons of Central Pennsylvania*. Check out her Slow Food Web site (www.slowfoodcentralpa.com) for seasonal details.

"We eat different things at different times of year—doesn't everyone? Like **ham pot pie** in the fall, after the hogs are butchered and the hams are cured. Venison in the winter, after hunting season. Fresh ramps and morels in the spring, if we're lucky and the weather cooperates.

"In the summer, it's a food fest of all sorts of local treats and we are decidedly corn, tomatoes, and zucchini dependent—not to mention the fruits—especially blueberries. Chicken and waffles is popular all the time; last night I made a version using pumpkin waffles. Apple, apple everything keeps us red-cheeked and bright-eyed—I could go on and on."

Merv Shenk told me there's a place called Celeryville, Ohio. Alas, like Kalamazoo, there is no celery in Celeryville these days, it was killed off by a fungus called fusarium. But there used to be celery, as you'd imagine, grown in the kind of lush muck soil that celery and leafy vegetables crave. Celeryville is a small town south of Norwalk and is home to the Ohio Agricultural Research and Development Center's (OARDC) Muck Crops Agricultural Research Station. OARDC is part of Ohio State University, and the station manager in Celeryville is Rick Callendar.

Curious about muck, I called Rick and he described soil types to me. The kind of heavy mineral soil that predominates in this country drains slowly. You get half an inch of rain in a thunderstorm, and it's two or three days before you can get back in and work. Muck, or muck soil, is much lighter and will drain in four or five hours. Muck is extremely rich in organic matter. A mineral soil might be 3 to 5 percent organic matter; muck can be over 40 percent, made up of broken-down vegetation from prehistoric bogs. The muck collects where land has flooded, and it needs to be in a well-drained situation. Satisfy these requirements and muck will give you bounteous crops.

Around Celeryville, people came to farm the muck. Where there once were more than forty families farming, there are now about four, growing crops in land heavily irrigated and drained using complexes of canals. Most anything will grow in muck, including the kinds of funguses that Rick Callendar investigates at his research station. You can get a crop of **radishes** in just twenty-one days, he says, and around here they grow a lot of cilantro, parsley, green onions, salad greens, turnip greens, collard greens, and the like.

QUICK BITE

Leeks are one vegetable that will thrive in muck soil. They're more popular in northern Europe than in the United States (see the Irish leek and oatmeal soup on page 200). Despite their giant green onion appearance, leeks have a subtle flavor. Braised, they are delicious; in a rich cheesy béchamel sauce with a lot of black pepper, even more so.

And Georgia Orcutt, coauthor of *Cooking USA*, speaks up for **ramps.** These are wild leeks beloved by the mountain folks in West Virginia. Ramps also grow all around New York State but aren't as widely celebrated there, she says. They're garlicky, strong, and fabulous with fresh-caught fish. There's an international ramp cook-off and festival in Elkins, West Virginia, every April.

Rick Callendar told me he often gets calls from people who have bought some land with muck soil on it. They want advice about how to grow stuff. Vegetables will grow fine in this soil, but a bigger challenge is the specialized machinery that farmers use to work it. Rick says he's seen farmers buy a piece of equipment and customize it thoroughly in their shop, like an American Chopper for farm equipment.

POTATOES

What's better to eat than a baked potato with a wedge of melting butter and some chives or scallions (spring onions)? How about some new potatoes scattered with rosemary and kosher salt roasted in olive oil in the oven? Or a helping of buttery mashed potatoes? Americans eat about 130 pounds of potatoes annually per head, in the form of spuds fresh and processed, the latter mostly French fries and chips. That's the most Americans eat of any vegetable. The popular aversion to carbohydrates has cut into potato sales in the last few years, but the next leading vegetable in the American diet is fully forty pounds a year behind, and that's the tomato (to the USDA, at least, the tomato is a vegetable).

Think of a potato in this country and more than likely you think of the state of Idaho—about a third of the nation's fall crop comes from here. If you buy a bag of Idaho potatoes, it's likely they're a variety called **Russet Burbank,** named for potato cultivator Luther Burbank, who played an important role in their development. The *russet* part of the name refers to the rough skin. The long, oval-shaped Russet Burbanks are starchy and low in moisture and are excellent for baking and frying, which accounts for their popularity. Smoother-skin varieties—like Green Giant's **Klondike Rose**—are better suited for boiling and roasting.

The city of Ashton, in the eastern corner of Idaho, is a gateway to Yellowstone. The Tetons lie to the southeast, and the city sits at an elevation of about a mile. It's this altitude that accounts for the fact that Ashton is a center for seed potato growing, the largest in the country. Farmer Clen Atchley explained why he grows seed potatoes for other farmers to plant rather than growing the crop himself. The higher elevation means a shorter season and smaller yields, but it also ensures a cleaner crop that has less disease. The reason for this factor is that Atchley's potatoes are some way from the largest potato farms, so it takes longer for insect-borne diseases to reach him.

I turned to Clen because I wanted to find out a little about growing potatoes. I asked if most Idaho potatoes are Russet Burbanks, and he said they were likely to be, though some producers had turned to the Norkotah, of which he's not a fan at all, saying it's more watery and less flavorful. Clen grows four varieties for seed: Russet Burbank; **Ranger Russet,** which is used strictly for French fries; a numbered variety (A93157-6LS) he's testing out; and a selection from the Russet Burbank that might produce better yields. Russet Burbank produces only about 50 to 55 percent "Number Ones" when other varieties might get to 90 percent. Number Ones are the top-notch individuals that go in bags for the supermarket. New varieties of potatoes are being developed all the time, but most die when you get a cellar full of them—they have a fatal storage problem. This new variety, however, was looking good so far.

Clen notes that other states might grow more esoteric varieties of potato, but it's mostly a volume business in Idaho. The J. R. Simplot Company, based in Boise, makes about three billion pounds of fries and hash browns for McDonald's, Burger King, and other fast-food chains (though not just from Idaho potatoes). Red- and yellow-fleshed varieties, even **Blue potatoes,** are grown here, but they're strictly niche crops. "Trouble is finding a market," says Clen. As for eating potatoes himself, Clen's not a great fan. He's around potatoes so much he gets sick of the sight of them. He says he can't look 'em in the eye anymore.

Clen Atchley and his wife, Emma, have three potato farms totaling about five thousand acres, together with a cattle operation, the Flying A Ranch. Clen's granddad moved out here from Tennessee in 1901, when there was still land available in the state for homesteaders. Potatoes obviously like the conditions here. You have to watch out for the weather, of course. Digging begins around September 15, maybe as late as the twentieth, as in 2006, but the weather can really turn in October, and potatoes don't like the cold. "You can get pounded," says Clen. But the water is easy to manage, because you have to apply water rather than worry about getting too much rain.

As for soil, the tubers like it volcanic. The Idaho Potato Growers Association ran a campaign that included the question "What Does It Take to Grow a Great Potato?" Answer: Take a volcano and wait a million years. Clen says he has some soil on his land that'll be good in about half a million years, once the rocks have worked their way out.

Potatoes are an expensive crop to grow, Clen reports. There's the land, the fertilizer, the labor, and the special equipment to take into consideration. After years of declining consumption, it looked like there might be a post-Atkins leveling off in 2006.

The weak dollar was helping, too, especially when it came to competing with the Canadians. But there're always the costs to cover first. And at $1,700 an acre, it means you can make money or you can get killed. Around here, Clen says, people don't have to go to Las Vegas to gamble.

JAMES CARVILLE'S FRENCH FRIES

Most of us like a good French fry, and I am no exception. About the most fabulous **French fries** I ever remember having were homemade by political analyst James Carville. James included his recipe in his book *Stickin'*, which I've adapted here, and thanks to him for that.

> Two pounds russet potatoes
> Oil for deep frying
> Salt (to taste)
> One brown paper bag

1. Take the russet potatoes. Don't worry if they sit around the kitchen a couple of weeks. The older the better, within reason. There's some chemical reason to do with starch that makes older potatoes fry better. I don't recall exactly what the reason is; just trust me. Peel 'em. (You can leave the skins on, if you prefer.)

2. Get a big bowl of iced water ready.

3. Use a good knife . . . Cut potatoes into quarter-inch strips (lengthwise).

4. Put 'em in the iced water for at least one hour, up to 36 hours . . .

5. Get oil up to 325 degrees. A good product is the DeLonghi Roto Fryer. Use that if you have one. Use peanut oil and add a couple of dollops of bacon grease for texture . . . Check with your internist. (I've done the fries in olive oil and never had a problem.)

6. Fry them at 325 for about ten minutes until they just turn golden. Do this ahead of time. Put the fries aside.

7. Five minutes before you get ready to eat, finish them off at 370.

8. Take a brown paper bag. Never use paper towels. Only idiots use paper towels. Put fries in the bag. Consistent with your blood pressure, add adequate but not too much salt. Shake 'em up real good.

9. Serve. Have some ketchup handy . . .

Serves 4

In the late summer, I read a story by T. C. Mitchell in the *Anchorage Daily News* about the vegetable-growing season that was about to come to an end in Alaska. Never having personally been to Alaska, nor having given this particular issue much thought, I was fascinated to read about all the produce that grows well out there. When I looked into the subject a little, my ignorance about Alaska turned out to be bottomless. Alaska is so enormous that any generalizations lie on weak ground, as, generally speaking, they tend to do. But it's safe to say that the seasons in Alaska are irregular, with a relatively brief spring and fall, a three-month summer, and a long, cold winter. But when vegetables are able to grow, the conditions are very good. The farmers don't need to use as many herbicides and pesticides as they do in the rest of the country, if they use any at all. Says T. C. Mitchell, "Vegetables are abundant and tasty due to the long hours of sun during the summer, and deep, rich soil. The vegetables grown here aren't much different than those in other places where truck farming is viable."

Herbs like **basil** and **sorrel** start to appear in early May, and crops keep coming through to late root crops like beets, carrots, and potatoes, which, if properly stored, can be kept almost through the whole winter. In the early fall, Alaskans will start going out to forage for wild-growing berries and mushrooms. Kirsten Dixon says that many women get together to gather berries that they'll preserve.

A FEW QUESTIONS FOR PAULA WOLFERT

Paula Wolfert, author of new-classic cookbooks like *The Cooking of Southwest France* and *The Slow Mediterranean Kitchen*, is a leading proponent of "slow food."

What do you like to eat in this country?

"I eat every day the wonderful food products we have here. With whole foods, farmers markets, and great Internet sites, no one should have a problem finding safe and delicious foods right here in the States."

What does the United States do best?

"There's never been a better time to live and cook in America. One typical American food I absolutely love is **John Cope's Dried Sweet Corn.** Check it out. They're based in Lancaster, Pennsylvania."

Are there any American dishes you can think of that lend themselves to the slow-food treatment?

"To my mind, the creation of **stale bread** (by leaving it out on the counter to dry so as to acquire texture and absorbency) is the ultimate form of 'slow cooking.' "

Order John Cope's Dried Sweet Corn: 1-800-745-8211 / www.copefoods.com.

SWEET CORN

In most of the country, fresh sweet corn is one of the delights of summer. The sweet corn brackets the season. At my house, we buy **Long Island sweet corn** all summer. In the few weeks after July 4, it isn't the best yet, though it's still wonderful to eat, with a scrape of butter and some salt. Then, suddenly, it's simply fantastic—until, equally suddenly, it's gone.

In Lancaster Central Market, in Lancaster, Pennsylvania, I'm buying some of the last of my year's sweet corn from Ruth Thomas of Thomas's Produce of Leola. It's just before Labor Day, and it's around this date that the farm switches from sweet corn to potatoes, as sure an indicator as any of the change of season from summer to fall. They'll dig potatoes (**Yukon Gold,** a yellow potato, and **Superior** and **Norwiss,** white-flesh varieties) from around Labor Day through the time of the first frost, and store them in the cellar through the winter.

I buy some of Ruth's **Argent** variety white sweet corn. It's the white corn people like around here, Ruth says, and I also pick up some small and

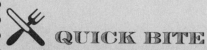

QUICK BITE

You have to buy sweet corn when you can from a farm stand. The corn may well have been growing in the field that day. The husks are a beautiful lush green and they squeak against the corn when you tear them off. Sweet corn has been bred to highlight the sugar. Off the stalk, the sugar in the corn starts to turn to starch, a process that takes about a week. The quicker you get to the corn, the sweeter it will taste.

delightful **Blake** peaches. Ruth says that everyone wants the same produce for Labor Day: corn, tomatoes, peaches, **watermelon, cantaloupe.** Sure enough, we pass a farm stand the next day and these five items are exactly what it is advertising.

Sweet corn is one of the few crops produced in every state. There are three distinct markets for sweet corn: fresh (corn-on-the-cob), for canning, and for freezing. Leading states for the more valuable fresh sweet corn crop include Florida, California, New York, and Georgia, while processed corn is grown in Minnesota, Washington, Wisconsin, and Oregon, among other states. The vast majority of corn grown in the United States is field corn, which is used for cattle feed—millions of acres of which carpet the land in Iowa, Illinois, and Nebraska.

There are regional variations in the sweet corn harvest. In Oregon, the bulk of the harvest starts later and finishes later, so the season runs from August through mid-October. In California, the season may run from June to October, but in the southern desert regions (Riverside and Imperial counties) there are distinct seasons: May–June and November–December. Florida sweet corn differs significantly from that in the rest of the country. The harvest runs January to July, with approximately a third of the crop picked in May, which is the earliest sweet corn you'll see in more northerly states.

For a few months a couple of years back, my family had a box of organic produce delivered each week from Urban Organic in Brooklyn. The system's easy: you can cancel the afternoon before if you don't need the stuff, and you can switch some of the items. The boxes range from the Little Box to a Super-Value Box, with 15–18 fruits and vegetables in the Value Box: lettuce, red chard, red potatoes, onions, peaches, plums, cantaloupe, and so on. Eventually, slowly buried under mounds of wilting chard, we gave up, but that said more about our inability, or unwillingness, to commit to cooking every night than about the quality of the produce, which was always good. Our friend Paula gets a box and systematically, and deliciously, uses every leaf within.

I always buy organic milk and eggs and often fruit, if I'm shopping in a supermarket. I'll also buy organic chicken as a rule. Look for the national standard USDA label. Some products are certified organic by Oregon Tilth, a nonprofit organization in Salem, Oregon. (Read about them at www.tilth.org, where the organic certification process is explained.) Check for organic produce where you live and compare prices and flavor. Eating organic is more expensive, for sure, and you have to decide if you're willing to pay a premium for knowing exactly what you're putting in your body.

Check Urban Organic's delivery area around New York: 1-718-499-4321 / www.urbanorganic.net.

ShopNatural in Tucson has a free local delivery area for its organic and natural products (natural is not the same as organic). The area is huge: Arizona, California, Colorado, New Mexico, Nevada, Texas, and Utah. The rest of us have to pay the freight: www.shopnatural.com.

PRAIRIE POTATO

At The Fort restaurant outside Denver, owner Sam Arnold has supervised an extensive menu that includes a lot of game meats blended with local ingredients with intriguing twists. There are frequent nods to the local history Sam Arnold is so taken with. The Fort's **Washtunkala Cast Iron Kettle,** for example, is based on an old Lakota recipe from South Dakota. It takes tips of buffalo tenderloin and mixes them in a stew with green chiles, onions, corn, and the **prairie potato.** The prairie potato resembles a black radish and goes by many names: the Indian breadroot, pomme blanche, and prairie turnip among them. It grows in places like South Dakota and Colorado. It's not commercially grown, so you have to go out and look for its carrotlike tops and dig it up yourself with a mattock.

The prairie potato was a staple for Native Americans. Just before The Fort opened, Sam was in South Dakota and met an elderly Sioux couple (the man was seventy-five or so). Sam told them he'd just built a replica of an old frontier outpost, something that would have a different cultural resonance for the Sioux. The couple wanted to check it out. They drove back to Colorado in the Arnolds' VW Bus and stayed six months. Sam learned some of the Sioux language and studied traditional herbal remedies. He says the man would take Sam out into a field and show him the plants that made up a natural pharmacy—this plant is for the heart, he'd say, that one's for cancer, and so on.

One plant that was harvested for centuries by native peoples was **wild rice**. Although its kernel looks much like a rice grain, *Zizania aquatica* is in fact a type of grass. (Cereals such as wheat, rice, and corn aren't strictly vegetables, either.) Wild rice grows by the sides of lakes, most commonly in the state of Minnesota, where for centuries members of the Ojibway tribes have taken their canoes out onto the water and have laboriously worked out the edible grains from the tall plant stalks. If you want to use these traditional harvesting methods to take the rice, you need a license in Minnesota. Wild rice is commercially grown and commonly available and has a wonderful and robust nutty flavor.

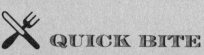

QUICK BITE

The Ostrich fern doesn't grow just in Maine, but its edible spring shoot, the fiddlehead, is most popularly known as the **Maine fiddlehead.** The coiled fresh growth of the fern is gathered over a short season, lasting maybe as little as three weeks in May. Eat steamed or boiled.

This company will send you fresh fiddleheads in season or canned Belle of Maine products the rest of the year: www.maine fiddleheads.com / 1-877-4-SHIP-ME (1-877-474-4763)

Wild rice is available from C&G Enterprises: 1-715-398-5921 / www.mnwildrice.com.

Minnestalgia, in McGregor, Minnesota, sells delicacies from the state's Northwoods region, including wild rice and wild rice pancake mix, and jelly made from tart **chokecherries, lingonberries,** and **wild plums:** 1-800-328-6731 / www.minnestalgia.com.

VEGETABLE SUMMARY

RUN, DON'T WALK, FOR . . .

▦ **Farm-fresh vegetables in season.** Ditto for vegetables as for fruit. Whatever you pick up at a farm stand or farmers market should be good.

▦ **Sweet corn.** The all-time number one farm stand food.

▦ **Potatoes.** It's time to explore the world of fresh potatoes again. Roasted in olive oil with parsnips and carrots and a lot of kosher salt and pepper, they can steal the show in winter. And homemade French fries really do taste better.

IF YOU'VE NEVER TRIED . . .

▦ **Leeks.** Will repay your attention many times over.

▦ **Wild rice.** Pricey, but a little goes a long way. An interesting nutty taste and a crop with a long Native American heritage.

3

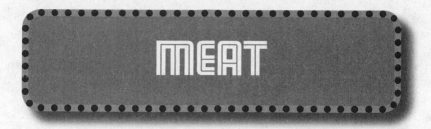

MEAT

*Americans have been great meat eaters from the beginning of their
history and still are. No other country in the world eats more meat per
capita, nor pays less for it in terms of proportion to total income.*
—Waverly Root and Richard de Rochemont, *Eating in America* (1976)

I f USDA statistics are to be believed, the average American ate eighty-
nine pounds of beef in 1976, a figure only to fall thereafter, perhaps
something a sociologist can explain in terms of the Carter presidency. In
2004, beef consumption reached sixty-three pounds per head. If we as-
sume it's around that amount today, if everyone took up their precise allo-
cation of beef, they'd be consuming five quarter-pounders a week, which
you could conveniently eat at the rate of one burger a day for the working
week. (Take the weekends off.)

There may indeed be some statistically average individuals who eat a
quarter-pounder every working day. Then there are millions of vegetarians,
vegans, and others who more or less avoid red meat because they have high
cholesterol, or because they feel that growing cattle for food takes up un-
conscionable resources of water and grain or because their faith forbids it
or because they're afraid of BSE (mad cow disease) or simply because they
don't like the taste of meat. Of course these people are counterweighed by

dedicated carnivores of equal numerical value for whom a quarter-pounder is little more than an *amuse-bouche*.

I imagine I eat less beef in a year than the American average. (For many, this is a question answered only slightly more honestly than when a doctor asks you to tot up how many units of alcohol you consume.) I probably should eat less than I do. I happen to have high cholesterol, but I did even when I was on an honest-to-goodness low-meat-and-dairy diet. I'm in the BSE danger zone, having lived in the United Kingdom in the 1980s and eaten beef in that period. Although this precludes me from giving blood in the United States, once the cause of acute public embarrassment for me, fear of BSE alone has never been enough to put me off. I know the ecological arguments, but I fudge my way out of them. Problem is, I enjoy beef. Even if I can walk past the door of a Ruth's Chris, I've developed an unhealthy regard for fine hamburgers that's going to be tough to shake.

Beef is the most popular meat in America, though it's a marginal tendency. Chicken runs a pretty close second, at 59 pounds consumed per capita a year, followed by the 48 pounds of pork. The USDA stats show turkey coming in fourth, at 13 pounds a year (much of that, I would imagine, in uneaten Thanksgiving leftovers). Lamb consumption is measured at a paltry 0.83 pound a head, barely more than a handful of loin chops and a genuine cause for national embarrassment. In a perfect world, I'd eat lamb three times a week at least— lamb shank, rack of lamb, lamb kebabs, lamb chops, roast leg of lamb, and so on.

When I called a gentleman in Oklahoma City to talk about beef and steak, the conversation turned to lamb, though not lamb in the form I was familiar with myself. I wanted to find somewhere in the American heartland

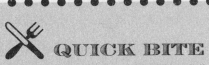

QUICK BITE

Beef is a seventy-eight-billion-dollar business in the United States, and Texas leads the country in the head count of cattle and of beef cows. While the United States is the largest beef-producing nation in the world, such is the national demand, the country is still a net importer of beef.

to represent the steak. The Cattlemen's Steakhouse in Oklahoma City, which has operated in one form or another since 1910 in an area called Stockyard City, presented good credentials. (The story goes that in 1945, rancher Gene Wade won the Cattlemen's Steakhouse from owner Hank Fry in a game of dice. Fry put up the restaurant against Wade's life savings if Wade could throw a pair of threes, which he duly did.)

QUICK BITE

In the stockyards in Forth Worth is the Cattlemen's Fort Worth Steak House, operating since 1947. The menu item that took my fancy here is the **Cattlemen's Bone-In Rib Eye Steak,** the rib eyes being among those items "Not to be ordered by those who object to heavy marbling."

Cattlemen's will *airmail* you steaks from their menu: T-bones, sirloins, porterhouse steaks: 1-817-624-3945 / www.cattlemenssteak house.com.

Dick Stubbs, the current owner, told me that Oklahoma City has the largest stockyards in the world. He also said that many of the restaurant's customers are stockyard workers, and you'd imagine they know their beef. Stubbs proudly told me how often Cattlemen's has won awards and been featured in national publications. His own favorite cut of steak is the **top**

WATCH OUT FOR . . .

Figuring out cuts of beef can be confusing. That's okay, because it *is* confusing, as the USDA concedes. You can look at your butcher's chart of the cuts of meat and ask what he means by "boneless top loin." This is what the USDA says:

"There are four basic major (primal) cuts into which beef is separated: chuck, loin, rib, and round. It is recommended that packages of fresh beef purchased in the supermarket be labeled with the primal cut as well as the product, such as 'chuck roast' or 'round steak.' This helps consumers know what type of heat is best for cooking the product. Generally, chuck and round are less tender and require moist heat such as braising; loin and rib can be cooked by dry heat methods such as broiling or grilling.

"Unfortunately, names for various cuts can vary regionally in stores, causing confusion over the choice of cooking method. For example, a boneless top loin steak is variously called: strip steak, Kansas City Steak, N.Y. strip steak, hotel cut strip steak, ambassador steak, or club sirloin steak."

butt—top butt sirloin—which has a little more flavor than other cuts, in his opinion. I ask what else he likes to eat, and Dick talks up the barbecue you can buy in town, which features a tomato-based sauce. As for a particular restaurant, he favors Earl's Barbecue.

There are fifteen types of steak on the Cattlemen's breakfast menu, but a higher proportion of eaters choose steak as the day goes on: 80 percent at lunch and over 90 percent at dinner. Every once in a while, Dick says with incredulity, someone will order a piece of fish. Dick's suggestion for visitors: the **Presidential Choice T-Bone Steak**—the sirloin plus the filet—which is exactly what Bush 41 had when he visited the restaurant.

━━━━━━━━━━

A few years ago, I was watching Julia Child and Jacques Pépin and their *Cooking at Home* series on PBS. In one segment, stately Child and her slightly puckish colleague dissected a beef tenderloin, removing the **Chateaubriand** from the thick end and working on the tournedos and then the filet mignon toward the narrower piece of the filet. (In their cookbook, Pépin explains how, as far as he's concerned, Chateaubriand can also come from the heart, or *coeur de filet*, of the tenderloin.)

Pépin and Child went on to the much more prosaic business of making hamburgers. The different approaches these two great cooking stalwarts took to their burgers neatly demonstrates that there's no right way, or wrong way, to make a burger. He likes a thick patty done medium-rare; hers is thin and rare. He prefers a Kaiser roll; she, a buttered hamburger bun. Julia seasons her meat with shallots, salt, and pepper; he adds salt and pepper, maybe, after the burger's cooked. She builds her burger iceberg leaf, thinly sliced red onion, ketchup, pickle relish, burger, cheese, bacon, and sliced tomato; while he goes iceberg, tomato, red onion, pickle, burger, ketchup, onion, and more lettuce.

Each looks equally wonderful. However you dress your burger, the key is in the meat. Here is Pépin and Child's very sound advice about buying ground beef for hamburgers to make at home: "Remember that fat is what gives flavor to meat: too little and the meat will be dry and you will lose much of the beefy taste. We both prefer a fat content of 20 percent. Julia buys chuck because she thinks it has better flavor."

━━━━━━━━━━

• • •

I ask Dick Stubbs, at the Cattlemen's in Oklahoma City, about something unfamiliar I noticed on the menu at his restaurant—**lamb fries.** I mention them, and Dick says, "You know what lamb fries are, don't you?" I had to reply that I'm from England and live in New York. So, sorry. No, I don't. Dick soon puts me right. Lamb fries are lambs' testicles that he serves cut into thin slices, dipped in flour and milk, and deep-fried. Dick says he sells about three hundred pounds of them a week. I ask what the provenance might be, and according to Stubbs, this sweet-tasting dish was first brought to the area by some Italian restaurateurs in the east of the state.

Dick Stubbs's description leads me to Pete's Place, an Italian restaurant in Krebs, a town of about two thousand near McAlester, toward the bottom right-hand (eastern) corner of Oklahoma. Joe Prichard is the third-generation owner of the restaurant. When he gets on the telephone and hears I'm calling from New York, he knows what the question is going to be about. Every now and again, someone calls up from out of town and wants to know about lamb fries. Joe is extremely good-natured about it. He tells me that his grandfather came to this country from Italy as a boy and started the family business. Joe has never found out how this unusual item made its way onto the menu.

Pete's Place serves lamb fries as an entrée. The lamb testicles are sliced very thin, breaded with cracker meal, then deep-fried and eaten with lemon, ketchup, or cocktail sauce, whatever you happen to favor. Pete's Place is a family-style restaurant, so your lamb fries come with salad, pasta and meatballs, ravioli, and garlic bread. Joe is quick to point out that not every restaurant in Oklahoma sells lamb fries. He's very familiar with Cattlemen's, though, and he reckons that between them, these two restaurants probably sell the majority of all lamb fries sold in the state.

More than the lamb testes, what really characterizes Pete's Place is its beer. Sure, Joe sells wine, too, but the restaurant is best known for its "Choc" beer, a cloudy, unfiltered wheat brew. The story is that the Italian immigrants who came to eastern Oklahoma to mine the coal learned about the brew from the local Choctaw Indians. Joe's grandfather had come to Krebs in 1903. He was known at the time as Pietro Piegari, but he changed his name to Pete Prichard when he started working in the mines at the age of eleven. Invalided out at twenty-one after an accident, Pete began serving Choc beer to the miners out of his house. He started fixing lunch to go with the beer and opened the restaurant in 1925. Oklahoma entered the union in 1907 as a dry state, and Prohibition ended here only in

1958 (meaning that anything stronger than 3.2 percent beer was banned before that).

COWBOY BEEF

I took my seat at supper.

Canned stuff it was, corned beef. And one of my table companions said the truth about it. "When I slung my teeth over that," he remarked, "I thought I was chewing a hammock." We had strange coffee, and condensed milk; and I have never seen more flies. I made no attempt to talk, for no one in this country seemed favorable to me. —*Owen Wister,* The Virginian *(1902)*

Philadelphia-born and Harvard-educated lawyer Owen Wister (1860–1938) went west (to Wyoming) in 1885. His novel *The Virginian* is narrated by an East Coast "tenderfoot" much like him and includes exquisite details of frontier conditions. (It's well worth reading, a fascinating account of the principles of rough-and-ready frontier justice.) Perhaps the Western-ers were all suffering from constipation, for there was very little in the way of fresh fruit and vegetables for a cattle driver to eat—pretty much everything edible that didn't walk around the land under its own steam had to be brought out in a can. It's not surprising that the readiest form of cowboy nourishment was the closest thing to hand: the cattle.

Like Wister, writer Dane Coolidge (1873–1940) was born in the North-east and educated at Harvard. But at the age of four, Coolidge moved to Los Angeles with his family (in 1877, L.A. County had a population of less than twenty-eight thousand) and grew up in California. Coolidge was a naturalist and a novelist. His nonfiction book *Arizona Cowboys*, published in 1938, includes a description of the 1904 Four Peaks cattle round-up in the Salt River Valley, near the fledgling city of Phoenix. The drive was carried out by a crew made up of eight Americans and eight Mexicans.

Coolidge writes that each morning, the crew would light a fire, unwrap the beef, and put the Dutch oven on the fire to cook their bread. They'd start up the coffee and the baking-powder biscuits, and there was always a pot of beans on the stove. Beans were good for you, Coolidge admitted, but were difficult to transport. The American hands weren't happy with-out stewed fruit, canned tomatoes, potatoes, onions, "and the rest," while the Mexican contingent could feed all its men for twenty cents a day. They'd live off beef, broiling pieces over the fire on the end of a stick. "At

QUICK BITE

A Dutch oven is the three-legged cast-iron pot that sits on an open fire or hot charcoal. These ovens are a relic of the country's pioneer heritage, but are still used widely. The International Dutch Oven Society holds a world championship every year in Logan, Utah, in which contestants have to prepare an entrée, bread, and a dessert in Dutch ovens. Valerie Phillips, food editor for the *Deseret Morning News,* in Salt Lake City, has been a judge in the contest and seen **stuffed Cornish game hens, crown rib roasts,** stuffed pork loin, and excellent rolls, cakes, and pies emerge from the simple cooking pot.

Check out the Dutch ovens at Dutch Oven Pro of Draper, Utah: 1-801-319-0778 / www.dutchovenpro.com.

Williams-Sonoma sells Le Creuset Dutch ovens designed for stovetop and oven cooking rather than over an open fire: www .williams-sonoma.com.

the end there would be no dishes to wash, except a few that could be scoured in the sand."

The beef that Coolidge writes about being unwrapped was prepared like this: The animal was killed and hung. The men would cut off strips of meat and cook them over the fire. Once everyone was fed, a large tarp would be draped over the carcass and the carcass would be left hanging overnight. In the morning, every man who left the camp would put his blanket on top of the beef. Returning from the day's work, they'd unwrap the meat before sundown and find it was still chilled from the night air.

A side of beef would keep four or five days lying out in the broiling hot sun; and when it began to get a little ripe they would slice all the meat off the bones, rub it with salt and ground chili-peppers and hang it in the sun to dry. A sack of this jerked beef came in very handy when we were moving out of fresh meat; and they can toast it over the coals, beat it to shreds on a rock and get a meal started in jig-time.

QUICK BITE

Alfred Henry Lewis (1855–1914) was a lawyer-turned-journalist and another writer who looked west for inspiration. Lewis moved from his hometown of Cleveland to Kansas City and traveled the frontier states picking up stories for his newspaper pieces and novels, including *The Sunset Trail* (1905), which gives us another example of western fare, this time in a restaurant.

On the day that Rattlesnake Sanders first beheld Miss Barndollar, he came into the dining-room of the Wright House seeking recuperation from the fatigues of a 60-mile ride. When he had drawn his chair to the table, and disposed of his feet so that the spurs which graced his heels did not mutually interfere, Miss Barndollar came and stood at his shoulder.

"Roast beef, b'iled buffalo tongue, plover potpie, fried antelope steak, an' baked salt hoss an' beans," observed Miss Barndollar in a dreamy sing-song. The Wright House did not print its menu, and the bill of fare was rehearsed by the waitress to the wayfarer within its walls.

In case you're concerned, "baked salt hoss" is corned beef, not a slab of a relative of Mr. Ed.

MORGAN VALLEY LAMB

If you live along the Wasatch Front, in Park City, or the Heber Valley, in Utah, Jamie and Linda Gillmor of Morgan Valley Lamb will deliver natural, hormone-free lamb straight to your door. Jamie Gillmor is the third generation of his family to raise sheep out on the open range of his mountain property. In 2001 he decided to start direct-marketing his lamb to restaurants and specialty stores, which involved creating new products like **Scottish lamb pies.** The pies came about when Gillmor partnered with Morrisons, a Utah company that'd been making pies for 125 years. The original recipe called for mutton; Gillmor and Morrisons make theirs out of premium-grade lamb. Jamie Gillmor told me he was working on an Australian-style lamb pie.

Gillmor sells his pies online, at farmers markets in Salt Lake and Park City, and in specialty stores like the British Pantry, in Salt Lake City. His lamb travels, too—Jamie told me that he recently sent a large shipment to the Sagamore, which is a grand hotel on a beautiful piece of land on Lake George in New York.

I asked Jamie how he likes his lamb. He enjoys messing around with it, making a braised lamb shank or a sirloin on the grill. Jamie loves **shoulder chops with potatoes, pulled lamb shoulder stew, ribs,** and so on. Jamie's got me salivating by this point, and I tell him how much I love lamb myself. I say I'm always commenting how little lamb you see in this country. Jamie thinks people are scared of cooking it. His theory is that a lot of ersatz lamb was sold during World War II and it was actually goat and old mutton, all greasy meat. So he now finds he has a harder time selling his meat in smaller towns to older folk, but he has great success with younger people, who perhaps are a little more willing to experiment. Jamie is doing his best to change people's tastes.

QUICK BITE

In Missoula, Montana, visit the Red Bar Restaurant and check out the lamb special, made from local meat. My wife, Kara, and I had a fine meal at Red Bar involving some steak and blue cheese on a trip checking out the stunning Glacier National Park. Missoula is a cool college town (University of Montana) with good bookstores where you can feed the mind. Visit them, and then tax the body by climbing up the hill in town where the big collegiate *M* is painted into the hillside facing the campus. *Brisk* isn't the word for it.

Jamie has worked his whole life in this business. He's spent many summers in the wild country in the mountains of northern Utah with the sheep. When he was a little kid, six or seven, he would cook up chops and potatoes out in the sheep camps on the range.

I ask Jamie about his name, saying I was more used to seeing *Gilmour* rather than *Gillmor*. Jamie told me that it used to be *Gillmore*, but his great-great-grandfather took the *e* off the end. It was he who gave eight or nine head of sheep to Jamie's grandfather. The grandfather started selling ducks he'd shot to hotels in Salt Lake City and then progressed to selling them lamb from his sheep. It's a real family business, one that Jamie's wife works in, too. This must be an advertisement for the product: when they were

married, Jamie's wife was a vegetarian but she quickly was converted to
eating lamb.

See www.morganvalleylamb.com for details of home delivery in
certain areas of Utah and for national shipping information. Even if
you think you don't like lamb, you owe it to yourself to give it a try.

ORGAN MEATS

*Leopold Bloom ate with relish the inner organs of beasts and fowls. He liked
thick giblet soup, nutty gizzards, a stuffed roast heart, liver slices fried with crust
crumbs, fried hencod's roes. Most of all he liked grilled mutton kidneys which
gave to his palate a fine tang of faintly scented urine.*

—*James Joyce*, Ulysses (1922)

So goes one of the most famous descriptions of food in literature. There
was a time when I regularly relished inner organs myself. My father loved
grilled **lamb's kidneys,** and I did, too. On a couple of memorable occasions he bought them "in their overcoats," meaning that the thick jacket
of fat surrounding the organ was still attached. Once the organ was cooked
(this was a process in which I wasn't involved), the dark meat of the kidney
was curled up around a gristled center. I'd bite down through the meat and
chew away, releasing what James Joyce would later tell me is the waste-
product flavor. **Braised liver** I liked even better than this, fried up in a pan
with onions.

It's a while since I've eaten either of these delights, though I have eaten
sweetbreads more recently, in New York City, at the Gramercy Tavern and
at Del Posto (**Lamb Sweetbreads** with Favetta and Lovage) and **Veal
Bone Marrow** with parsley and capers at Lupa. There's an essential meati-
ness to these carnivorous delights, and I mean that literally.

CURED MEATS

For my birthday one year, six of us went to Mario Batali's Babbo Ristorante
Enoteca, in New York City's Greenwich Village. I had my eye on the cured
meats, specifically the **testa (head cheese)** and **lardo.** Of the six of us,
only my friend Ivan and I tried the lardo and testa. Lardo is described by
the restaurant as house-cured pork fatback. That's pig fat to you and me.

QUICK BITE

Erik Cosselmon is executive chef at Kokkari Estiatorio in San Francisco. Kokkari features Greek cuisine. (Kokkari is the name of a small fishing village on the Greek island of Samos.) Erik prepares **Greek-style testa,** and here's how. Take a pig's head and cut the bones of the head so you can remove the brain after cooking. Cure in brine for three days. (Add the pig's feet to the brine if you like.) Take the meat and chop it. (Some choose to grind the meat.) Cook the meat with onion, garlic, and spices like clove, bay leaf, mustard seed, and fennel and make a broth using gelatin. You can serve the testa in a terrine, or wrapped in a towel or in a sausage casing.

The testa was thinly sliced and a delicate sensation for the mouth. Our waiter said the lardo was flavored by what the animal had eaten. Indeed, it was nutty to the tongue and just sublime.

There is a scientific explanation for the lardo's flavor, as Peter Kaminsky explains in his book *Pig Perfect*. Ruminants such as cows digest food twice, and in the process the fat they eat is transformed into hard, hydrogenated fat. A pig doesn't have the second stomach of a cow, so the fat remains soft and retains its original flavor. Kaminsky explains, "If the fat tastes good, so will the meat." In the case of lardo, if the fat tastes good, the fat tastes good.

A couple of times, my friend Ivan and I have visited Batali's less formal establishment, Otto, a wine bar and up-scale pizzeria. Each time we tried more cured meats, some of the great small plates, a quantity of good Nero d'Avola (red wine from Sicily), and, the day it was the special, a **pizza**

QUICK BITE

Our friend Joe Surak introduced a group of our friends to the manifest delights of the dry-cured meats from the Calabria Pork Store on Arthur Avenue in the Bronx, a locale famous for its Italian American food. Arranged on a platter were *sopressata, salami,* and *capicola*—pungent air-dried meats shot through with intense and complicated meaty flavors. Sublime, and a perfect accompaniment for the fabulous risotto Joe whipped up for his guests.

QUICK BITE

My friend Sheryl told me about **chipped-chopped ham** (or chip-chopped ham), which is very, very thinly sliced ham, very familiar to her growing up in Erie, Pennsylvania. She also mentioned **ring bologna** (which is what it sounds like: bologna formed into a ring of sausage), which could be eaten fried. Sheryl's aunt used to make **ham salad** using ring bologna instead of ham (ring bologna, relish, and mayonnaise). Another local deli food would be **ham loaf** (meat loaf made of ham), cooked with rings of pineapple on top, which was big at church suppers.

with guanciale, which is salted pork cheeks, a small explosion of taste, with the salt hitting you first, then the fat. We have also enjoyed the cured meat selections at Lupa, where Mario Batali is a partner: **proscuitto di Parma, coppa, soppressata,** testa, **veal tongue,** and so on. Each has a singular joy: the paper-thin, melting proscuitto; the robust coppa, which is cured pork shoulder; the darker, harder soppressata, the warm testa dusted with fennel pollen; and the meatier veal tongue prepared with a hint of orange. Later, in one meal, we had a superb, spicy **lamb sausage.**

Across the country from Mario Batali's restaurants, Mario's father, Armandino Batali, has embraced the noble cause of cured meat. After one career in the airplane business, and after his son had found his success, Armandino spent time in Italy learning how to make salumi (and salami.) *Salumi* is the broad term for Italian cured meat, of which salami, or salame, is but a small sausage subset.

In 1999, Batali senior opened Salumi in Seattle. Among the most alluring meats are **Salumi salame,** which has a touch of ginger, **salame with mole, finocchiona** (a Tuscan salami flavored with cracked fennel, black pepper, and a touch of curry), and coppa (pork shoulder cured in sugar and salt, spiced with cayenne or chili pepper), **lamb "prosciutto,"** and **lomo** (boneless whole pork loin cured and air-dried).

For $150, you can buy a cured ham and "adopt" it, participating in its transformation into a full-fledged proscuitto. Every now and then, you can come in and help in the processing, and after a year or so you take your ham home.

 For those outside the Seattle area, Salumi has a few meats for shipping, as well as mole and Salumi salami: 1-877-223-0813 / www.salumicuredmeats.com.

Peter Kaminsky describes the sensation, or sensations, of eating a fine ham with poetic flair. **Country ham** is prepared with loving attention, first cured in salt, then smoked with a hardwoodlike hickory or maple, and finally stored to age like wine. This process marries the techniques the settlers and the Native Americans used to preserve meat: Europeans packed meat and fish in salt for storage, while the native peoples used drying and smoking methods. Kaminsky writes of the tremendous bouquet released by the first slice of a country ham:

As the ham comes in contact with your tongue, the punch of salt pushes forward wave after wave of subtler notes—smoky, floral, fruity. Finally, as your teeth come together and you breathe out, you smell the return, only deeper, of that initial aroma of flesh and sweet decay. You would think this last might be off-putting, but in the right balance, it is a heady perfume, just this side of rancidness. (Pig Perfect)

QUICK BITE

I have to thank Bethany Fong, a manager for the Sodexho Company in Hawaii, who reminded me of the triumph of the world of processed meats, Spam. Bethany says, "I know, it's made in Minnesota, but Hawaii just happens to be the greatest consumer of Spam, and we know how to cook it in every possible way—**Spam Musubi,** Spam omelet, **Spam as ham,** Spam burrito, Spam dip, Spam fried rice, or just straight out of the can. (Yes, I do know people who have done that before.)"

Gourmet Web site www.chefshop.com was offering "smoked to order" bone-in ham last time I checked. As well as artisanal vinegars, fresh fish from Alaska and Hawaii, fresh fruit from Washington State, and tempting-looking creations called Maui Ribs.

GAME MEATS

By the close of 1883 the last buffalo herd was destroyed. The beaver was trapped out of all the streams, or their numbers so thinned that it no longer paid to follow them. The last formidable Indian war had been brought to a successful close. The flood of the incoming whites had risen over the land; tongues of settlement reached from the Mississippi to the Rocky Mountains, and from the Rocky Mountains to the Pacific. The frontier had come to an end; it had vanished.

—Theodore Roosevelt, The Wilderness Hunter *(1893)*

There can have been few more enthusiastic outdoorsmen than Theodore Roosevelt. In the years before he entered public service, and after his first wife, Alice, died in childbirth in 1884, Roosevelt retreated to the Dakota Badlands and worked his ranch. He roamed the great interior, here and in Montana and Wyoming, and he wrote about the wild game he observed (and hunted for food) in *Hunting Trips of a Ranchman* (1885) and *The Wilderness Hunter*. It's interesting to leaf through these books and glean some appreciation of the natural bounty of the country at the time. This is no chore, either—TR was a terrific writer, and his energy makes modern brush-clearing chief executives look positively lazy.

THEODORE ROOSEVELT'S (EDIBLE) GAME

- Curlew: "very good eating," writes TR.
- Grass and golden plover: "delicious eating"; Plains plover: "good eating."
- Prairie fowl, or grouse: "very good eating from about the middle of August to the middle of November."
- Blue grouse: "furnish dainty food to men weary of venison."
- Sage fowl: "excellent eating in August and September."
- Black- and white-tailed deer: "most delicious eating."
- Prong-horn, or antelope: "equally good all through the year."

- Big-horn, or mountain, sheep: "Mountain mutton is in the fall the most delicious eating furnished by any game animal. Nothing else compares with it for juiciness, tenderness, and flavor; but at all other times of the year it is tough, stringy, and worthless."

- Buffalo: "The so-called hump meat—that is, the strip of steak on each side of the backbone—is excellent, and tender and juicy. Buffalo meat is with difficulty to be distinguished from ordinary beef."

- Elk: "Elk tongues are most delicious eating, being juicy, tender, and well-flavored; they are excellent to take out as a lunch on a long hunting trip."

- Black bear: "Excellent . . . tasted like . . . a young pig."

- Grizzly bear: "We tried eating the grizzly's flesh but it was not good, being coarse and not well flavored."

- White goat: "Old white goats are intolerably musky in flavor."

- Moose: "The flesh of the moose is very good; though some deem it coarse. Old hunters, who always like rich, greasy food, rank a moose's nose with a beaver's tail, as the chief of backwood delicacies; personally I never liked either."

QUICK BITE

There are plenty of opportunities around the country for hunters to bag game and take it home and eat it. South Dakota is renowned for its **pheasant** hunting. At AAA South Dakota Pheasant Hunting, there is a bird processor on the premises. Birds are cleaned, packed, and stored until you leave. (In our family, there is a piece of lore in which my father came home from work with a brace of pheasants someone (not he) had shot and given him whole, still full of shot, as a present. "Here," he said, handing them to my bemused mother.

Shop for pheasant, quail, ostrich, elk, buffalo, alligator, rabbit, and more at MacFarlane Pheasants of Janesville, Wisconsin: 1-800-345-8348 / www.pheasant.com.

Lawrence Johnson is executive chef of Briarhurst Manor, in Manitou Springs, Colorado. The manor dates from 1876, the year Colorado became a state, and was built by Londoner Dr. William Bell in the style of a fine English country home. Bell came west after the Civil War and founded the town as a spa and resort, and was so successful that Manitou Springs was once known as the "Saratoga of the West" after the long-established New York vacation destination. Chef Johnson knows the history of the manor and how Dr. Bell arrived by wagon with his new wife, Cara, from England in 1872. With them the Bells brought Antonio, their Italian-born, English-trained chef. When he works, Lawrence puts himself in the mind-set of Chef Antonio, who came to the New World with his Old World traditions and recipes. As he traded with the Ute Indians, Antonio was heavily influenced by the Native American accents he found in his new home.

Chef Johnson also blends these culinary cultures. He prefers the term "Rocky Mountain cuisine" to what has been styled "Colorado cuisine." Johnson pairs game like deer, bison, elk, snake, and trout with indigenous produce grown on the property and from nearby farms. A wide array of fruits and vegetables are cultivated at the manor—seven kinds of apples and two of grapes; pears, elderberries, and black raspberries; purple, white, and red potatoes; sorrel, watercress, and horseradish. Starting in the springtime, when the apple blossoms and baby apples come out, Chef Johnson likes to go out into the garden and see what looks good to cook with that particular day.

Chef Johnson will prepare **wild boar** marinated in a smoked herb infusion (there is an herb bed in the manor garden), grilled, topped with green chile, and served with **cheddar cheese and dark chile mashed potatoes.** While I am trying to taste these dishes in my head, Chef Johnson starts talking about his signature **Red Mesa Barbecued Mole Lamb.** Johnson takes a whole hind shank, cooks it in red chile mole sauce, and finishes it off on the barbecue. "Best lamb in the world," says its cook—and who am I to demur?

Lawrence Johnson was born in Minnesota and moved to Colorado be-

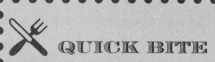

QUICK BITE

I ask Chef Johnson about the snake dish he serves. The chef takes western diamondback rattlesnake meat and prepares a **Rattlesnake Tamale.** I want to know what the flavor is like, and Lawrence tells me it tastes like . . . turkey, a light turkey that is richer and rather more accented than chicken.

fore he was a year old. He enjoys the rugged, outdoor Colorado lifestyle and is a keen turkey hunter. No wild turkey bagged by the chef is going to end up in the restaurant, where all the meat is properly USDA inspected. **Wild turkey** tastes like "Turkey times three," Johnson says. "Dark, intense and rich." But you have to baby the thing in preparation and be careful not to overcook it.

Briarhurst Manor sells a lot of bison, the meat most popularly associated with Colorado. For a time, Chef Johnson had a Buffalo Kidney and Liver Pie on the menu. Buffalo organs are very rich—too rich for the contemporary palate, as it turned out. A more manageable **Tenderloin of Buffalo** goes down very well, says Lawrence, and he also features a **Maple and Whiskey Shellacked Plains Bison** on his menu, a mix of the Old World and the New inspired by his Italian predecessor more than a hundred and thirty years ago.

Ellen Sweets of the *Denver Post* guided me to some other meat-laden Denver venues. Ellen says, "If you want authentic, what-they-were-eating-way-back-when, you want Buckhorn Exchange. It holds the city's first liquor license (1893). As long as you're not squeamish about dead animal heads on the wall, you'll be fine." And here on the menu are the familiar game meats: for lunch, medallions of elk and buffalo served as part of two famous East Coast sandwiches, the Reuben and the cheese-steak. (See page 275 for a more traditional Reuben, and chapter 16 for the Philly cheese-steak.) Rattlesnake is also featured, as a supper appetizer (mari-

QUICK BITE

Venison, if kept to the proper time, is the most tender of all meats, but care is necessary to bring it to a fitting state for table without its becoming offensive; a free current of air materially assists in preserving its sweetness, while a close, damp atmosphere is destructive to this as well as all other kinds of meats.

—Mrs. M. E. Porter, *Mrs. Porter's New Southern Cookery Book and Companion for Frugal and Economical Housekeepers* (1871)

In Vermont, writer Marialisa Calta tells us that venison chili or **venison stew** is served at "any number of game suppers . . . the biggest is the Bradford Game Supper, which serves more than a thousand people."

nated in red chile and lime with a chipotle pepper cream cheese), along with nonindigenous fried alligator tail served with seafood cocktail sauce.

Elk, **quail,** and game hen are among the dinner entrees, together with dry aged **New York strip steak** that you can order for the table: four pounds for five guests, with sides, for a hundred and sixty dollars.

If you go to the Buckhorn Exchange, says Ellen Sweets, "be sure to try the Rocky Mountain oysters . . . heh-heh-heh." They're presented as "**Rocky Mountain Oysters**

QUICK BITE

Check out the menu at The Gun Barrel Steak & Game House in Jackson Hole: Velvet elk, which is pan-seared elk tenderloin; a thick, mesquite-grilled elk chop; and a number of buffalo items, such as bison carpaccio, buffalo ribs, and buffalo sirloin.

with horseradish dippin' sauce." Rocky mountain oysters, or prairie oysters, are, of course, calf or bull testicles that are usually prepared by being coated in flour and fried. You're either going to be okay with that or you're not. Many of us will eat a hot dog without wondering what's in it, but there's no processing between you and the mountain oyster. True fans can take part in a Testicle Festival in September at the Rock Creek Lodge in Clinton, Montana, where two and a half tons of testes are consumed and where sundry adult activities take place in the bracing air of the great outdoors.

In the early sixties, advertising executive Sam Arnold found in a Denver library a couple of drawings of Bent's Old Fort, a fur-trapping station that operated from 1833 to 1849 near where the town of La Junta stands today, to the southeast of Denver. The fort was right on the border of land claimed by Mexico and was used as a staging post in the Mexican War, before it was abandoned. A West Pointer visiting the fort when it was operational drank some river water and fell ill. While he was recuperating, he drew detailed pictures of the fort from different perspectives. Seeing these old sketches, Arnold was taken with the castlelike structure and the fort's two round towers, set at diagonals to each other. His wife asked if he'd like to live in a place like that, and Arnold went ahead and built his replica 160 miles from the site of the original.

The Fort Restaurant came to be when the Arnolds discovered that they couldn't get a loan to build just a house but could if they added a restaurant. The thirteen-thousand-square-foot structure was constructed with eighty thousand forty-five-pound adobe bricks, and the restaurant

QUICK BITE

I bought myself an eight-ounce pack of ground **ostrich** at the local Whole Foods. At home I halved the meat and shaped one of the four-ounce pieces into a patty and cooked it as recommended in a frying pan with a little olive oil. The meat is tremendously lean, so it exuded very little fat. So little fat that the meat may stick to the pan if you're not paying attention. As for the taste, don't think of an ostrich as a giant chicken. Its flesh is red meat with a good sharp flavor, much like beef, and there's no real gaminess to it at all. My ostrich meat, from Blackwing, was marketed as a healthy alternative to chicken (promising 81 percent less fat and 50 percent fewer calories than chicken) that tastes like beef, and indeed it does.

For Blackwing antibiotic- and hormone-free meat and organic meat—ground ostrich and elk, quail, duck, guinea hen, and more: 1-800-326-7874 / www.blackwing.com.

opened for business on February 1, 1963. Sam Arnold is a keen food historian and the author of *Eating Up the Santa Fe Trail*, which includes old frontier recipes, not just of the pioneers but of trappers, Native Americans, Mexicans, and soldiers. (Gunpowder-flavored whiskey anyone?) Arnold says that life was tough for the mountain men but a lucky few at Bent's Fort ate off Limoges china and drank French and Spanish wine shipped in by wagon train. "It wasn't all blood and guts out here," he says.

Like Lawrence Johnson, Sam Arnold gets a lot of his meat from outside the state. Deer comes from Texas; the elk from New Zealand, where it is a smaller animal than the American elk, the wapiti. Sam Arnold goes pretty much whole hog with his buffalo. Rocky Mountain oysters, of course, along with a twenty-ounce steak, roast bison marrow bones (four split femurs served as an appetizer); bison sausage; braised bison tongue, served with toast and caper aïoli, barbecued ribs, and so on. Sam himself likes a buffalo consommé and has enjoyed the liver and kidneys, the liver raw following Native American fashion. In October, The Fort holds what it calls the "Awful Offal Dinner," where such organ delights can be sampled, fully cooked.

Although he's now very much a man of the West, Sam Arnold was born in Pittsburgh and attended Yale, class of 1947, one year behind George H. W. Bush. Sam studied English literature, and he recited for me the prologue of Chaucer's *Canterbury Tales*, with impressive cadence: "Whan that Aprille with his shoures soote / The droghte of Marche hath perced to the roote . . ." At school, Sam made up a song, "I'll Be Down to Get You in a Taxi, Honey," and set Chaucer's words to it as an aide-mémoire. He sang that for me, too.

After Yale, Sam decided to go west and moved to Santa Fe in 1948, but it proved to be a tough town in which to make a living, and he moved to Denver in 1950, where he worked in advertising. He was running an agency when the restaurant opened, and as he shifted his attention to The Fort, the ad business gradually went into mothballs. It took years, Sam says, for The Fort to make money, and you could have bought it from him cheap back then.

Now, The Fort is a roaring success. In 1997, the G8 summit was held in Denver, and the leaders of the Western world—Clinton, Chirac, Kohl, Yeltsin, Blair and co.—ate at The Fort. Sam Arnold liked Tony Blair and enjoyed Boris Yeltsin, who helped himself to a buffalo tenderloin off the grill before dinner. The leaders could choose from entrees of buffalo, lamb chops, trout, and quail. Unsurprisingly, the security was intense. For one night, the fort that Sam Arnold built was at the same time the safest and the most dangerous place in the world.

REINDEER, CARIBOU, DALL'S SHEEP

Because you can't sell wild game in restaurants, you'll find meat from the plentiful local game in Alaskans' home kitchens. The exception is reindeer. Reindeer were introduced into the country from Lapland at the turn of the century, and several cooperatives produce reindeer meat out on the tundra. If it's mixed properly, T. C. Mitchell says, reindeer sausage can be very good.

Kirsten Dixon cooks with reindeer mostly in the fall and early winter. She describes it as a delicious and fine meat that's perfect for anyone who might be squeamish about game. She prepares a small **tenderloin** that is about two and a half pounds in weight, pan-searing it perhaps, with herbs and spices. After finishing the meat in the oven, she'll slice it on the bias (at a slight angle) and serve it with a wild berry sauce to add a real Alaska flourish. She also makes a **Black Bean and Reindeer Chili,** which features the fascinating combination of chipotle chiles and reindeer sausage.

When it's buffalo-hunting season on the range behind the lodge, hunters might pay for a night's stay with some meat. It is possible to get a special permit to hunt bison up by Fairbanks, T. C. Mitchell says, and even tundra-living musk ox.

As for other game meats, Dixon likes **caribou,** which is like elk, or New Zealand red-tailed deer, lean and not particularly gamey. Kirsten's daughters, who are now in their twenties, had never eaten beef until they were nine or ten. They grew up eating **moose,** and the first time they had beef they thought the meat was rancid. The moose is a big beast: it's possible to take seven hundred pounds of meat from each animal. Moose has a leaner, stronger taste than beef.

The **Dall sheep** (or Dall's sheep) is like a mountain goat. Kirsten was hesitant to try it at first but found it delicious and light. She'll also eat **ptarmigan** and **spruce grouse.** Everything she eats is in consideration of how it is taken and the appropriate season. Personally, she doesn't care to eat duck or goose or, as some back-country people like, **bear.**

Wapiti *is the Shawnee word for the American elk, a large grayish-brown deer that roams the mountains of the Pacific Northwest. My dad's side of the family is largely of the Yakima Nation, and they would hunt for elk each fall. From them we would receive elk meat. The steaks are a bit tough, but with a lot of flavor. My mom liked to use it for stew. The slaughterhouse my cousins took their elk to also made elk pepperoni sticks, which were the only one I had tasted until a bad middle school Slim Jim experience.* —Dana Cree

---

GATOR MEAT

Edwin Froelich has been in the gator business for forty years. Froelich tells me he was the first farmer to sell legal alligator meat in the state of Florida, and he now ships tens of thousands of pounds of it each year. After a long period finding his feet, Edwin's business has been good for about twenty years. In 1981, a large restaurant in Fort Lauderdale came to Edwin to see if he could supply some gator meat. The restaurant had been serving green turtle meat, but trade in that delicacy had been outlawed and the place wanted a similarly exotic replacement.

Edwin Froelich wasn't in a position to do business with the restaurant, not if he wanted to make any money. The Florida Game and Freshwater Fish Commission said that you could give gator meat away but you couldn't sell it. Froelich had an order for three thousand pounds of meat he couldn't sell. Froelich was able to get a onetime permit to sell the meat, but the restaurant came back the next year and wanted to buy everything he had. Other establishments said they were interested. Florida's nuisance trappers, who take animals who get too near to people, wanted to sell their meat, too, the regulations changed, and the processing and supply of gator meat became established.

If you haven't seen it, **alligator** is a white meat. Raw, it's not very distinct, with just a little pink in it sometimes. When it's cooked, it's all white, and Froelich says it takes seasoning well, like chicken or veal. The meat is high in protein while low in fat and cholesterol. It is also very versatile. Froelich says you can deep-fry it, kebab it, steam it, barbecue it, grill it, bake it, and make chili and hamburger out of it. Froelich himself has eaten so much of it he doesn't pay it much attention. Personally, he likes it deep-fried in thin strips. He takes it with a little cocktail sauce and makes like it's shrimp.

Exotic Meats of Bellevue, Washington, sells gator meat, among a lot of interesting fare, at its store and online: alligator tail steak and sausage, kangaroo, wild boar ribs and bacon, and **yak steaks:** 1-800-680-4375 / www.exoticmeats.com.

Froelich harvests his gators when they're four and a half to five feet long. *Harvesting* alligators means you take them out of the pens they're raised in. How do you catch an alligator? According to Mr. Froelich, you roll up your pants, take off your shoes, and step into the pen. You need to make sure there's at least a foot of water where you're taking the gator. The animal will skulk underwater, where he thinks he's hidden. When a gator is out of water he'll get nervous, and when he's nervous that's when he's liable to bite something, namely, you. With the animal safely submerged, you go in and get your hand round the jaws with a couple of fingers positioned over the eyes. Then you pick him up by one of his hind legs. Easier said than done, Mr. Froelich.

Froelich decided to raise gators himself. Having started gator farming, Froelich faced the challenge of getting his animals to breed. Froelich knew a man who ran a scientific outfit who had seen his alligators establish only eight successful nests in thirty years of research. The two men put their heads together and designed a system of pens. They mixed up a bunch of females and a bunch of males. The gators produced one functioning nest the first year and three the next. Within three or four years the operation was yielding about a thousand hatchlings a year.

Froelich says the guys at the Game Commission didn't believe he was raising the gators himself. They suspected he was taking young animals from the wild and building fake nests to raise them in. A couple of officials came down to inspect the nests to see if they could tell if they were fake. As they approached one site, a big female rose up out of the water, reared up, and chased the inspectors away from the nest. Later Froelich joked with the officials that it had been easy for him to build the fake nest but he'd had a heck of a job training the gator to protect it.

Edwin Froelich was born in West Palm Beach County and has never lived in a city or a town. His two-thousand-acre ranch is in an area known as Christmas, about 25 miles from Orlando, which, Froelich says, is coming out to meet him. He figures he'll be fine because there's a thick wooded area by the St. John's River bordering one part of his ranch and a game reserve wrapped around the rest. In his lifetime, Froelich has eaten a lot of stuff, not just alligator. Whatever it is, he'll eat it if it doesn't eat him first, he says. He's tried 'coon, 'possum, even **armadillo.** Armadillos used to be all over the farm, and he'd shoot them as pests. According to Froelich, the armadillo also makes excellent eating. To prepare an armadillo, you debone it and fry up the meat like a veal cutlet. The taste is like very young pork, he says, but not as greasy.

MEAT SUMMARY
RUN, DON'T WALK, FOR . . .

- **Lamb.** I love lamb. I'll always look forward to a plate of **lamb chops** at my favorite neighborhood restaurant: Gennaro, on Amsterdam Avenue in New York. Wherever you live, do yourself this favor and eat some lamb.

- A platter of **cured meats.** Homemade testa will just light up your mouth.

- Once a year (at least), you deserve a good **steak** from a restaurant that knows its meat.

IF YOU'VE NEVER TRIED . . .

- ▦ **Ostrich.** Low fat and high taste—what's not to like? (**Buffalo**, too, and **yak**, apparently.)

- ▦ **Kidneys.** In honor of *Ulysses*.

- ▦ **Veal bone marrow** and similar. It's a mark of respect to try as many parts of the animal as possible.

4

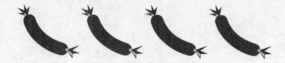

SAUSAGE

There are more than two hundred different kinds of sausage on the American market; it is a safe guess that German-Americans make a majority of them . . . Germany, after all, is perhaps the world's leading concocter of sausage; many of the types found there have been transferred almost unadulterated to the United States.
—Waverly Root and Richard de Rochemont, *Eating in America* (1976)

More Americans trace their ancestry back to Germany than to any other country. At the last census, about 1 in 7 Americans, 42.8 million people, did so. Where the original German immigrants gathered across America, you're more than likely to find the sausage they brought with them. Root and de Rochemont mention Milwaukee, a German-settled city, where there were fifty sausage manufacturers operating around the time they published their book. Thus, there is the American **Braunschweiger** (aka Braunschweig, or Brunswick, sausage), a smoked pork liver sausage, and **bratwurst** (a pork sausage from Thuringia that became a pork and veal sausage here), together with **knackwurst** (aka knockwurst), **bockwurst, weisswurst,** and so on. There are also **wieners** (originally Wienerwurst) and **frankfurters;** the terms are often used

QUICK BITE

Sausage is a very basic food. Every ethnic group that eats meat has stuffed animal membranes with meat and spices, and many types of these live on as relics of the homeland. Tubed meat has endless uses, and it pops up all over this book. It's a split mettwurst that appears on a hamburger; chorizo, inside a breakfast burrito; sliced pepperoni, on a fine Neapolitan pizza; and barbecued link sausage that is one of the cornerstones of Texas barbecue.

interchangeably despite the fact they are referents to two quite different places: Vienna and Frankfurt.

If you want to know anything about sausage, including how to make it yourself, consult Bruce Aidells, founder of the eponymous sausage company and author of books like *Bruce Aidells's Complete Book of Pork: A Guide to Buying, Storing, and Cooking the World's Favorite Meat* and *Bruce Aidells's Complete Sausage Book.* I bought some of the Aidells sausage varieties—**habañero and green chile** (smoked chicken and turkey sausages) and **Cajun-style andouille** smoked porkers—and cooked up a bunch.

The packaging suggests all sorts of ingenious uses—cook with pasta, use in tacos in place of ground beef, dice into a potato soup, and so on; but I stuck to the tried-and-trusted method of sautéing in a little butter in a skillet. My friend Bud and I ate a few of them for lunch on **wheat salad** rolls with English mustard and sautéed onions and yellow and red peppers. I couldn't get hold of any of my favorite brew of the moment: Burlington, Vermont, brewery Magic Hat's **No. 9 ale,** a sublime study in apricot, so I took a bottle of their **Fat Angel** with my lunch.

The andouille sausage was robust and fulfilling, not unnecessarily spicy or harsh. The habañero was terrific, a pleasantly surprising taste grounded in the big chunks of green chile within. Look at the ingredients and you'll find that this sausage holds no end of delights to go along with the chicken and turkey: Fire-roasted green chiles! Cilantro! Tequila! Jalapeños and habañeros! What's not to like here?

I'm also eager to try the **chicken and apple,** the **pesto** (a turkey-and-chicken sausage with Romano cheese and garlic), and the **sun-dried tomato** (another turkey-and-chicken-based sausage).

Check out the Aidells store locator: www.aidells.com/sausages/ where.

Koegels, near Flint, Michigan, is a good example of the German influence on American food. Albert Koegel learned his trade in Germany before moving to the Flint area to establish the business in 1916. Koegel's manufactures a full range of sausage. They make a smoked pork and beef hot dog sausage called a **Koegel's Vienna;** a pork and pork-liver braunschweiger; a spiced pork holiday bockwurst and **Pickled Red Hots,** which are smoked beef and pork frankfurters blended with hot chili pepper and packed in vinegar. Koegel's sausage is available in stores throughout Michigan and in some parts of Ohio and Indiana, and at Angelo's Coney Island restaurants, in Genesee County, Michigan.

QUICK BITE

In the ethnic neighborhoods of the Midwest a wide variety of kielbasa can be found—from lightly-spiced fresh versions to coarse-textured smoked sausages with plenty of garlic, spices, and pepper.
        —Bruce Aidells, *Bruce Aidells's Complete Sausage Book* (2000)

From novelist Adam Langer: "**Polish Sausage** at Jim's Original Polish in Chicago—the original Maxwell Street stand has been bulldozed to make way for new University of Illinois developments, but the sausage is still available nearby. It is quite possibly even less healthy than anything on offer at Hardee's but also a hundred times more delicious."

So in all this talk of franks and other German sausage, don't forget the rest of Europe. From Poland comes the **kielbasa,** which represents a many and varied sausage family in its own right but which is known in the United States mostly in the form of the smoked ring. In a similar vein is the Hungarian **kolbasz,** a pork sausage with a lot of garlic and paprika. **Boudin noir** is a French blood sausage that's been a mainstay on the menu at New York Meatpacking District eatery Florent for years. For breakfast, eat it served over apples and onions.

🛒 Koegel's has an online store locator that tells you where their products are available. They'll also sell you sausage online: www .koegelmeats.com.

BRATS

Wisconsin is bratwurst country. There are brat festivals here: In Sheboygan in the first week in August, for example, where the Johnsonville Company sponsors Brat Days. Madison has a four-day Bratfest, billed as the world's largest, where about eighteen miles of brats may be consumed over Memorial Day weekend. Tailgating with brats is a tradition for sports fans, most notably Packers fans at Lambeau Field, in Green Bay. Brats have their own rules that purists will claim you must apply: Don't use yellow mustard; use **German-style Düsseldorf mustard** instead. Don't cook your brat in beer. Don't put a sausage on a hot dog bun, and so on.

My friend Bud came into possession of some genuine **Wisconsin brats,** ordered through Mars' Cheese Castle, in Kenosha, and originating from the Usinger Sausage Company of Milwaukee. Bud fixed the brats in his apartment in New York City. I was concerned about violating the list of brat dos and don'ts, so I called Nolechek's Meats in Thorp, Wisconsin, for some tips. This is a store that sells fresh and smoked bratwurst among numerous sausage products. (Nolechek's will also process the deer you shot for you.) Some of the brats sold here are taken to Packers games to be tailgated. Nolechek's said we could grill our brats, or parboil them and then brown them.

🛒 Smokehouse meats, Wisconsin cheese, baked goods, gift boxes: Mars' Cheese Castle: 1-800-655-6147 / www.marscheese.com.

🛒 Fresh and smoked meats and sausage and cheese at Nolechek's: 1-800-454-5580 / www.nolechekmeats.com.

Without any advice from me, Bud had decided to start off the brats in a slow cooker. While Bud was at work, the brats simmered away in a can of **Boddington's** beer, the cream of Manchester, United Kingdom. We met up at his apartment, and Bud transferred the brats to a frying pan and browned them with onions and butter. We ate the sausage in genuine **S. Rosen's Brat & Sausage Rolls,** which originate in Chicago. We assumed these would be acceptable to the brat police. But throwing dirt in the face of convention, we used fancy French mustard, not the German kind. The brats were very good, with the seasoning well to the fore. They were peppery rather than herby. Having been plumped up in beer and then browned in a pan, they were crisp outside and juicy within. Fleshy cylinders of goodness.

 QUICK BITE

Spicy Italian sausage is endlessly adaptable because you can mix and match hot and sweet sausage according to your taste. It's great braised and crumbled into pasta sauce or paired with meatballs in a lasagna layered with ricotta, pasta, leaf spinach, and basil. One of my favorite dishes with Italian sausage is **Orecchiette with Broccoli Rabe and Sausage,** as per the recipe in the *Rao's Cookbook.* When the dish is dashed with red pepper flakes and fresh Parmesan or Pecorino Romano, your mouth becomes a happy playground bombarded with flavors and textures: hot, sweet, bitter, creamy, chewy, leafy. The dish is also a nicely balanced nutritional plateful, especially when accompanied by a glass of red wine.

BANGERS

A couple of days before eating the brats, it happened that I had eaten a good few English sausages—known as **bangers**—at a Guy Fawkes Night party. Each November 5, the English celebrate the foiling of a plot to blow up the Houses of Parliament in 1605 by setting off fireworks and burning a "Guy," an effigy representing the Catholic plotters. The bangers I ate in New York were from Myers of Keswick, a store in Manhattan that sells a wide array of old-fashioned English food. The traditional English banger is a pork sausage that roasts up very nicely in the oven. I was encouraged by these bangers to buy some of my own to eat on December 26, a holiday called Boxing Day in the United Kingdom (which has nothing to do with pugilism but refers instead to medieval practices of collecting tips from your masters once a year in special boxes).

Myers of Keswick is jammed with British products I would never

QUICK BITE

From Scotland comes the seemingly sinister **haggis,** the mythic dish associated with Burns Night (January 25), when Scots commemorate their national icon, poet Robert Burns. I've twice eaten haggis on Burns Night in the company of expatriate Scots. The first time, served on the territory of the auld enemy (England), was definitely "traditional" haggis, made from the pluck of a sheep (its lights [lungs], liver, and heart) ground with oatmeal and spices, stuffed into a sheep's stomach, and boiled. It's served with **tatties and neeps:** mashed potatoes and Swede (Swedish turnip), which tastes good with a heavy dusting of freshly ground pepper.

A haggis is in fact a giant sausage, and I remember being taken by the overwhelming spiciness of it. American-made haggis is probably ersatz: it's very unlikely that it will include all the sheep's organs, because the FDA has declared lung tissue "unfit for human consumption."

normally have bought when I lived in London but that are irresistible to me when I see them over here. Which is why I don't go to Myers of Keswick very often. (Don't let this stop you, however.) Propelled by atavistic urges last time I was in, I bought a packet of Tunnock's wafers (Scottish caramel biscuits), together with two cans of microwavable spotted dick (sponge pudding with raisins), which at the time of writing sit uneaten in a kitchen cabinet. I picked up a tin of Bird's instant custard powder and a box of Jaffa cakes, which are chocolate-covered cookies with a soft orange jelly filling (half of which sit, ossified and uneaten, in another cupboard). None of these items were what I was in the shop for. The charming Scottish woman who filled my order indulged me as I bought pounds of Cumberland sausage, bangers, pork pies, steak and kidney pies, Scotch eggs, and sausage rolls, cleaning the store out of many of them.

It turned out, of course, that I over-ordered wildly at Myers for the small gathering we assembled. I had a lot of fun cooking. I enjoyed making a couple of versions of the classic British **trifle,** spreading raspberry jam on pieces of pound cake and layering them with raspberries, real custard, and whipped cream. (One trifle had alcohol soaked into the cake; the other didn't.) I cooked up the **Cumberland sausages** and bangers in the oven, boiled (far too many) potatoes for the mashed potatoes, and made Jamie Oliver's **Onion Gravy** (balsamic and red wine vinegar, butter, beef bouil-

QUICK BITE

It is thanks to the British that America's premier sausage maker found his vocation. But it was nothing that inspired him in a positive way. Bruce Aidells used to live in London, in the area called Barons Court, and he worked in Lincoln's Inn as a scientist at the Imperial Cancer Research Fund. Aidells told me that when he ate pub food he would find out first-hand what breaded filling does to a sausage. The horrors of bad British sausages persuaded him to try his hand at making them himself, and he founded the Aidells Sausage Company in 1983.

lon, and red onions) from *Jamie's Dinners*. You can't miss it: it's the first recipe in the book.

I have to say—and no one is more modest about his cooking and with better reason than I—the sausage and mash with onion gravy, taken with a cold pint of Guinness, was fantastic. Roasted in the oven, the sausage will develop a sticky carapace as the casing browns in the fat released by the sausage meat. You have to make sure to turn the sausage a few times, but not before it has got good and brown along the side facing down. That surface will harden. It's best to take a bite when the banger is just as hot as you can stand it. Keep your lips clear and set your teeth into the thing and find the steaming, still-pink but cooked core. Whether you've made a fancy gravy or not, you need a good portion of **Colman's English Mustard** into which to lightly dunk the banger. There's a reason why sausage, in all its forms, is so popular. It's just good eating.

SAUSAGE SUMMARY

RUN, DON'T WALK, FOR . . .

- **Bangers and mash.** Homemade, with Jamie Oliver's onion gravy and a lot of Colman's English Mustard, this dish transcends its origins.

- Real **Wisconsin brats,** cooked any way you like. Just good eating too.

▦ Bruce Aidells's **Habañero and Green Chile Smoked Chicken and Turkey Sausages**. I'll eat anything with habañero and green chile, and these sausages aren't just anything.

IF YOU'VE NEVER TRIED . . .

▦ **Real haggis with tatties and neeps.** Eat, enjoy, and don't think about it.

▦ **Boudin noir** and any blood sausage. See above.

5

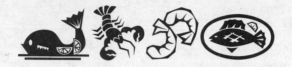

FISH AND SEAFOOD

*Probably the busiest time the girls of the Bear Flag ever had
was the March of the big sardine catch. It wasn't only that the fish
ran in silvery billions and money ran almost as freely. A new regiment
moved into the Presidio and a new bunch of soldiers always shop around
a good deal before they settle down. . . . The men from the sardine fleet,
loaded with dough, were in and out all afternoon. They sail at dark
and fish all night so they must play in the afternoon.*

—John Steinbeck, *Cannery Row* (1945)

An aphorism that can be well applied to all food works best for seafood: there's no such thing as too fresh. Let's illustrate. A friend tells a story about a party he went to in Seattle, a city known for its seafood. The host asks of the assembled company, "Anyone want crab dip?" "Sure," someone replies, so our obliging host leaves the room. When he reappears a minute or two later, he's not carrying a dish of dip, but he is wearing a wet suit. "I'll be right back," he says, or words to that effect. Off he goes, down to Puget Sound, which is right there on his doorstep. He pops in the water, picks up some crab, comes home, and makes the dip. How fresh do you want your seafood to be?

Few of us are lucky enough to be able to cater to our friends quite like this. In the Pacific Northwest, however, there are plenty of places that will provide the service for you. Hsiao-Ching Chou at the *Seattle Post-Intelligencer* told me about a couple of them. The first is the Willows Inn on tiny Lummi Island, a couple of hours' drive north of Seattle, the last stretch being a five-minute ferry ride from Bellingham. In the summer, Washingtonians make weekly pilgrimages up here for the **spot prawns.** Spot prawns are big, as big sometimes as the palm of a hand, with large heads and sharp barbs on the tail. When it comes to our eating them, they have an ephemeral quality, with sweet, crisp flesh that starts to deteriorate as soon as the prawn leaves salt water. Before long, the meat has turned to mush. It is possible to buy frozen spot prawns, but by far the best way to eat them is straight out of the water. They're tough to eat, but "they are amazing," Hsiao-Ching says. "I can't believe how good they are."

The proprietor of the Willows Inn is Riley Starks. On Sunday evenings in the summer months (May 1 through August), Riley and his wife, Judy Olsen, host "Prawns on the Deck," where you come and relax with a margarita while your prawns are cooked. They're prepared simply: cooked in olive oil with some coarsely chopped garlic. Riley buys the prawns from a neighbor—Leo's Live Seafood—and keeps them alive in large tanks until Sunday. Guests can look in the tank and pick out their own dinner.

QUICK BITE

*The tiny native Olympia oysters eaten with a toothpick are a delicious novelty but nothing beats a really fresh **Puget Sound Oyster** grilled over coals until the shell pops open, then drowned in warm garlic lemon butter with a splash of Tabasco sauce. Best when you pick out the oysters yourself, or if you buy them from the stall at the Shelton OysterFest in October.*

—Susan Volland, author of
Love and Meatballs (2004) and Cooking for Mr. Right (2005)

The chef at the Willows Inn is Craig Miller. Riley provides his chef with the choicest and freshest salmon by catching it in his own reef nets out on Legoe Bay. Reef-netting is cumbersome and labor intensive. So much so that Riley Starks says there are perhaps no more than eleven full reef-netting gears (concerns) left, three in the San Juan Islands, of which Lummi Island is the most northerly. Most salmon fishing that doesn't involve a rod and a reel uses methods like drift nets, which chase after the fish. But reef net rigs are stationary—you don't go after the fish; you wait for the fish to come to you. On the Leo's Live Web site there's a sequence of photographs that shows how the two boats that have the gear strung between them work together to capture the fish. The salmon are taken alive. Only premium fish are kept; everything else is thrown back.

As far as Riley Starks is concerned, **reef-net-caught salmon** is a far superior fish to one taken any other way. Hooking and reeling in a salmon puts the fish under considerable stress, which causes it to produce lactic acid. The acid builds up in the flesh, adversely affecting the flavor. Japanese fish buyers will test for lactic acid in tuna, and its presence can make a difference of thousands of dollars in the market value of a single fish. Salmon caught in a reef net and bled out in salt water simply tastes cleaner and better. At the restaurant, the salmon might simply be roasted in a wood oven with salt and pepper or prepared as a **ceviche with dill and jalapeño.**

Riley Starks, who was born in Port Townsend in Washington, is a confirmed booster of his region. He says Lummi Island is in a rain shadow so it gets less precipitation than famously soggy Seattle. Riley points out that this is also world-class oyster country. He recommends local supplier Taylor Shellfish, who will ship you oysters, including the famous, and once rare, **Olympia oyster.**

QUICK BITE

*The Puget Sound is a huge oyster-producing area, the favorite being the petit Olympia oyster. These silver-dollar-size mollusk crops are maintained and harvested in the Hood Canal, and in the Puget Sound down around Olympia. They became part of a dish called **Hangtown Fry,** which consists of scrambled eggs, oysters, and bacon. Legend has it that a condemned man at the time of the Gold Rush asked for the most expensive things in San Francisco to be made into his last meal. And those ingredients included eggs and oysters.*   —Dana Cree

For oysters, manila clams, mussels, geoduck, and more: 1-360-432-3300 / www.taylorshellfishfarms.com. The **geoduck** is a large burrowing clam that abounds in Puget Sound. It can live more than a hundred years and get up to seven pounds in weight. Most are one to three pounds.

The locally ubiquitous **Dungeness crab** is named for the town on the Olympic Peninsula, which is itself named after Dungeness in the county of Kent in the United Kingdom. The English version is a seaside town best known for being home to two nuclear power stations, Dungeness A and Dungeness B. (What would you rather be famous for, a tasty crustacean or a nuclear power plant?) Eat Dungeness crab, or anything else, at Seattle's Dahlia Lounge, a long-time favorite in the city where, at its original location in 1997, my wife waited patiently for me while I watched TV until the last out of game seven of the World Series was recorded.

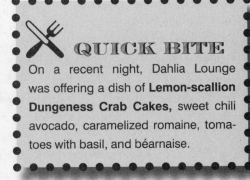

QUICK BITE

On a recent night, Dahlia Lounge was offering a dish of **Lemon-scallion Dungeness Crab Cakes,** sweet chili avocado, caramelized romaine, tomatoes with basil, and béarnaise.

While the best-known crab is a resident of the West Coast, the country's favorite crab dish is the crab cake, indelibly associated with Baltimore. Crab cakes are often served in appetizer-size portions, but the Crackpot Restaurant in Towson, outside of Baltimore, serves a twenty-ounce **"pounder crab cake,"** which comes in blackened, Mexican, and Hawaiian varieties, among others.

Snaking through Puget Sound to the north of Seattle is Whidbey Island, where the Penn Cove Mussel Festival is held in Coupeville each March. The festival includes a recipe contest, with the 2006 winner for **Mussels Tarragon.** In Coupeville, go to The Oystercatcher Restaurant, a local pub, where you can eat fresh **steamed mussels.** The local **Penn Cove mussels** are large, sweet-tasting mollusks about three inches long. They're available wholesale from the eponymous Penn Cove Mussels along with the Mediterranean variety, which are more commonly found in warmer waters farther south. This is a family business whose owners know what they're doing and care about their work, says Hsiao-Ching Chou.

———

The state of Alaska has more coastline than any other U.S. state, and fishing employs more workers than any other private industry in the state. The dollar value of the fish caught here is perhaps 40 percent of the U.S. total. The great Pacific fisheries come together here in waters that are very cold and free of pollution. This last, Kirsten Dixon points out, is a theme of the state and of all the food produced here—it's wild and likely to be mercifully untainted.

T. C. Mitchell adds, "Of course, what we do have here that very few other places, if any, have is wild, good, safe seafood, from salmon to crab, to sea cucumbers. Alaska has taken great pains to protect seafood habitats. There are failures, occasionally, but by and large, eating a fish out of our waters will suit you and your body well."

———

The sea cucumber isn't a cucumber at all but an *echinoderm*, like the sea urchin and starfish, an ancient sea creature that has existed for more than four hundred million years. At some point humans discovered we could eat the sea cucumber, something I have done knowingly only once, at the wedding banquet of my friends Deborah Kwan and Erik Cosselmon in San Francisco. The dish in question was **Sea Cucumber and Abalone over Greens,** one of a number of fantastic traditional Chinese preparations (for more of which, see page 323). Although the sea cucumber has a skeleton (an endoskeleton), it is has a jellylike texture, and I remember the gelatinous mouthfeel of the thing more than any strong taste.

The abalone is a mollusk that attaches itself to a rock with its foot. Sadly for the abalone, the foot has proved very tasty to humans, who have pried so many abalone free of their homes that they are in danger of disappearing from the wild. Harvesting is severely restricted in California (you can take only a few abalone of a specific size below a certain ocean depth in particular months, using deliberately primitive tools). Abalone are fabulously expensive: a quick check online found vacuum-packed steaks (one pound) with shells that could be shipped to you overnight for $105.

The Abalone Farm: 1-877-367-2271 / www.abalonefarm.com.

Kirsten Dixon points out that it's illegal in Alaska to farm salmon, so any and all Alaskan salmon you're going to buy will be wild. On the East Coast, when a chef buys Atlantic salmon, he or she can order custom-made fish (all the same size; all the same color) because practically all of it is farm-raised. As well-informed shoppers know, there are also certain health and environmental issues thought to be associated with farm-raised salmon that should be taken into consideration. "Wild" salmon now bears a heavy premium in stores as a result.

> ## QUICK BITE
>
> I ask Caprial Prence in Portland where the best salmon comes from. "Oregon, of course. But Alaskan king is wonderful also." So how do you like your salmon? "I like it best grilled, then smoked. [Husband] John does an amazing smoked salmon."

The city of Seattle serves as a portal for Alaska salmon that is sent here, then around the rest of the country and across the world. Fisherman come to Cordova, at the mouth of the Copper River, to look for king salmon as the fish find their way back to the river to spawn. The sport season is from mid-May to mid-June, but salmon is fished commercially throughout the year.

Copper River salmon is available from any restaurant in the Pacific Northwest and by mail from Prime Select Seafoods, in Cordova. Fish designated simply "Copper River salmon" might be any one of the five salmon species, from the best king or chinook, through the milder, summer-running sockeye, or red, then the coho, or silver, salmon to the small pinks

QUICK BITE

In June, in the middle of the salmon season, I picked up a piece of Copper River salmon in New York City at the Wild Edibles stand in Grand Central Market. Just under a pound and a quarter of fish cost about thirty bucks. I wasn't able to find out whioh typo of salmon this was, beyond the fact that it had swum in the Copper River, but it was a smallish fish, with a bright red tinge to the flesh. Lightly baked, it made a delightful summer dinner. The taste was real essence of salmon—very strong.

Wild Edibles fresh fish and seafood: 1-877-295-3474 / www .wildedibles.com.

(humpies) and keta, or chum, which has the least oil and consequently the least flavor and which might end up being fed to the dog teams.

For fresh and freshly frozen salmon, halibut, and cod, try Prime Select Seafood: 1-888-870-7292 / www.pssifish.com.

Rarer than the **Copper River king salmon** is the **Yukon River king salmon.** What makes the Yukon fish so appealing is the very high fat content, which means that the flesh is very rich and sumptuous. The fish have to build up a great deal of fat in their bodies so they are able to traverse the long Yukon River—they have to swim up to two thousand miles from the Bering Sea to the spawning grounds upriver. As a result, the taste is different from that of Copper River king salmon, and it's too intense for some people. T. C. Mitchell says also to look out for "what's called a **White King** that is very succulent. They're not rare, but not easily found either. A local sushi chef [Peter Park of Peter's Sushi Spot] covets them and serves it to special guests when he gets one."

In the cold, clear Alaskan waters, **halibut** can live long enough to attain enormous sizes. In England, when I thought of a flatfish, I'd probably think of a whole sole dressed up and laid out on a plate. But in Alaska, hundred-pound halibut aren't particularly rare, and monsters up to eight

QUICK BITE

*One of my first vivid childhood memories is of salmon, from Seattle's Ballard Locks, standing in front of the windows that expose the fish ladder watching these magnificent creatures fight their way upstream. Each year my father and uncle would spend long weekend days fishing, and occasionally they'd bring home a salmon. My father would call from the marina and my mother would set up the Little Chief home smoker. She would prepare a brine for the salmon that used a lot of brown sugar, as I remember. The fish would spend around four hours out of the water before it made its way into the brine. The next day it was in the smoker on our front porch, the alder chips changed frequently by my mother. My favorite dish was my mother's **smoked salmon spread.** She'd mix the salmon with cream cheese and a hint of horseradish, lemon juice, and chopped herbs. It was such a hit with our friends and family that one woman asked for some as her wedding gift.*   —Dana Cree

feet long and 450 pounds in weight have been recorded. Kirsten Dixon says she often buys halibut by the side, as in a side of beef, which in this instance might mean forty pounds of fish. Occasionally, she'll buy a small whole fish, but she uses it for stock. She says halibut is a very versatile fish. It has a delicate, suggestible flavor but will hold up to the rough treatment of barbecuing. In Alaska, it's an inexpensive fish and is used by everyone. You can dress it up and dress it down, Kirsten says, make a **chowder** out of it, or something more formally plated and delicate. She likes to prepare it in an adapted Asian style, with Thai seasonings. Halibut is also meaty enough to be broiled up and served with creamed spinach in a steakhouse, a dish I've enjoyed once or twice.

Kirsten Dixon has written a couple of cookbooks: *The Winterlake Lodge Cookbook* and *The Riversong Lodge Cookbook*. Her Web site is packed with sumptuous recipes, including a preparation for halibut, **Alaskan Halibut and Reindeer Sausage Pizza,** and also an alluring **Russian Salmon Pie,** also known as

Coulibiac, or Koulibiac, which includes onion, mushrooms, cabbage, a hard-boiled egg, and rice along with the salmon, all sitting expectantly under a puff pastry crust. Kirsten has her own recipe for **Baked Alaska,** which originated in its most well known form at Delmonico's restaurant in New York in the 1870s, and which Kirsten says appears in Alaska most often on the cruise ships that visit the state.

━━━━━━

Alaska is also well-known for **king crab,** which Kirsten describes as "large and intriguing." They're "just flat good eating" for T. C. Mitchell. There are three different kinds of commercially fished king crab: golden (or, confusingly, brown), blue, and red, the last of which yields the giant legs that are so prized, and so pricey. In Alaska, there's shrimp and mussels and oysters, too. "So we eat pretty well on fresh seafood," he says.

SARDINES

John Steinbeck's *Cannery Row* was published in 1945 when the Pacific sardine he wrote about was well on its way to being almost completely fished out. At the time, it was a significant industry; about a quarter of all fish landed in the United States were sardines. By the early fifties the industry was pretty much gone, and the fish has significantly recovered only in recent years. It might be that sardine populations ebb and flow with changing climatic conditions, and the fact that people are eating more of sardines' main predator, the anchovy, has helped the previously downtrodden sardine. Whatever the reason, sardines have been reappearing among catches of squid and mackerel. (**Squid** is now the most valuable California catch.)

Sardines are a fantastic fish—flavorful, healthy (rich in great Omega-3 oils), and freer of heavy-metal contaminants than larger, longer-lived fish. I love grilled fresh sardines. If you're buying them yourself, it's important to get your sardines as fresh as you can, because they degrade quickly. I am certainly not against a can of sardines, the poor relation, every once in a while.

Look at the Web site for the Monterey Fish Market, whose retail store is in Berkeley, for interesting pieces on all the locally available fish, including sardines: www.montereyfish.com.

WATCH OUT FOR . . .

In 2004 the Food and Drug Administration and the Environmental Protection Agency issued a consumer advisory on methylmercury levels in some fish. Waterborne mercury becomes methylmercury that fish absorb. It builds up at different rates in different fish. The advisory stressed that eating fish and shellfish was part of a healthy diet but that methylmercury could be harmful to unborn babies and small children. So women who might become pregnant or are pregnant, nursing, or feeding a young child might wish to follow these guidelines:

1. Do not eat shark, swordfish, king mackerel, or tilefish, because they contain high levels of mercury.
2. Eat up to twelve ounces (two average meals) a week of a variety of fish and shellfish that are lower in mercury.

   ◆ Five of the most commonly eaten fish that are low in mercury are shrimp, canned light tuna, salmon, pollock, and catfish.
   ◆ Another commonly eaten fish, albacore ("white") tuna, has more mercury than canned light tuna. So, when choosing your two meals of fish and shellfish, you may eat up to six ounces (one average meal) of albacore tuna per week.

3. Check local advisories about the safety of fish caught by family and friends in your local lakes, rivers, and coastal areas. If no advice is available, eat up to six ounces (one average meal) per week of fish you catch from local waters, but don't consume any other fish during that week.

Follow these same recommendations when feeding fish and shellfish to your young child, but serve smaller portions.

For more information, see www.cfsan.fda.gov/~lrd/pestadd .html#mercury.

OYSTERS

There are three kinds of oyster eaters: those loose-minded sports who will eat anything, hot, cold, thin, thick, dead or alive, as long as it is oyster; those who will eat them raw and only raw; and those who with equal severity will eat them cooked and no way other. —M. F. K. Fisher, Consider the Oyster (1941)

I haven't eaten nearly enough oysters to know with any certainty where I stand on the question of what type of oyster eater I am. I just haven't eaten nearly enough oysters. A dish of **smoked oysters** from a water-side eatery in Virginia I remember much better than the restaurant itself. (This was years ago.) My happiest oyster experience was made more memorable because it was so unexpected. Together with our friends the Magees, we were driving along Route 25 past the vineyards on Long Island's North Fork. It was a rainy evening and we were making our way to Greenport for dinner. Suddenly we spied a sign on the roadside: CHAMPAGNE AND OYSTERS. Instinctively, Bob Magee, the driver, veered off the road into the Lenz Winery, which lay just beyond the sign. It wasn't really a tough decision for Bob: he loves champagne, and his wife, Paula, loves oysters.

And the oysters were fabulous. We ate three kinds of Blue Point oysters from local waters: **Robins Island oysters, Orients,** and **Mystics.** Paula went around the station many times. There were enough oysters to sample them with lemon, with cocktail sauce, with nothing. The last is best, for the liquor (much of which is the oyster's blood) needs no augmentation. It seems a waste just to let the beast slide straight down your throat without so much as a hello. Chew on it a little, and the oyster's full delight is revealed. It's just like eating the ocean.

QUICK BITE

Treat yourself and a few good friends to a seafood **Plateau** at the Blue Ribbon Restaurant on Sullivan Street in New York City (and it is a treat—this isn't a cheap dish). All the shellfish is super fresh—scallops, oysters and clams, giant prawns, a couple of blue crabs, and a small lobster. The Plateau is served with true style, a towering two-level contraption holding trays full of ice on which rests the glorious shellfish. With a glass of cold white Bordeaux, this is summer eating at its very best.

I talked with Karen Rivara, who farms oysters on the Peconic Bay in eastern Long Island and whose Orients and Mystics I have eaten with joy. Karen said she prefers simply a drop of lemon on her oyster. "I like to taste the complex flavors from the sea that change with the season, the location of the harvest, and the species," she says. Karen says the best place to buy oysters in the shell is any local seafood market that will let you see the harvest tags so you know where and when the oysters were harvested. And what are her personal favorites?

"As a rule I like our Mystics the best. Orients are my second favorite for local oysters. We have very few of them—most of our oysters are Mystics, lucky me! Oysters from Martha's Vineyard are also very good. They are nice on a plate with our Mystics and Orients, then you can taste three distinctly different, high-quality, delicious oysters."

I wanted my oyster vocabulary to be bolstered. What are some of the characteristics of American oysters?

"Saltiness (brininess), sweet (like bay scallop meats), butter, seaweed, cucumber, metallic, marshy, to name a few."

Can you remember the first time you ate an oyster? My friend Rick attended Oyster Bay High School in Oyster Bay, Long Island, a town that grew up on oysters. Rick remembers back to 1975. "The climax of our science class that year was a boat trip, skippered by Butler Flowers of Frank M. Flower and Sons, a company that still exists today. He drove us around the bay, and we dredged up various 'baylife' from the bottom, for study.

"Well, of course we pulled up a load of oysters, which Mr. Flowers quickly opened with a knife I remember being short and sharp, and he offered them around. Most of us wouldn't eat the oysters except one classmate, who had brought with him a bottle of hot sauce. He eagerly slurped them down, heaping verbal abuse upon us in between swallows. My young manhood was challenged, so eventually I gave one a try. This was my first oyster, and I must confess it was a mixed experience. The texture of the oyster was a real challenge to my fifteen-year-old palate, but the briny-buttery flavor was outstanding. Every time I've had oysters since, I think of each swallow as the taste of my hometown."

There's good reading to be had with the oyster too. M. F. K. Fisher's *Consider the Oyster* is the last word in cooking them, while Mark Kurlansky has used the bivalve's pearly shell as a prism through which to view the history of New York City. *The Big Oyster: History on the Half-Shell* details the oyster's front-row place in New York history from its pre-Colonial superabundance to the moment in the last century when the city's over-powering growth outdid the local waters' ability to sustain oysters enough for New York's massive appetite. For a brief period, though, oysters domi-nated local cuisine:

> *The New York of the second half of the nineteenth century was a city overtaken by oystermania. It was usual for a family to have two oys-ter dinners a week, one of which would be on Sunday. It was one of the few moments in culinary history when a single food, served in more or less the same preparations, was commonplace for all socio-economic levels. It was the food of Delmonico's and the food of the dangerous slum.*

FISH AND SEAFOOD SUMMARY

RUN, DON'T WALK, FOR . . .

- Fresh **sardines**—grilled, just great.
- **Oysters,** preferably eaten under a tent in summer with a glass of champagne in your hand, but lesser circumstances will suffice.
- A plateau of **mixed fresh seafood,** or whatever you want to call it.
- **Copper River salmon.** If you can't get to Alaska for this wonder-ful fish, they have ways of getting it to you.

IF YOU'VE NEVER TRIED . . .

- **Oysters.** Or oyster, singular. One of those things you just have to try once. Chewing helps alleviate that disconcerting slimy sensa-tion.
- **Sea cucumber.** Like nothing else I've ever eaten, and take that how you will.

6

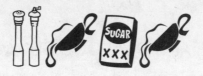

SAUCES, CONDIMENTS, AND PRESERVED FOODS

Ketchup derives its name from the Indonesian fish and soy sauce kecap ikan.
The names of several other Indonesian sauces also include the word kecap,
pronounced KETCHUP, which means a base of dark, thick soy sauce.

—Mark Kurlansky, *Salt* (2002)

For a time I would mention this book project to anyone within earshot and often get a lead to follow up. When my back doctor said, "Isn't there somewhere they mix ketchup and mayonnaise?" I looked into it. I thought this practice was probably ubiquitous and not associated with one particular place or another. My wife said that when she was growing up, the ketchup/mayo combo was called Doug Welsh dressing, after one of her brothers who made it. I used to double-dip limp, greasy chips (English fries) in separate puddles of generic British ketchup and mayonnaise when I lived in London. (Fries and good mayonnaise, on the other hand, are one of the great gifts of European cuisine.) But it turns out that in Utah, **fry sauce** (as in a sauce for fries, not fried sauce) is a distinct condiment, in the commercial form of Original Fry Sauce from the Arctic Circle chain of restaurants.

The first Arctic Circle was opened in Salt Lake City in 1950 by Don Carlos Edwards, the owner of a local barbecue place. There are now twenty-six company stores and fifty-seven franchise restaurants selling the chain's popular Black Angus Ranch Burgers in eight states, but mostly in Utah and Idaho. According to the company Web site, Bob Edwards invented fry sauce, which is "tomato concentrate, lemon juice, eggs, and a whole bunch of other ingredients." The last of these are a secret, but they don't include anything pickle-related, so this isn't **Thousand Island Dressing** under another name. (I was surprised to learn that the "thousand islands" in Thousand Islands Dressing refers to a region of upstate New York where the dressing originated.) You can have fry sauce slathered on your burger in situ, and twelve-ounce bottles of Original Fry Sauce are for sale in the restaurants or online.

For details on ordering fry sauce, visit www.arcticcirclerest.com.

Utahns have clearly developed a taste for the stuff, and also for various homemade fry sauces, the basic constituents of which are ketchup and mayonnaise with various spices thrown in. Kathy Stephenson, who writes about food for the *Salt Lake Tribune*, says you will find fry sauce all the way down to St. George, in the south of the state, but not as far away as Las Vegas, which is a hundred miles farther on.

I called Hires Big H, in downtown Salt Lake City, one of a family of Utah drive-ins. They confirm that they put their own Fry Super Sauce on the burgers, and most people do take it. I like the sound of a **Hires Golden H,** a cheeseburger with lettuce and tomato and three onion rings, the whole daubed with fry sauce ($4.25). The Cotton Bottom Inn, which is a tavern—meaning it can sell beer—told me they didn't add fry sauce to their signature **Garlic Burgers.** (It would be pointless, because the dish consists of "a half-pound burger with a lot of garlic.") I like the sound of the garlic burger even more than a burger with onion rings, though it might best be eaten alone.

· · ·

Much human ingenuity, together with what must have been generations of trial and error, has gone into finding processes, like those involved in making ketchup, to treat fresh food to prevent it from spoiling. Introducing sugar or an acid like vinegar can have this effect. The most ancient method is the addition of salt, which retards the multiplication of the bacterial organisms that cause food to go bad. Cheese, for example, emerged as a vehicle for preserving milk and butter through the use of salt.

Mark Kurlansky's book *Salt* chronicles the central place of the mineral in world cultures and how the food we eat now was shaped by salt's most useful properties. You can follow the development of fermented and salted fish sauces, which may well have appeared independently in the ancient West, in Greece and Rome, and in the East, in China, where soybeans were added to the fish and then fermented on their own—hence soy sauce. Much later, in England, sauces made from salted anchovies were used, and by the eighteenth century these sauces were called ketchup, katchup, or catsup, after the Indonesian word. Worcestershire sauce (or Worcester sauce, as it's called in the United Kingdom), created in the 1840s, also originated in Asia. Kurlansky recounts how tomato ketchup was created in America sometime around the end of the eighteenth century, with the first published recipe surfacing in 1812.

Many sauces, such as Lea & Perrins original **Worcestershire Sauce** and Arctic Circle Fry Sauce, have a secret ingredient. In the case of Worcestershire, it must be among the "Natural Flavorings" listed on the label. Although the recipe for the sauce used on a Big Mac is popularly thought to be a secret, if you look through the McDonald's Web site, you'll find a list of the ingredients in "Big Mac Sauce." There are twenty-six in all, starting with soybean oil, pickles, and distilled vinegar, and running through to extractives of paprika, turmeric, and calcium disodium EDTA, aka calcium disodium ethylenediaminetetraacetate. (This is what's known as a "sequestrant," a commonly used food additive that stops metals from oxidizing fats and thereby spoiling your dinner.) Thus will regular people be foiled in their attempts to make the sauce themselves when they look in the panty and find they're right out of calcium disodium ethylenediaminetetraacetate.

I like ketchup as much as the next person and I use a lot of **Tabasco sauce,** sometimes to my wife's consternation. On eggs, I can go either way. I like some hot sauce with scrambled eggs and a little ketchup with an omelet, but I switch it around every once in a while and occasionally will reach for both. That set me to thinking (or a simulacrum of the same): Why don't they make hot ketchup, ketchup with hot sauce? Well, needless to say, they do! Heinz, even, and with Tabasco, in something called, I think, **Heinz Ketchup Kick'rs Hot & Spicy,** with Tabasco. This I have never seen in a store, though now I will search for it closely. It's a personal annoyance when companies willfully misspell a word and Kick'rs takes the cake. Why no *e*? I know there are other Kick'rs—mesquite and garlic flavors—but Ketchup Kicker reads perfectly well to me.

An entire realm of novel ketchups is opened wide on a Web site called KetchupWorld.com. This is one of those Web sites you look at and say to yourself, who knew? The ketchups are helpfully organized by type: sugarless, organic, tomato-free, gluten-free, hot n' spicy, and international (there are German, Dutch, South African, and Jamaican ketchups). And there's more than just the Kick'rs in the hot ketchup category; other sauces include **KetchHot Habañero Ketchup** from Pennsylvania, which was awarded first place for ketchup in the 2005 Scovie Awards. The Scoville scale is used to measure the heat in a pepper, hence "Scovie." Check out

QUICK BITE

Lafcadio Hearn's 1885 *La Cuisine Creole* includes a recipe for **Superior Tomato Catsup.** Scald and strain a bushel of tomatoes. Add a pint and a half of salt, four tablespoons of ground cloves, four tablespoons of cayenne pepper, a quarter of a pound of allspice, a tablespoon of black pepper, a head of garlic cloves, and a half gallon of vinegar. Boil until it is reduced by half, then bottle.

(A bushel, I find looking in my dictionary, is a dry weight measure equivalent to four pecks. A peck is a dry measure of eight quarts, while a quart, as a dry measure, is listed in my source, helpfully, as one-eighth of a peck. And a dry quart isn't quite the same as a wet one. There are standard bushel/weight equivalents associated with agricultural produce, and a bushel of tomatoes, according to the Georgia Farm Bureau, is fifty-three pounds in weight.)

www.fieryfoods.com/scovies/list for winners in all categories. The 2006 ketchup winner (ketchup is in the condiment bracket) is **Big Rick's Chipotle Ketchup,** out of Wichita, Kansas, another Web site worth finding, for its barbecue sauces and salsas.

KetchupWorld: 1-866-KETCHUP (1-866-538-2487) / www.Ketchup World.com.

Big Rick's: 1-800-964-7425 / www.bigricks.com.

Mustard is both a plant and an ancient condiment that's been around for thousands of years and is made using the crushed-up seeds of the eponymous plant. The ne plus ultra of mustards is without question Colman's English Mustard, made since at least 1814 in Norwich, in the

QUICK BITE

In the L.A. Farmers Market, check out the store called Light My Fire, which is given over entirely to hot sauce, which you can slather over your breakfast eggs. The bottles are arranged according to a homemade heat scale: 1–4 is wimpy, 5–7 nice 'n' spicy, 8–10 is a pleasant burn, followed by 10+, ++ etc., as you rise up the Scoville Scale into rank irresponsibility. Here there were more sauces than I had ever seen, or could have imagined are produced, some with X-rated names and labels. "**Smack My Ass and Call Me Sally**" is a favorite from the PG-13 table.

Looking around on the Internet for a friendly port of call from which to order hot sauce, I alighted on Austin's Tears of Joy Hot Sauce Shop. They have Smack My Ass and Call Me Sally, a native of Florida, for $9.25. Their best seller is their own **Tears of Joy Tequila Lime Hot Sauce**: ". . . crisp and tangy with fresh lime juice and fiery with jalapeños and African bird pepper."

Contact the Tears of Joy Hot Sauce Shop: www.tearsofjoy sauces.com.

lovely county of Norfolk, in the east of England. Unless world events have made a dramatic turn since this book was published, Norfolk isn't part of the United States. But I make no excuses for including Colman's mustard in this book because I love it. The white-vinegary taste of standard American yellow mustard doesn't do it for me, I'm afraid. As far as I'm concerned, it always pales in comparison. (If pressed, I'll say **Annie's Naturals Organic Yellow Mustard** has a good bite to it.)

Colman's, as it's colloquially known, is an invigorating and colorful condiment. Carefully applied, it adds a potent punch to most savory foods. It's great, for example, added to the cheese sauce for a decidedly grown-up mac and cheese. My father would always load up a few teaspoons' worth of Colman's on the side of his plate for the Sunday lunch of roast beef or lamb, together with hillocks of salt and pepper and a river of **homemade gravy** (made by deglazing the roasting pan and adding a gravy mix or flour). My mother would often comment that it was in the unused dollop of mustard always left on my father's plate that Mr. Colman made his fortune.

The most common use for Colman's is the irresistible if slightly dominating note it adds to any deli meat and/or cheese sandwich. A traditional American sandwich made out of whatever meat and cheese you can find in the fridge (turkey, ham, and Provolone, for example) on whatever bread you have (say, sliced whole wheat) with a slather of Hellmann's (Light) Mayonnaise is immeasurably enhanced by a generous application of Colman's English Mustard. The possibly bland and eminently predictable is made fresh and exciting, and may even leave you with tingly sensations.

Colman's is available in the original powdered form and also in more common premade paste in glass jars. The powder allows you to mix the mustard to your own specifications. You can make it as strong as you like, although it will overpower everything it touches after a certain point, including you. Thank goodness you can buy Colman's mustard in many good food stores in this country and also over the phone or by fax from Myers of Keswick (see pages 85–86). You can also order it through the Ketchup-World Web site.

There is an American shrine to mustard, the famous Mount Horeb Mustard Museum in Mount Horeb, Wisconsin, brainchild of Mr. Barry Levenson. The museum, packed with yellow delight, is open seven days a week, ten to five. It sponsors National Mustard Day the first Saturday in August and has a Web site from which you can order any or all of about five hundred varieties. For an intriguing gift, consider one of their mustard clubs. Three different mustards will be sent to a lucky friend or relative at an interval you select: quarterly, bimonthly, or even monthly. Can you eat that much mustard?

Mount Horeb Mustard Museum store: 1-800-438-6878 / www .mustardmuseum.com.

Mustard fans should also investigate the Napa Valley Mustard Festival, held in February and March, when the valley is yellowed by the brightness of the wild mustard plants. The festival includes a World-Wide Mustard Competition, in March at COPIA, the American Center for Wine, Food, and the Arts, in Yountville. There are fifteen categories of homemade mustard judged, like sweet-hot, honey, coarse-grained, and garlic. Barry Levenson, of the mustard museum, is involved in judging the entries.

Pickling produce in a briny, vinegary solution is another preserving method. The most popular vegetable to pickle in this country is the cucumber, usually the Kirby variety. The word that describes the preservative process is now used to describe this specific food. These are the main types of pickle:

- **Dill.** Sour, whole cucumbers pickled with dill seed and/or fresh or dried dill.
- **Kosher dill.** As above, with garlic added. (The name often refers to the presence of garlic so it may or may not be certified kosher.)
- **Sweet dill.** Can be made sweet by adding sugar during pickling.
- **Sour.** Very sour, long-cured for weeks in spicy brine, creating sour taste. A New York favorite.
- **Half sour.** As above, but less so because of shorter immersion.
- **New pickle.** A cucumber removed from the briny solution after a couple of days rather than the weeks a sour pickle is pickled. Still crunchy.
- **Bread and butter.** Sweet, sliced cucumbers, pickled with onions, seasoned with sugar and spices like mustard seed, celery seed, turmeric, and cloves.

You can pick your pickle to suit your mood: sweet, sour, and in be-tween. I like the hopeful, up-tempo snap of a new pickle. The pickle is closely associated with New York City and the Lower East Side, where pickle vendors once flourished. Now there is Guss' Pickles on Orchard Street, another Guss' Pickles in Cedarhurst, New York, and also The Pickle Guys, the last two of which will sell you a pickle (and other pickled vegeta-tion) by mail-order. You pay your money and take your pickle.

Guss' Pickles: 1-800-620-GUSS / www.gusspickle.com.

The Pickle Guys: 1-888-4-PICKLE / www.nycpickleguys.com.

Check out the International Pickle Day held annually on the old pickle-centric Lower East Side of Manhattan, on Orchard Street in Sep-tember. Organizers highlight the international flavor—it's about more than just pickled cucumbers: "Pickle adventurers will see that pickles can be radishes, tomatoes, okra, cabbage, fish, meat, carrots, beans, onions, eggs, limes, mangoes, peaches, beets—any food preserved in brine."

So there's a whole world of pickled food for us to explore. Take the **Pickled Green Tea Leaf Salad** at the Myanmar Restaurant in Falls Church, in the D.C. area. Monisha Primlani says, "I cannot describe to you what is in this dish, because it is so foreign that I could not venture to guess." The Burmese food ("unbelievable cuisine") featured at this unas-suming location boasts unusual flavors to a Western-trained palate—stuff like **jackfruit,** which I tried out of a can and whose salty-sour tase I just couldn't reconcile with anything I knew. As Monisha puts it, "The tastes from this restaurant are downright invigorating."

Then there is the world of canning. A couple of generations ago, people canned their own food in Mason jars as a matter of course if they had ex-cess produce available. The idea is to heat whatever foodstuff you're work-ing with, once you've sealed it into its storage jar, in order to kill off whatever organisms are present. The heating creates a vacuum that pre-vents microbes from getting in. The amount of acid present in certain foods, such as tomatoes, makes them easier to store because the acid kills off bacteria without the presence of heat. Some foods, such as berries, are better stored as a preserve; others, such as cabbage, are better pickled (hence sauerkraut).

Visit the Jam and Relish Kitchen at Kitchen Kettle Village, in Intercourse, Pennsylvania, where you'll get a good look at the range of foods that can be canned, and be able to watch a group of Amish women at work in the kitchen doing the canning. The hostess of Kitchen Kettle Village is Pat Burnley, who grew up in the house that's now the village restaurant and who started a canning business with her husband, Bob, in 1954. The village is a collection of stores, restaurants, and attractions in the center of Intercourse, one of the best-known stops in Pennsylvania Dutch Country. There's a bakery, a shop selling local meat and cheese, a candy store, and a **kettle korn** outfit. (Kettle korn is the local popcorn wickedly seasoned with sugar and salt. I bought a huge bag of it at the railroad museum in Strasburg and couldn't stop eating it.) There are also a lot of craft stores (more than thirty stores in all) and even a bunch of guesthouses where you can stay the night. It's quaint but unpretentious and very well done. My family went on a buggy ride while I proceeded to the jam and relish kitchen on Pepper Lane.

What you notice first when you walk in the store is the group of women in the back making the product. The store sells more than seventy types of jams, jellies, preserves, sauces, salsas, and spreads, and they're all made here, out in the open for everyone to see. Today's batch was **Seedless Black Raspberry Jam**. The food is cooked in stainless-steel kettles, and a jar's worth is shot every two seconds into a glass container, which is then plunged into 185°F water, which creates the vacuum. Later the jars are all checked, and any that haven't formed a good seal are discarded.

You can test most of the products on offer. Dip into an open jar and spread your salsa on an oyster cracker. It's easy to overstimulate your taste buds here: I went from **Jalapeño Jam** and **Hot Red Raspberry Preserve** (made with dried Chile de Arbol peppers) through **Pepper Jam, Pickled Beets,** and **Horseradish Mustard** to **Fig Jam, Rhubarb Jam,** and **Damson Plum Jam**. It was all good, and I bought some mustard, some **Black Bean Salsa,** some of the seedless black raspberry preserve, and a jar of **chow chow**. Chow chow is a relish/salad similar to the Italian *giardiniera*. The Kitchen Kettle version is made of beans (green, kidney, wax, and lima), onions, carrots, cauliflower, pepper, and so on, and fulfills the local liking for sweet-and-sour dishes. It is quite sweet, but great to eat with cold chicken (or by itself out of the jar). There's also a **Hot Chow Chow** made with habañero flakes that I tried, and it's genuinely hot.

This is a very enjoyable place to shop—we also bought a doormat and some knickknacks for the kids at the jam and relish kitchen, and made it back to the car only after stopping at the Lapp Valley Farm Ice Cream stand and buying a couple of servings of their most delicious homemade ice cream.

 Order Kitchen Kettle products from 1-800-732-3538 or from www .kitchenkettle.com.

Also check out the Amish Mart out of Geneva, Indiana, at www .amishmart.com.

✗ QUICK BITE

Another way to preserve food is to dry it. I bought a two-ounce pack of dried raspberries at one of the fancy Wild By Nature stores (an offshoot of Long Island's King Kullen). At $6.99 for two ounces, they weren't cheap. The lurid red berries looked like something you might glue onto a piece of artwork at a preschool craft fair, but they tasted great—of the intense, sharp essence of raspberry. These were **Just Raspberries** from the Just To-matoes company of Westley, California. The company says that all it does with the fruit and vegetables it sells is remove their water. Nothing's added to the freeze-dried foodstuff, hence the name. Bell peppers, corn, garlic mushrooms, onions, peas, apples, bananas, blackberries, blueberries, mango, pineapple, strawberries. Even persimmon. Many of the products are organic and they keep for a long time, especially out of the sun.

Order from 1-800-537-1985 / www.justtomatoes.com.

Back in Colonial America it was a practice to make "butter" from very ripe fruits such as apples, prunes, plums, peaches, pears, grapes and at times even cherries. If no sugar or honey was available, the fruit often furnished the sweetness of this favorite spread.   —James Beard's American Cookery (1972)

You will see a lot of **apple butter** around Lancaster County, and Kitchen Kettle Village has apple, peach, pear, and pumpkin versions. There is an annual apple butter festival in Berkeley Springs, West Virginia, where vats of the stuff are made and passersby can help in the important work of keeping the butter stirred to prevent scorching.

Apart from discussing chowder preferences, another way to start an argument in New England is to brag on your state's maple syrup. American maple syrup production is dwarfed by that of Canada, but Vermont makes the most in the United States, followed by Maine and then New York State. **Vermont maple syrup** comes with language that sounds like an *appellation d'origine contrôlée*. "Vermont Pure Maple Syrup," announces the small jerry can I bought in Burlington. "Sealed in Accordance with Vermont Law. Natural Maple Color and Flavor. Nothing Added—Nothing Deducted." Vermont clearly takes its syrup seriously. The state even chose a scene of a person collecting sap from a couple of maples to adorn its state quarter. (Which other states depict food or produce on their quarters? Georgia and Wisconsin, so far. Idaho's quarter, released in 2007, doesn't have a potato, as some might imagine, but a peregrine falcon.)

 QUICK BITE

Kirsten Dixon mentions **birch bark syrup** as an unusual Alaska specialty. It's still quite rare, but more birch trees are being tapped in the state. The syrup is very different from that of the maple. It's very sweet, Kirsten says, with a distinctive piney flavor. It takes about a hundred gallons of tree sap to make one gallon of birch syrup, which is more than twice the amount of maple tree sap required to make a gallon of the better-known maple version. The Alaskan Birch Syrup Makers Association has codified rules for its Pure Alaskan Birch Syrup so you know what to look for. This is a rare commodity—only two thousand gallons or so are produced each year.

BirchBoy.com (1-877-769-5660) has a big selection of birch and other unique Alaskan syrups. The company makes syrup from the fruit of the **salmonberry** plant, which is a kind of raspberry, from the tips of the **Alaskan Sitka spruce**, from **wild red elderberries**, and more.

Bob Pastorio, cook and radio host, talks about the Highland Maple Festival in Highland County, Virginia, held each March (see www.high landcounty.org). Here, "Maple-sugaring (a new compound verb) takes place. Every little country church, service organization, and civic group is out selling food. Each has staked out a particular kind of thing— doughnuts (with maple glaze, hot to order); pancakes (and everything else) . . . with maple syrup; local fresh trout (caught that day); dinners with the (sometimes strange) fixin's; candy (maple, of course); and lots of other offerings." Bob lives in the Shenandoah Valley. "It's a place that conjures romance," Bob says, "an unhurried rural image and a kind of solid-earth living. It is all (slightly) true in its surprising, evocative power. And there's good food. Essentially, robust farm food served in family-run places and a perpetual run of church suppers open to the public."

SAUCES, CONDIMENTS, AND PRESERVED FOODS SUMMARY

RUN, DON'T WALK, FOR . . .

- ▦ If you're a canner, you'll do all this at home. If not, head to Kitchen Kettle Village and try something of everything you fancy.
- ▦ A New York City **new pickle.**
- ▦ Your own favorite hot sauce: **Tabasco** brand **Habañero Sauce.** Simple but effective.

IF YOU'VE NEVER TRIED . . .

- ▦ **Chow chow.** Sounds banal, tastes great.
- ▦ **Colman's English Mustard.** There's nothing banal about this bright yellow fire raiser.

7

CEREALS AND BREAKFAST FOOD

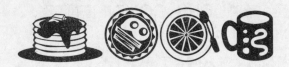

"You got donuts in the bag?" I said.

"Oatmeal-maple scones," Quirk said.

"Scones?"

"Yep."

"No donuts?"

"I'm a captain," Quirk said. "Now and then I like to upgrade."

—Robert B. Parker, *Cold Service* (2005)

At the risk of sounding like a weak stand-up comic, what is it with cops and donuts? It's an old joke, says John T. Edge in his book *Donuts: An American Passion*, and "the gags are just about spent." Well aware of the stereotype, Robert B. Parker's popular Boston private eye (no first name) Spenser finds that on this occasion, his friend in the Boston Police Department has bought scones. The inference here, of course, is that Quirk believes the scone is a superior article to the donut, certainly a classier one. In this I'd have to disagree.

I'm assuming that this fictional exchange is taking place in the morn-

ing, but I'm more familiar with the scone as an afternoon food. It is traditionally part of a British Victorian afternoon tea served midafternoon with
little sandwiches with the crusts cut off. The scone is also the centerpiece
of a cream tea of clotted cream and jam. **Clotted cream** is a specialty of
the English county of Devon, made from cream that has been heated up
and cooled. A yellowish crust forms on top of the cream, which is super-
concentrated and rich. You can't help thinking of other, medical, associa-
tions for the word *clotted* when you eat it. By and large, people don't have
formal tea anymore in Britain, though you can get it at Harrods and other
upscale eating establishments. This is how the scone is served for tea at
the Ritz: freshly baked raisin and apple scones with Devonshire clotted
cream and organic strawberry preserves.

You can order clotted cream in this country online, from the
oxymoronic-sounding Web site www.britishdelights.com.

Alas, I find it impossible to take high tea or cream tea seriously, and the
scone with it. So you can keep your scone, Captain Quirk. In this country,
sensible people won't have the hang-ups about scones that I do. Essentially,
scones are a sweet biscuit and easy to fix at home.

*Although they are similar in ingredients and technique, scones are sweeter and
richer than biscuits, with a crisp exterior and a tender, creamy crumb. They are
traditionally accompanied by an array of jams and preserves.*
    —*John Phillip Carroll,* The Baker's Dozen Cookbook *(2001)*

As for donuts/doughnuts, very rarely I'll take a Krispy Kreme donut
for breakfast. Plain **glazed** is as far as I've gone recently, though I did once
accompany someone to a drive-through Krispy Kreme outside Nashville,
where he bought a box of twelve, including some of the chocolate-glazed,
custard-filled variety. If you're going to drive to pick up your donuts, it
seems churlish to do anything other than go hog wild on them.

My favorite donut place is Bob's Coffee and Donuts in the Los Angeles
Farmers Market. The first time I went to Bob's, I asked the guy serving me
what was good to try, and he suggested an **apple fritter** to go with my coffee. It was some of the best $2.10 I'd spent in a long time, and most of that
went toward the coffee. The fritter was large, crispy, and sweet, with a dark
caramelized frosting that was like a crust around the apple center. You
could say it was a giant sweet apple French fry, and I have no idea how

many calories it might have contained. I can't stand writing about it—I want one right now. I saved the little wax paper bag Bob's donuts come in, so I'll stare wistfully at that for a while . . .

The second and third of Bob's apple fritters that I tried at a later date were just as good as the first. I also tried the gleeful **Raspberry Bismarck,** which is a large glazed jelly donut and Bob's **beignet,** from which powdered sugar cascades as you eat. Two of the Bismarcks, two apple fritters, and a cup of coffee cost $4.65, a minuscule price to pay for such joy. The apple fritter is eighty-five cents, for goodness sake.

The extent of my donut eating can be measured by the fact that Bob's in Los Angeles is my favorite donut place and I live in New York and have been to the store maybe five times. I expect you have more donut experience than I do. I eat even fewer muffins. As far as I can see, they usually manage to be both bland and cloying, a fatal combination. If there's a choice between a muffin and nothing at all, I'll have nothing. I will eat a commercial English muffin, like **Thomas' Multi-Grain English Muffins.** (An English muffin is something like what's called a **crumpet** in the old country, though not exactly the same. There's no need to go into that here.)

Anyone stuck for ideas for breakfast-menu planning at home might consider turning to *What Shall We Eat? A Manual for Housekeepers*, published by G. P. Putnam & Sons in 1868. The book provides menus for breakfast,

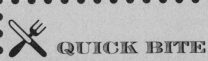

QUICK BITE

Our Rhode Island correspondent Delores Custer is a fan of the **cake donuts** sold at longtime (since 1968) R.I. favorite Allie's Donuts in North Kingstown.

QUICK BITE

Fancy a fancy donut in the desert? Kristen Cook of the *Arizona Star* recommends the warm **cinnamon-sugar donut** with vanilla custard and berries at Montana Avenue in Tucson. (Okay, it's a dessert, but who's counting?) Crunchy on the outside, soft and pleasantly dense within, "It's like the best inside-out custard doughnut ever made," Kristen says. It's eight dollars, but for that, the donut comes complete with its hole.

dinner, and tea (aka lunch and dinner) for every day of the year. The book's lofty promise is "to suggest to ladies, without the trouble of thinking, what is seasonable for the table, each day of the week, and how it shall be cooked." Always one to seek an avenue that saves on excess mental energy, I checked out the book's breakfast advice.

> *It should be what will best fortify a man for the labor of a long day, and should consist of palatable solids. In a chill climate like America, wine is a mistake, even with French cookery; if strong it diminishes business keenness; if weak, it imparts no warmth.*
>
> *Every variety of cold meats, game, potted meats, and fish, tongue, boar's head, pickled poultry, etc., are suitable, and with bread form a desirable meal. Omelets, sardines, and roes of different fish, hot buttered cakes, etc., make the eater heavy for the day.*

Palatable solids proliferate in the menus that appear in the book. Variations on **sausage toast** seem to have been popular (sausage toast being fried sausages spread on toast). In the book, see also ham toast, kidney toast, and German toast (leftover meat chopped with eggs, parsley, and gravy, then spread on toast and coated with bread crumbs.)

My other 1868 breakfast favorites:

- Breaded veal cutlet
- Cold snipe
- Calves' brains fried in butter
- Baked calf's head
- Stewed eels
- Liver hash
- Lamb's head
- Cold grouse
- Mutton kidneys, fried
- Stewed terrapin
- Stewed larks
- Giblet soup

We can only hope our nineteenth-century cousins weren't drinking wine when they were tucking into any of this stuff.

• • •

Cold grouse aside, there are two or three foods I do actually eat in the morning on a regular basis: oatmeal and breakfast cereal. (Weekends I may well go for a bagel. See page 136.) I expect the same is true of most Americans, who, somewhat harried and pressed for time at this time of day, grab a bowl of something on the way out the door. Oatmeal is yet another food that means something similar in the United Kingdom to what it does in America, but not quite the same. There, oatmeal is finely ground oats, the consistency of cornmeal. The oats used for breakfast are called porridge

---

WATCH OUT FOR . . .

Whatever you eat for breakfast, try to make sure you eat something. More important, if you have kids, definitely make sure they have some breakfast before they head to school. Multiple studies point out the benefits of breakfast. Kids who eat breakfast tend to eat better as a whole and get more of their recommended levels of vitamins and minerals. They'll also be better placed to maintain a healthy weight. Well-fed kids may well perform to a higher standard in school because they're more likely to be able to concentrate. There are plenty of ideas out there for quick, healthy breakfasts for kids. I like these one-minute Beat-the-Clock breakfast ideas from the American Dietetic Association (www.eatright.org):

◆ **Fruit and Nut Oatmeal.** Add dried cranberries and almonds to instant oatmeal, and microwave for sixty seconds.

◆ **Shake It Up, Baby!** Whir low-fat milk, frozen strawberries, and a banana in a blender for thirty seconds. Have a whole wheat bagel on the side.

◆ **Banana Dogs.** Spread peanut butter in a whole grain hot dog bun; add a banana; and sprinkle with raisins.

◆ **Breakfast Taco.** Sprinkle grated Monterey Jack cheese over a corn tortilla; fold in half; and microwave for twenty seconds. Top with salsa.

oats. My mother eats **porridge** made with water and adds milk and salt, which is definitely worth trying if you haven't done so.

Types of oatmeal (we're back in the United States) are differentiated by the process the oat grain is subjected to once the hard outer hull has been removed. The resulting oat groat, as it is called, can be chopped into two or three pieces. These are pinhead oats, or steel-cut oats, and might be called porridge oats, Irish oats, or Scotch/Scottish oats. If groats are rolled, they're rolled oats. Quaker Oats' Old Fashioned Oats are rolled oats, and Quick Oats and Instant Oats are still rolled, they're just rolled thinner. The original oat, and its inherent healthy goodness, is the same in each case. Each type of oat requires different amounts of cooking—the more processed the oats, the less time they need to be cooked.

QUICK BITE

While staying on the Shenks' Stone Haus Farm Bed and Breakfast, in Manheim, Pennsylvania (see page 43), my family was treated to Angie Shenk's homemade breakfasts. I especially liked the **baked oatmeal**. There are plenty of recipes for this dish on the Internet, all including the basic ingredients of sugar, eggs, baking powder, and oil that make baked oatmeal so different from its semi-liquid cousin. In its Pyrex dish, it is crusty atop, then cakelike, then gooey on the bottom. I found it went wonderfully with the Shenks' **home-canned pears**, which were firm, sweet, and just delicious. There are a couple of pear trees behind their barn that Angie says you can absolutely ignore and will still reliably provide fruit. Angie Shenk's **shoo-fly cake** was stunningly good, too. (Shoo-fly is so called because cooks would have to shoo flies away from it.)

Morality joined marketability in the whole wheat flour cult founded by a revivalist clergyman, Sylvester Graham, in the 1830s: his was the first American doctrine of global appeal since the Declaration of Independence.
        —*Felipe Fernández-Armesto,* Near a Thousand Tables *(2002)*

Remember when you look at the lurid display of breakfast cereals in your local supermarket that the original American cereals were designed to be as bland as possible. Sylvester Graham (1794–1851) believed that much of what people ate and drank was bad for them: meat, alcohol, coffee, tea, and tobacco were overstimulating and prompted unhealthy sexual appetites. He had a special antipathy to popular bleached white bread and promoted his own whole wheat flour, hence Graham bread and the name of the still-popular graham crackers. From Graham's flour a man called James Caleb Jackson (1811–1895), operator of the Jackson Sanitarium in Dansville, New York, developed a granulated cereal he called Granula.

In Battle Creek, Michigan, another sanitarium operator and vegetarian activist, John Harvey Kellogg (1852–1943), created a cereal he also called Granula, then Granola, when Mr. Jackson sued him. Sometime in the last decade of the nineteenth century John Harvey and his brother, Keith Kellogg, made the first corn flakes in another of those semi-mythic culinary accidents. A visitor to Kellogg's sanitarium was Charles William Post (1854–1914), who invented a cereal he dubbed Grape-Nuts. In 1906, Keith Kellogg started the Battle Creek Toasted Corn Flake Company to manufacture corn flakes for the masses. Kellogg's, the company, is still based in Battle Creek, and C.W. Post has a factory there, too. Battle Creek is cereal city, home of Kellogg's Cereal City USA, which is to Battle Creek what Hershey's Chocolate World is to Hershey, Pennsylvania.

WHEN WAS YOUR FAVORITE CEREAL CREATED?

Cereal	Manufacturer	Released
Grape Nuts	Post	1897
Corn Flakes	Kellogg's	1906
All-Bran	Kellogg's	1916
Wheaties	General Mills	1924
Rice Krispies	Kellogg's	1928
Cheerios*	General Mills	1941
Raisin Bran	Post	1942
Frosted Flakes	Kellogg's	1958
Lucky Charms	General Mills	1962
Froot Loops	Kellogg's	1963
Cap'n Crunch	Quaker Oats	1963

*Cheerios were originally called Cheerioats.

I just went to see what cereal we have in our kitchen cabinet. Perhaps you can glean some profound insight into a family by looking at the cereal they buy. Our selection speaks (perhaps) to a lot of good intentions and a couple of nods to practical reality. Or perhaps just indecisiveness. Here's what was in our kitchen:

- Multi-Grain Cheerios
- Honey Nut Cheerios (two boxes)
- All-Bran Bran Buds (two boxes)
- Kashi Heart to Heart Honey Toasted Oat Cereal
- Rice Krispies
- McCann's Irish Oatmeal
- Ambrosial Granola Apricot Almond Granola (for my birthday breakfast)
- Frosted Flakes (a third-less-sugar version)
- Trix

I'm a big fan of Kashi whole grain cereals. Check out www.kashi .com to shop online and for stores selling its products.

Many of us develop a strong attachment to particular brands of breakfast cereal. At one of Cereality's Cereal Bar and Cafes you can order brand-name cereals mixed up to your own specifications with toppings like malted milk balls, fruit, and nuts. You can also take this cereal home by the boxful. Cereality has its own cereals, too, as well as lines of breakfast bars and parfaits. This might sound like a college student's dream—all cereal all the time—which explains why the first restaurant was set up on the campus of Arizona State University in Tempe in 2003 and another near the University of Pennsylvania in Philadelphia. But the third location is in the Loop in Chicago, where, Cereality co-founder and CEO David Roth tells me, a customer is more than likely to be a business executive sneaking the bowl of Cinnamon Toast Crunch he's not allowed to eat at home.

David Roth has a business background he describes as eclectic. He trained as a psychologist and worked on issues like depression and substance abuse in the workplace. Roth also set up a magazine called *Palate and Spirit,* which focused on culinary travel, and he was later associate publisher at Fodor's Travel Guides. Then, as a consultant, he worked with organizations on reconnecting them with their customers. Companies itch for consumers to establish emotional ties with their products, and David wound his way round to breakfast cereals, an entire category of foodstuffs with built-in connections to growing up, the family, and other emotive subjects.

Cereality's foundations are based on the premise that 95 percent of Americans like breakfast cereal. But it's a lot more sophisticated than simply lining up boxes of Wheaties and Froot Loops. David says if you ask people if they like cereal, 95 percent of them will say yes. If you ask them if they like, say, Cap'n Crunch, four out of five are going to affirm. Then ask how they like to eat it, and people get more animated. One will say they love their cereal crunchy, so it digs into the roof of their mouth. The next might rhapsodize about slicing bananas on top and leaving the milk to soak in. The third will attest to always eating their mixture of raisin bran and Cheerios in their pajamas, just before bed. Cereality has drilled down to this level of attachment and provided customers with the means to replicate their cereal experience anytime they like.

David Roth cites a number of business influences, primarily the book *The Experience Economy*, by B. Joseph Pine II and James H. Gilmore, and the models of Howard Shultz, who at Starbucks has been able to parlay a couple of cents' worth of coffee beans into a coffee that costs upward of four dollars, and of Steve Jobs and iTunes. Then he mentions the prominent place cereal played in *Seinfeld*—cereal boxes are visible in Jerry's kitchen cabinets. So Cereality is selling an eating experience, with its "Cereologists" selling you cereals in their pajamas in rooms with Crate and Barrel furniture. The whole idea is that it's Always Saturday Morning (this is one of several names and phrases the company has trademarked).

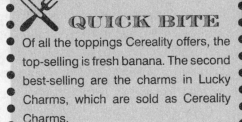

QUICK BITE

Of all the toppings Cereality offers, the top-selling is fresh banana. The second best-selling are the charms in Lucky Charms, which are sold as Cereality Charms.

Cereality has found willing partners in the major cereal manufacturers. The company is also working with the Dodge arm of Daimler-Chrysler on a Cereality Sprinter, which will sell cereal on the street like an ice cream truck. The company is working its way through thousands of franchise applications.

Cereality will put blends together in a box and sell you fifty, or however many you want. There are eight Signature Blends: **Health Kick,** containing Nature's Path Optimum Power and Kellogg's Special K with dried cranberries and walnuts; and **Frost Bites,** consisting of Kellogg's Frosted Mini Wheats and Kellogg's Frosted Flakes with malted milk balls and coconut. In each "My Cereal. My Way." box you'll get a Cereality Sloop, the combination spoon/straw created by cofounder and chief creative officer, Rick Bacher.

David Roth grew up on Long Island, where he usually ate oatmeal, cooked with milk, with brown sugar, butter, or raisins for breakfast. At the Cereality locations, they use special ingredients to flavor their oatmeals. Their **Banana Brown Betty,** for instance. The **Chocolate Banana** oatmeal has Nutella stirred in with three kinds of chocolate chips and fresh banana. Now David says he's very fond of organic cereals, such as **Nature's Path Corn Flakes,** which he likes to eat with banana. It stays crunchy in the milk, he says, and you can really taste the corn. Roth used to have a sugar allergy and isn't what he'd describe as a cereal fanatic.

While you can create your own cereal at Cereality, David Roth says that most first-time customers try one of the blends, like **Life Experience,** made with Life cereal, banana, almonds, and honey. Kids get the concept right away. David Roth says they think any kitchen is cereal plus milk anyway, so they step directly up to the counter and order just what they want. Roth happily describes the diversity of his customers: truckloads of suburban families in Philadelphia coming back every weekend, guys in sweats, chic students. He asks me if I can characterize what sells the most at the college campus locations and in Chicago. Predictably I get it wrong: college kids fixated on their bodies eat healthy cereal, while the traders in Chicago eat sugary cereal for the energy. Whatever you like, it's yours. As Roth says, if you love cereal, this is cereal heaven.

CEREALS AND BREAKFAST FOOD SUMMARY

RUN, DON'T WALK, FOR . . .

- Anything from Bob's Coffee and Donuts in Los Angeles, especially an **apple fritter.** Even the coffee's good.
- Angie Shenk's **baked oatmeal.** As served at the Stone Haus Bed and Breakfast in Manheim, Pennsylvania.
- **Kashi Heart to Heart Honey Nut Toasted** Cereal. My favorite this week. Next week, who knows?

IF YOU'VE NEVER TRIED . . .

- **Oatmeal** (aka porridge) made with water, with milk and salt added. Change things up one day—you may be surprised.

- **Breakfast on weekdays.** You should because it's good for you. (This is a public service announcement for my daughter.)

- The **Cereality** experience.

8

THE BAKERY

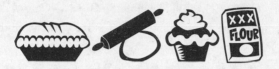

Marie took out a pan of delicate little rolls, stuffed with stewed apricots, and began to dust them over with powdered sugar. "I hope you'll like these, Mrs. Lee; Alexandra does. The Bohemians always like them with their coffee. But if you don't, I have a coffee-cake with nuts and poppy seeds. Alexandra, will you get the cream jug? I put it in the window to keep cool."

"The Bohemians," said Alexandra, as they drew up to the table, "certainly know how to make more kinds of bread than any other people in the world. Old Mrs. Hiller told me once at the church supper that she could make seven kinds of fancy bread, but Marie could make a dozen."

—Willa Cather, *O Pioneers!* (1913)

Entire lengthy *Eat This!* volumes could be written on the tasty little pastries and other baked goods that come with a regional or ethnic story to tell, and that's before we even begin to consider bread. Bread has traveled a circle from handmade through mechanized and back again, and it's now one of the premier artisanal foods in the country. Alas for me, bread was ruined for all intents and purposes by visits I made to Paris in my twenties. Low on funds, I'd mostly eat bread, cheese, and tomatoes with red wine out of jugs that had plastic caps (but which was perfectly good). In the morning my oversize bowl of café au lait would have its own bread to dip in. Fresh French baguettes are it for me, and the rest is just bread. So I do not live by much bread at all, let alone bread alone.

First up in the bakery, pastries. Let's say that Willa Cather's characters, pioneering immigrants in Nebraska, were talking about the **kolache,** a pastry, usually fruit-filled, that is a well-loved symbol of Czech (Bohemian) heritage. The kolache is celebrated in Czech festivals across the state of Nebraska—in Omaha, Lincoln, Wilber, and Prague, population 362. (You might see the Hungarian **kalache** on your travels, too.)

Czech immigrants found their way to other states than just Nebraska and they celebrate there, too. Yukon, Oklahoma, for example, has a festival each October. The kolache is very popular in Texas—Caldwell, Texas, has a big kolache festival in September. In that state you can find this usually

QUICK BITE

Italian pastry shops are national institutions, of course: Mozzicato DePasquale Bakery and Pastry Shop in Hartford, Veniero Pasticceria and Caffé in the East Village in New York, and Vaccaro's Italian Pastry Shop in Baltimore, to name but three. In New Haven, Libby's Italian Pastry Shop is just down the street from Pepe's and just a little farther down from Sally's, the two great New Haven pizza parlors. Inside, Libby's looks a little like the gate area of an old East European airport, but the kids loved the **chocolate gelati** we picked up after feasting on pizza. We also loaded up on **cannoli,** a piece of **ricotta cheesecake,** and a small box of Italian cookies. These are reliably good and popular treats.

Mozzicato: 1-860-296-0426 / www.mozzicatobakery.com/store.asp.

Vaccaro's: 1-410-685-4905 / www.vaccarospastry.com.

Veniero: 1-212-674-7070 / www.venierospastry.com.

sweet pastry adapted to hold savory fillings. Take a look at the variety offered by Robert Ahrens at his Kolache Shoppe, in Austin, alongside the standard fruits: cherry, apple, peach, apricot, pineapple, strawberry, blueberry, raspberry, and prune. From Bacon and **Bacon and Cheese** you can work your way along the meat register to Sausage; Sausage and Cheese; and **Jalapeño Sausage and Cheese,** a real Texas twist on a classic.

At one time, there were more Hungarians living in the city of Cleveland than in any place outside of Eastern Europe. Some grocery stores there still have a machine to grind the poppy seeds that are commonly used on East European pastries. This nugget of information led me to Michael Feigenbaum, owner of Lucy's Sweet Surrender, a scratch Hungarian pastry shop in the Buckeye Road district of the city.

QUICK BITE

Since my days as a juvenile stamp collector, I have known that Suomi is what Finns call Finland. So the Suomi Restaurant in Houghton, Michigan, must have something to do with the Finnish influx. I call and reach the owner Paula Rocco. Rocco is not, as she acknowledges, a Finnish name, but her maiden name is Heikkinen, which is. The Suomi serves some Finnish specialties: **Pannukakku,** which is an oven-baked breakfast pancake. It's made thin, somewhat like a crepe, and can be served with blueberries. **Nisu bread** is a sweet bread made from a sugary dough that can be the base for rolls with fruit fillings or for a Finnish French toast. The bread is characterized by the addition of cardamom. How this Indian spice made it into Scandinavian baked goods, Paula didn't know, and I can't guess.

Michael Feigenbaum grew up in Cleveland, in the Shaker Heights region, which borders Buckeye Road. As a youngster, Michael was very familiar with the dozen or more Hungarian bakeries in his neighborhood. After high school, he went to culinary school in California and was a baker in the Bay Area. When he decided he wanted to move back to Cleveland, Michael answered a classified ad about a bakery. He says he didn't know there were any bakeries left in Buckeye Road, but it turned out there was one: Lucy's. Michael's company at the time was called Sweet Surrender, so when he bought the bakery from Lucy Ortelecan in 1994, the current name suggested itself.

On one of his trips to the New Jersey shore, my friend Bud picked up some Tastykake products. Tastykake has been a Philadelphia institution since 1914—this product line has been long tried and tested. **Butterscotch Krimpets** (iced sponge cakes) were introduced in 1930. We ate these, **Chocolate Kandykakes** (little chocolate cakes covered in chocolate with a cream filling), and a Tastykake **Cherry Pie.** Bud said that the father of someone he knew from his time living in Philadelphia had been involved in developing the quick-release packaging for the pies, and we were happy to confirm it worked effectively. The pie filling had that oversweetness of commercial pie, at least to my taste, but the other cakes belied their superficial resemblance to Wing Dings (or whatever they're called), one of which I ate once. As Bud promised, the Tastykakes tasted pretty good.

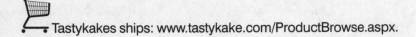 Tastykakes ships: www.tastykake.com/ProductBrowse.aspx.

Lucy's Sweet Surrender was helped by a couple of assists early in its life. First, the bakery was featured in Alison and Margaret Engel's popular book *Food Finds* (well worth checking out), which details sources of regional eats. Then the Food Network came calling. Michael Feigenbaum says that stretching strudel dough, a key feature of Hungarian baking, is very dramatic to watch and so it makes good television. The channel repeated the segment frequently, and the mail-order business took off. Now, Lucy's sells a lot of pastries over the Internet. As Michael puts it, there are ex-Clevelanders all over the country with ties to the city and relatives in the cemetery.

Michael's own background is Polish and Ukrainian, with family who came to Pittsburgh and Cleveland at the turn of the century. His wife, Marika, is Hungarian, from a small town in Transylvania that is officially part of Romania.

I urge everyone to look at Lucy's Web site, but it might be wise to postpone your visit until you've eaten. You know what they say about shopping when you're hungry. The pastries look just fantastic, as do the cakes and rolls and, for that matter, everything else. The **Dobos Torte,** for example.

QUICK BITE

We stopped off at Yeh's Bakery in Main Street in Flushing for some Chinese baked goods. The little curried pork pastries only just made it home. The **green tea cake,** a rolled cake with a light creamy vein through it, was light and lovely. We picked up a small glazed **red bean paste moon cake** for the Moon Festival, which is in late September or early October, whatever is the fifteenth day of the eighth month by the Chinese lunar calendar. This is a very rich cake you might want to eat in small pieces, and it may or may not contain the traditional delicacy of a salted duck's egg yolk. Ours did not.

This is a seven-layer cake made with caramelized sugar that Michael Feigenbaum says is very elaborate to make, requiring a special set of baking trays. Or **Zserbo,** another layered pastry made in a long sheet with jam between the layers. This grows in the pan, creating a huge sheet cake. There are **nut rolls, poppy rolls,** and all manner of strudels. Lucy's makes savories, too, like the **Pogacsa,** a pastry made with a yeast dough similar to that of a croissant, three layers of which are spread with bacon and pork fat, and which bakes like a small biscuit. Fortunately for us, we have our own Hungarian pastry shop (called the Hungarian Pastry Shop) in my neighborhood in Manhattan, to which we can take a stroll and get our **strudel** fix. (Cherry always hits the mark.)

Lucy's Sweet Surrender ships nationwide: 1-216-752-0828 / www.lucyssweetsurrender.com.

How many novels can you name that popularize a cake, or a food of any kind? Owen Wister's *Lady Baltimore* describes **Lady Baltimore Cake**—the first mention of the cake in print. "Each year at Christmas time hundreds of white boxes go out of Charleston to all parts of the country bearing the tall, the light, the fragile, the ineffable Lady Baltimore cakes." The cake is quite basic, but it is filled with walnut and vanilla filling and has a nutty frosting.

Kathleen Purvis of the *Charlotte Observer* told me about **twelve-layer cakes** from Robeson County, North Carolina: "There's a restaurant called Fuller's [Fuller's Old Fashion BBQ] in Lumberton that is owned by a Lumbee Indian family," she writes. "They make a [chocolate] **six-layer** version of the twelve-layer cake that still captures the spirit of the thing."

For a New York taste of Southern cake, visit Rack & Soul, a recent barbecue/soul food place that has opened up in my neighborhood, for a giant slice of **Red Velvet Cake.** Indigenous to the South, this is an occasional migrant to other parts of the country. A large slab of moist cake with sweet icing is probably not what you need after a plate of ribs or pulled pork (or, in my case, a plate of ribs *and* pulled pork—both are very good here), but it might well be what you like.

Cincinnati is a city with a profound German influence. **Schnecken,** which are cinnamon rolls, are popular here. *Schnecken* is German for "snails," so called because the whirled shape of the roll resembles a snail shell. These rolls are rich. Polly Campbell of the *Post* says they are "like butter with bread in it." In 2006, a local Schnecken favorite, the Virginia Bakery, closed but the Cincinnati-based chain Servatii took over the location. Schnecken are also on the bill of fare at Shadeau Breads, which is located in a Cincinnati neighborhood called Over-the-Rhine. How's that for German-influenced?

Lizzie Kander's *Settlement Cookbook* came out of Milwaukee, and so it's filled with German recipes: for Schnecken, Kuchen (yeast-based cakes), Kipfel (cakes), and **Kugelhopf** (kitchen rolls). There's also a recipe for Bohemian Kotlachen, a relative of Willa Cather's kolache. Here is the recipe for

QUICK BITE

Gooey Butter Cake is a St. Louis specialty that is popularly believed to be the result of a culinary accident. The cake is gooey because the cook, perhaps a German baker working in the 1930s, mixed up his measures in preparing the batter. But he liked what he made anyway, and the cake lived on.

Auf-Lauf: "Line a pudding dish with stale cake or macaroons. Cover with fruit (apples, peaches, pears) and sugar. Heat on the back of the stove. Cover with sponge batter (six yolks, six tablespoons of sugar, six egg whites, almonds) and bake. Or add the batter to baked apples."

The many hobbyists who make bread at home, in conditions resembling those of early agrarian society, without exact means of measuring quantities, temperatures and timing, know how easily the process can go wrong, and how exact the baker's judgment has to be.
—*Felipe Fernández-Armesto,* Near a Thousand Tables

Historian Felipe Fernández-Armesto tells us that wheat's emergence as the world's most important cereal was not a foregone conclusion. The presence of gluten in wheat gives it the properties that eventually allowed the creation of bread. But for anyone who's tried it at home, making bread out of flour, water, and yeast is never an easy transformation to effect, even when we're armed with the most precise instructions and expensive equipment. Quite how we figured out it would work at all, and who did it first, we'll never know.

Bread came to the Americas with the Europeans. The native peoples did what they could with maize and got along fine with it. As Raymond Sokolov tells us in *Why We Eat What We Eat*, cornmeal lacks the same properties as wheat flour. It has no elasticity (because it lacks gluten) and won't rise even in the presence of yeast. The settlers adapted native corn recipes to make dishes like Indian pudding, **corn and molasses,** and **corn pone.** And they adapted Indian breads into various settler cornbreads: hoecake, **ahcake, spidercake,** and the best known, the thin cornmeal pancake called the **johnnycake** (which you'll also see spelled as "Johnnycake" or "Johnny Cake." The name is explained either as a corruption of "journey cake" (meaning it was a convenient food to take on a trip) or of "Shawnee cake," after the tribe who taught the whites how to make it. Sokolov believes the Shawnee are the more likely source.

Food stylist Delores Custer mentioned johnnycakes to me. They're found all over New England, and with a particular fervor in Rhode Island. The provenance of the corn is a key factor in a good johnnycake. Relatives of Delores's grind their own cornmeal from heritage corn that Native Americans grew and sell it at the farmers market in South Kingston held May to October on the campus of the University of Rhode Island. Another Rhode Island source is Gray's Grist Mill, in Adamsville, right on the Massachusetts border. There's been a mill here since perhaps 1700. Gray's Grist Mill uses white cap flint corn for its johnnycake cornmeal.

———————

Old cookbooks include numerous recipes for cakes of various kinds, many of which are more like fry breads or biscuits than sweet cakes. *What Shall We Eat?*, from 1868, suggests for tea or lunch **Oleycooks** (from Washington Irving, it says). Combine flour, a pint of milk, a quarter of a pound of butter, two eggs, a tablespoonful of brewer's yeast, a half a cup of sugar, and a little salt and nutmeg. Stand overnight till very light, and fry in boiling lard.

There is an odd little pamphlet in the New York Public Library called *18 Colonial Recipes* that is bound into a volume with a mismatched group of sundries and which includes no publishing information. Herein is described a dish called "Oly Koeks" made of flour, butter, eggs, milk, mace, and yeast. "An old Dutch receipt," the legend claims.

Also championed in this little book are "the justly favored **Waffles** of Flatbush."

Receipt handed down through four generations for the Waffles always to be had in Flatbush at any High Tea among the old families.

One Pound of Sugar
One Pound of Butter
One Pound of Flour
Ten Eggs

Bake in window pane waffle-iron and when slightly cool, sprinkle with powdered sugar. From Flatbush, Long Island.

———————

We continue everywhere to buy the packaged monstrosities that lie, all sliced and tasteless, on the bread counters of the nation, and then spend money and more money on pills containing the vitamins that have been removed at great cost from the wheat.   —M. F. K. Fisher, How to Cook a Wolf (1942)

My criterion for good bread is simple: it must stand by itself, perhaps with only the addition of a little sweet butter. Good bread has a look, a smell, and a texture that tells you it is "handmade."

—*Alice Waters,* Chez Panisse Menu Cookbook *(1982)*

Bad bread is not difficult to recognize. More than likely it comes in a plastic wrapper with a twisty tie and when you squeeze the loaf, it's soft, and when you let go, it re-forms suspiciously to more or less its original shape and size. Good bread is not like that. In the world of fine handmade bread that has blossomed in the last twenty-five years, perhaps the acme is the Acme Bakery in Berkeley, California. Steve Sullivan used to be the baker at Alice Waters's legendary Chez Panisse restaurant in Berkeley. (It was Sullivan's bread Waters was describing in her 1982 *Menu Cookbook*.) In 1983 Sullivan founded his own company. Acme bread is also available at the company store in the Ferry Plaza Farmers Market, which opened where the unlamented Embarcadero Freeway used to run.

The Bay Area, particularly San Francisco, is well known for the self-starting **sourdough** bread variety. (Sourdough is made using a live starter rather than dry yeast.) Bruce Aidells says this is an area that takes its bread seriously. There are a dozen or so great bakeries, including Acme, Metropolis (Berkeley), Semifreddi (Berkeley and Emery), and Della Fattoria, in Petaluma. Della Fattoria describes some of the bread-making process and how it can be painstaking, if exquisitely simple. The ingredients might be organic flours, a natural starter, pure well water, and coarse gray sea salt from Brittany. The bread is baked in wood-fired brick ovens. The day before the oven is needed for baking, a fire is burned for twelve hours and

 QUICK BITE

Maria Hunt on pecan rolls at Hob Nob Hill in San Diego: "Hob Nob Hill is a diner that's been in operation since the forties. One of the coolest things about it is that it's directly under the landing path for Lindbergh Field [San Diego's airport] so all these planes are constantly roaring overhead. Inside, it looks as you'd imagine, and most of the waitresses are ladies that call you hon. They are well known for their **pecan rolls,** aka sticky buns, that are spiral yeast rolls covered with sticky brown sugar caramel and pecans."

then swept out. The bread cooks in the retained heat the oven gives off over the next eight hours.

San Francisco's Boudin Bakery, which represents San Francisco's sourdough bakers with an exhibit at Disney's California Adventure, will ship sourdough to you or a friend as part of a bread club: www.boudinbakery.com.

SOME QUESTIONS FOR TARA DUGGAN ABOUT PAN DULCE

Tara Duggan writes the "Working Cook" column for the *San Francisco Chronicle* and is the author of *The Working Cook: Fast and Fresh Meals for Busy People*. Tara wrote a story featuring bakeries like La Mexicana, in the Mission District, where people stream in for coffee and baked sweet bread from four-thirty in the morning on. They get a diverse clientele, but for Mexican and Salvadoran people, these bakeries—*panaderias*—offer a taste of home. *Panaderias* make a great variety of baked goods: rolls that are like baguettes (Mexican *bolillos*), *churros* (long cinnamon-dusted donuts), and all kinds of *pan dulce,* sweet pastries made with shortening, margarine, or lard, rather than butter. For All Saints' Day (November 1) and All Souls' Day (November 2), when the Day of the Dead is commemorated, *panaderias* bake special *pan de muerto,* "bread of the dead," which is flavored with anise and orange with skull-and-crossbone decorations.

I had some questions for Tara:

Are *panaderias* particularly a Bay Area specialty?

"The *panaderias* in the Bay Area are modeled after *panaderias* in Mexico and, occasionally, El Salvador. Though I'm not sure I'd call them a Bay Area specialty, the region does have a really great selection of the bakeries, with a concentration of classic family-owned ones on Twenty-fourth Street in San Francisco, some of which have been there for decades."

What are your favorite *panaderias?*

"My favorites . . . have historic charm, they have a big selection, and they stick to higher standards in terms of ingredients. My absolute favorite is La Mexicana; after that I like La Victoria,

Dominguez (especially Sunday morning *churros*), and Pan Lido (Salvadoran)."

What are your favorite types of *pan dulce*?

"Salvadoran *pasteles* [fruit- and meat-filled pockets] and **quesadillas** [made with cheese, sour cream, rice flour, and eggs], ***churros, puerquito,*** or ***cochinito*** [pig-shaped molasses cookies], *empanadas* [pastry pockets with apple, pineapple, pumpkin, and custard fillings], and any custard-filled pastries."

QUICK BITE

Fry bread is a Native American specialty. There are numerous recipes (see www.manataka.org/page180.htm for a bunch of them). All involve a dough that is rolled out and fried in oil. Gwen Walters suggests the Fry Bread House in Phoenix.

The bread is made in house, then fried and topped with a multitude of toppings. The most common is topped with red or green chile, beef, tomatoes, lettuce, and cheese. It is served open-faced, but fold it over like a taco (sometimes it is called a Navajo Taco) and eat it, with juicy chile dripping down your chin. So very, very good. There are lots of places that serve fry bread, including stands at our State Fair every year. Another favorite topping is just a sprinkle of powdered sugar and a drizzle of honey. Tastes very similar to homemade donuts or beignets . . . just divine.

THE BAGEL

The bagel came to the United States with Jewish immigrants from Eastern Europe. But caveat emptor: around the country, what is described as a bagel invariably turns out to be a big piece of bread shaped like a doughnut. A real New York bagel is boiled and then baked to elicit a crunchy crust around the softer interior. In good bakeries they come in different varieties: plain, salt, egg, cinnamon/raisin, **sesame,** onion, garlic, poppy, and my favorite, the all-things-to-all-people choice, the **everything bagel.**

There should be cream cheeses to go with the bagel (veggie, smoked salmon, jalapeño, tofu, etc.) and some smoked fish that includes salmon. Once in a blue moon, I'll have a bagel, lightly toasted, with light cream cheese, slabs of tomato, thick slices of red onion, a piece of smoked salmon and capers, along with a big glass of OJ and a cup of coffee.

As with many things in New York, there is a tedious debate about who makes the Best Bagel. When H&H was the nearest bagel shop to where we lived, that was where we went. H&H has a citywide reputation, though the bagels are said to be sweeter than most, and that does seem to be the case. When we moved uptown, Columbia Bagels, just north of 110th Street, was close to home and proved to be very reliable. Alas, Columbia Bagels is gone, making way, along with its immediate neighbors, for an apartment building.

Find out for yourself how good a New York bagel is: H&H ships its bagels: 1-800-NY-BAGEL / www.handhbagel.com. For a true New York experience, pair your bagel with some smoked fish (salmon, sturgeon, sable) from the world-famous Zabar's: 1-800-697-6301 / www.zabars.com.

Now we go to Absolute Bagels on Broadway between 107th and 108th streets. The bagels are very good, too, superior, even. The bagels are not too big, a fault that plagues many bagels. They're about four, four and a half inches across and an inch-and-a-half tall. The bagel is not exactly round: where it was conjoined to its neighbors on two sides, it is slightly flatter than on the two rounder sides. There is a lot of crunch to the crust and then chew to the interior, which is just what you want. In the best New York tradition, the bagel master and proprietor, Sam Thongkrieng, who trained at another prime bagel establishment, Ess-a-Bagel, is an immigrant from Thailand.

CUPCAKES

There are four birthdays in my family and a good few have been celebrated in recent years with a **cake** from the Cupcake Café. For years the café stood on Thirty-ninth and Ninth Avenue in Manhattan, until it moved across the street to larger premises. My wife loves good cupcakes. To her, they're little vehicles of happiness. The very word alone makes her smile because they're so closely associated with childhood, with her own and with our kids'. Other cupcake places in New York have their adherents. There's Billy's in Chelsea, and the Magnolia Café in the Village, which is now a stop on the *Sex and the City* coach tour. I find their frosting too sweet, but that's just me—they have thousands of devoted customers.

Ann and Michael Warren opened the Cupcake Café in 1988, and although the neighborhood has changed greatly in the intervening years, there's still a little bit of the devil in Hell's Kitchen back behind the ugly bulk of the Port Authority Bus Terminal. You have to invest some time in your cake, because you must call ahead and then show up at the bakery and pick it up (no delivery), but no subway journey is more pleasurable than one when you've found a seat and you ride home clutching a Cupcake Café box to your knees.

I was in the area with my friend Dan and I said I needed to stop in to pick up some cupcakes for research purposes. You go ahead, Dan said, determinedly. I had a cup of coffee and a big, messy **jelly donut** that left powdered sugar all over my face before I checked out the cupcakes. You don't need a fancy showcase for the little works of art they turn out at the Cupcake Café. Dan's resolve had crumbled instantly and he was choosing between the cakes decorated with irises and those with roses. They weren't for him, he assured me.

The large **cupcakes** I picked up at the Cupcake Café were $3.25 each. They're a couple of inches across, and I guess you could say they'd serve two, but it requires an extraordinary feat of self-abnegation to eat just half of one. Before you eat the cake, look closely for a second at the floral arrangements that make up the decoration. There is an effect of shading and gradation of color on the frosting that give life to the petals and leaves. You feel bad, for a second, cutting into what looks like a *tableau vivant,* and then you bite into it. The buttercream icing is impossibly luxurious and the cake dense and substantial. If you look in the Café's recipe book, you'll see that frosting a ten-person cake takes, among other things, two and a half pounds of butter, and that one of the ingredients of the cake is buttermilk. But no mind—this is a special occasion, right?

The larger cakes come in many combinations of cake, filling, and frosting. A nine-inch cake, which serves twelve to twenty, starts at fifty-five dollars. The Cupcake staff tells you how to care for your cake—don't carry the box by the string, for starters. The advice includes taking the cake out of the fridge an hour before you want to eat it. But the way I like to eat the cake after the party is to slice it right out of the fridge. When it's been chilled overnight you can cut the cake in almost translucent slices about half an inch thick. Rationed like this, you can make it last perhaps one day more.

THE BAKERY SUMMARY

RUN, DON'T WALK, FOR . . .

- A **birthday cake** from the Cupcake Café in New York City, or the bakery you trust near you. If it's not anyone's birthday, a cupcake or two will have to do.

- A warm **everything bagel** with cream cheese, smoked salmon, capers, red onion, and tomato. If the bagel's still warm, no need to toast.

- Real handmade bread.

IF YOU'VE NEVER TRIED . . .

- A nationally representative dish from a bakery from one of the countries of Eastern Europe. It's a sweet little piece of heritage. (For me, any **strudel** will do.)

- San Francisco sourdough.

9

ICE CREAM AND CANDY

Oh, that inimitable combination of textures! That symphony of flavors!
And how they offered themselves to the heat and wetness of the mouth—
the sensation of the crisped rice drenched in melted chocolate, chomped
by the molars into the creamy swirl of caramel. Oh, woe and pity
unto thee who never tasted this bar! True woe! True pity!

—Steve Almond, on the late,
lamented Caravelle bar, *Candyfreak* (2004)

My friend Doug and I were standing in front of Carl's ice cream joint in Fredericksburg, Virginia, wondering out loud what we were going to have. On a hot sunny day the bright, white stand was positively gleaming. Even the painted concrete blocks on the patio were shining hard. On top of Carl's stand is a big ice cream cone pointing proudly heavenward. CREME—SHAKES—SUNDAES, it says on the blue sign. There are only three varieties of frozen custard to choose from, and we couldn't decide. One of us pondered aloud how long Carl's had been around. Right at this point, a woman about our age walked up, and she knew exactly what she wanted. "Well, I've been coming here since I was this tall," she said, holding her hand as close to the ground as she could without bending her knees. So it's good? we asked. Oh, it's good.

It turns out that Carl's has been around since 1947, and the Electro Freeze machines you can see through the window squeezing out custard are of a similar vintage. Carl's is open from Presidents' Day weekend to just before Thanksgiving. The lines can get long apparently, but they move fast, processed by the crew of four working quickly in the close confines of the storefront.

Carl's calls its custard "ice creme" and it comes in vanilla, strawberry, and chocolate flavors. A dish is $1.37 and a pint $3.95, which is less than we pay for a small cup of extruded frozen whatever-it-is sold out of ice cream trucks and delis in New York City. The first dish I had was **strawberry ice creme**. It was dense and rich, so much better than all soft-serve products I'd ever tasted and more than competitive with any ice cream. I tried the other flavors, and ditto. You can buy sundaes (pineapple, maple nut, etc.), shakes, and malts, but I'd see no reason to deviate from the order of the ice creme on the menu: **vanilla**, then strawberry, then **chocolate**, daily or weekly or whatever you fancy.

What is frozen custard? It's similar to ice cream but it is made with egg yolks and has less air blown into it. This accounts for the rich taste and thick consistency. The folks at Andy's Frozen Custard in Missouri are happy to talk some trash. "To compare [frozen custard] with ice cream would be like comparing potted meat to a premium slab of USDA prime beef." Ouch.

Story is, eggs were first added to frozen dessert by Archie and Elton Kohr at a stand on the Coney Island boardwalk in 1919. There are Kohr Brothers stands in ten states, many in the Northeast, including clusters on the boardwalks of New Jersey in Ocean City and three in Wildwood, New Jersey.

While Carl's sports three flavors of custard, at the three Kopp's Frozen Custard stands around Milwaukee there is a flavor of the day, as well as floats, sundaes, sodas—pretty much every application of frozen custard you can think of and more you couldn't dream up in a hundred years. You can go online (www.kopps.com) and browse through the month's flavors:

Orange Dream (orange and vanilla swirls), **Malted Peanut Butter Pleasure** (malt-flavored custard with peanut butter and chocolate ribbons), Tiramisù, Lemon Raspberry Shortbread, Grasshopper Fudge, and Rum and Coca-Cola (made with real rum and real Coke).

Kopp's, which has been around since 1950, is also well known for its burgers.

 Kopp's will ship you ten pints of custard (with some hot fudge and a package of pecans), second-day FedEx: 1-414-961-2006 / www.kopps.com.

Andy's Frozen Custard started in Osage Beach, Missouri, in 1986 and now has franchises through Missouri, and also in Jonesboro and Rogers, Arkansas; Bolingbroke, Illinois; and Tyler, Texas. Andy's features its version of action-packed desserts, like a **James Brownie Funky Jackhammer**—"Andy's Frozen Custard blended with creamy peanut butter & brownies and filled with hot fudge! Oooooh! It's GOOD!"

Meanwhile, citizens of St. Louis swear by a Concrete from Ted Drewes Frozen Custard. Ted Drewes started selling ice cream in St. Louis in 1930, and the business is now run by Ted Drewes, Jr. There are two Ted Drewes stores (and only two), with the main one on Chippewa, which is the old Route 66. Ted Drewes custard comes in many flavors—peanut butter cup, lime, peach, banana. This stuff is famously thick—if handed to the customer upside down, it will not fall out. Concretes, or sundaes, include

✗ QUICK BITE

When my brother-in-law Craig and his wife, Heather, took a vacation in Hawaii, I asked them to pick out one *Eat This!* destination. Craig reported back, "Hawaii's best treat is the 'Shave Ice' at Jo Jo's in Waimea. They call it 'shave' ice, not 'shaved' ice, and it comes in sixty flavors. They offer up to three flavors on each cup of shave ice. They start out as separate flavors and then melt together by the time you're near the bottom. My **pineapple/cherry** combo rocked. On a hot Hawaiian day, the people were lined up out the door. Good stuff. You'll need to put the island of Kauai on your places-to-visit list, it's pretty much paradise."

Hawaiian Delight (pineapple, banana, coconut, and macadamia nuts) and **All Shook Up**, a nod to Elvis (peanut butter, cookies, and bananas), **Strawberry Shortcake** (shortcake, strawberries and whipped cream), and the oddly named **Sin Sunday** (tart cherries and hot fudge). It's worth pointing out that Ted Drewes will also sell you a Christmas tree around the holidays.

Ted Drewes ships large orders of custard by next day DHL: 1-314-481-2124 / www.teddrewes.com.

It's the summer as I write, and ice cream is one of the great seasonal treats. The last couple of Augusts, my family established a late-afternoon routine by which we'd go to the Magic Fountain ice cream stand on Route 25 in Mattituck, New York, after spending time at the beach. Wet and sandy, we'd sit outside the Magic Fountain and eat our ice cream in quiet appreciation. Other than the occasional experiment, which was always regretted, our order was the same: one medium **lemon ice cream** in a cup; one vanilla chocolate soft ice cream swirl in a cup; one small **birthday cake mix** in a cup; and one **soft chocolate cone with rainbow sprinkles** placed upside down in a medium cup so my daughter, Lindsay, could eat it with a spoon. I'm sure you have your favorites. Sometimes it's good to celebrate the familiar as much as the new.

I'm very glad that I chanced upon the lemon ice cream the first time we visited the stand, because Magic Fountain lemon ice cream is wonderful: lemony but not too sharp, rich, and very refreshing. As a kid on a European holiday, I had a fresh-squeezed *citron pressé,* and it opened my eyes to the wonders of real lemon. So I've always liked lemon sorbet, when it's made with real lemon, and it's why I love the lemon ice cream

QUICK BITE

Get me away from home and I'll eat ice cream. I believe I'm correct in saying I've never eaten a hot fudge sundae within walking distance of where I have been living, or a subway or London Underground ride or cab journey away, for that matter. But take me to Florida, and I'm there eating a **Hot Fudge Sundae** at the Ghirardelli Soda Fountain Shop in Miami Beach, and loving every bite. Eating vanilla ice cream with hot fudge and whipped cream is the kind of thing you should do only on vacation.

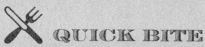

QUICK BITE

My friend Rick is a passionate devotee of **coffee ice cream**. He tried a small cup from Bennett's Ice Cream in the Los Angeles Farmers Market and pronounced it "superior." The **green tea ice cream** went down very well here with me. A small cup of **bubble gum ice cream** yielded my son, Sam, five gumballs, which I thought was an excellent haul.

at the Magic Fountain. I don't really want to eat it anywhere else; it would seem disloyal.

Away from the Magic Fountain, no member of my family would ever turn down a Carvel **Brown Bonnet** (the one with chocolate ice cream is the one I prefer). For anyone who doesn't know, a Brown Bonnet is a cone whose pointy ice cream warhead has been dipped in chocolate. One bite of a vanilla Brown Bonnet and all my wife's childhood summers and trips to Carvel are instantly invoked, though she regrets they don't dip them in front of you, as of yore—at least at the store we go to.

QUICK BITE

From my publisher's office, Jennifer Fragleasso confesses, "I'm an ice cream snob. I only eat at the Brooklyn Ice Cream factory, here in New York City. Otherwise, I save my appetite when I travel home to Connecticut for the best ice cream, which comes complete with the farm atmosphere (cows included)." At home, Jennifer visits the Gran-Val Scoop in Granville, Massachusetts. "My brother and I make the twenty-minute drive over the border every time we're home visiting my parents in the summertime. It's the most amazing **homemade ice cream**. And it doesn't get more authentic when you walk out of Scoop and can see (and smell) the cows right there on the farm."

Gran-Val has been a farm since 1903 and has sold its ice cream since 1990. They use produce from the farm for flavors, including maple syrup, wild blueberries, and peaches. The Brooklyn Ice Cream Factory is right by the ferry stop from DUMBO, in Brooklyn, to Manhattan and a convenient spot for dessert after a visit to Grimaldi's Pizzeria (see pages 353–55).

Amy Traverso is a New Englander living on the West Coast. She is food editor for *Sunset* magazine in San Francisco. Amy suggested New England ice cream locations plus bonus donuts and apple pie.

◆ A **brownie sundae** from Sundae School in Orleans, Massachusetts (Cape Cod)
◆ **Mapple walnut ice cream** from Kimball's in Jaffrey, New Hampshire
◆ **Cider donuts** from the Cold Hollow Cider Mill, in Waterbury, Vermont
◆ **Mile-High Apple Pie** from the Mountain Creamery, Woodstock, Vermont

Marialisa Calta is a writer, columnist, and the author of *Barbarians at the Plate: Taming and Feeding the Modern Family*, and she has some ice cream ideas in Vermont: "**Creemees** (also spelled 'Cremees' and, I think, 'Cremies' . . . pronounced 'Kree-Mees'), the Vermont name for soft-serve ice cream. It is sold all over the place in summer. Especially of note are Maple Creemees. I know that they are excellent at Morse Farms Sugarworks in Montpelier and the Bragg Farm Sugarhouse in East Montpelier. Burr Morse, at Morse Farms, also makes amazing maple-kettle corn (popcorn popped with maple syrup . . . this is not a New England tradition, as far as I know, but it's damn good!)."

Marialisa also suggests ice cream from the Strafford Organic Creamery, in Strafford, Vermont. "Oh. My. God" is what she says about that.

Jane Tobler works in food PR in Washington. Into the ice cream ring, she threw the hat of Graeter's, a favorite she happily recalls from her days in Oxford, Ohio.

No visit to Ohio is complete without an empty stomach and a sweet tooth, so you can stop by Graeter's ice cream. Yum! One of the best things about Graeter's ice cream is that they make their own fabulous chocolate and are generous with it in their ice cream. Chocolate chip ice cream isn't chocolate chip, it should be called chocolate chunk.

Growing up in Cincinnati, my girlfriends and I would split a pint of **Black Raspberry Chip** *or* **Mocha Chocolate Chip** *and give thanks for the great veins of chocolate that we found inside. "I found the mother lode!" Fights would break out over who had rights to the largest piece, but they were always amicably settled. Heck, there was always more ice cream to eat. You have to go and get some.*

The Graeters were a family of German immigrants who started their ice cream business in Cincinnati in 1870. Now they have stores around Cincinnati, Columbus, and Dayton and over into Indiana and down to Kentucky. Graeter's uses what they describe as a "French Pot process," which folds the ice cream and doesn't whip air into it. This accounts for its denseness. As for flavors, there is, presumably in honor of the state of Ohio, the **Buckeye Blitz**, comprising chocolate/peanut butter ice cream with peanut butter cookie dough pieces and chocolate chips. **Toffee almond** and **double chocolate chip** speak for themselves. The Graeter's "Signature Flavor" and bestseller is Black Raspberry Chip.

 Graeter's ships its ice cream: 1-800-721-3323 / www.graeters .com.

 QUICK BITE

My friends Meredith and David wanted to make sure I had mentioned Kopp's frozen custard (check) and Graeter's ice cream (check). There was one place I had overlooked, though: the Purity Ice Cream Company in Ithaca, New York, a favorite of Meredith's brother. Online, Purity ("serving central New York since 1936") touted some tasty-sounding combos: **Finger Lakes Tourist** ("rich chocolate ice cream studded with white chocolate chunks and hazelnut pieces"); **Sleepers Awake** ("robust coffee ice cream with fudge swirl and lots of chocolate chunks"); and **Boomberry** ("our velvety vanilla ice cream loaded with fruit—black cherries, blueberries, strawberries, and raspberry puree").

In Chicago, Adam Langer recommends **Palmer House Ice Cream**—available as one of a variety of flavors on the titular cone at Rainbow Cone on Chicago's South Side. Available only in summer. The Rainbow Cone is made up of five flavors, one of which is the Palmer House, a mix of cherries and nuts in vanilla. The other flavors are chocolate, pistachio, strawberry, and orange sherbet. Adam also speaks well of Mario's Italian Lemonade, on Taylor Street, where for ices the **melon** flavor is among the best.

Adam is among those who mention **Frango Mints**—the specialty of Marshall Field's

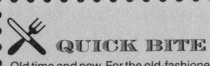

QUICK BITE

Old time and new. For the old-fashioned soda fountain experience, try the homemade **ice cream** at Bauder's Pharmacy in Des Moines. On the same street, at Zanzibar's Coffee Adventure, they'll whip you up an **Eggs Expresso**: that's a couple of eggs and cheese agitated into a soufflé-like concoction using the steamer from the espresso machine.

department store on State Street. Though they're no longer made in Chicago, they still taste the same, which is a good thing. But not only are Marshall Field's Frango mints not made in Chicago, but Marshall Field's isn't even Marshall Field's anymore. It's become Macy's, which I thought was the name of a store in New York. Frango mints actually originated in Seattle, before Marshall Field's bought the company that made the mints in 1929. (In 2006, just before the name was retired, *The Marshall Field's Cookbook* was published. This was the first department store with a restaurant, and it was well known for its food. For example, there was/is the **Marshall Field's chicken salad**, which gained a life beyond the store. Recipes for the salad differ, but they include some or all of the following: homemade mayonnaise, sour cream, pecans, and strips of bacon for the sandwich garnish.)

Food publicist Ellen Malloy, based in Chicago, also likes Frango Mints, and Garrett popcorn: the **Caramel and Cheese** mix.

*In Chicago the first thing that comes to mind is ice cream at Margie's where they make the most delicious **hot fudge** I've ever tasted.*

—*Jonathan Eig, author of*
Opening Day: The Story of Jackie Robinson's First Season

. . .

QUICK BITE

Joanne Weir is the James Beard Award–winning author of *From Tapas to Meze* and *Weir Cooking in the City*, among other books, and star of the television series *Joanne Weir's Cooking Class*. She loves the **vanilla soft-serve ice cream** at Picco, which is a pizzeria in Larkspur, California. You can get the ice cream with a drizzle of **California olive oil** and a sprinkling of salt. "So California," says Joanne. "Picco is a find," she says. "Amazing margarita, or marinara, pizza by a great chef, Bruce Hill. A fun place and truly San Francisco."

My wife, Kara, goes on business trips a few times a year. She likes to shop for souvenirs and bring back stuff for the kids, which explains why our daughter has an Arkansas Razorbacks football that shouts "Pig sooey!" when you throw it to the ground. Recently she went to Nashville and bought me a couple of local items: a six-pack of **GooGoo Supremes** and a **Pepper Patch Jack Daniel's Tipsy Cake.** ("You can taste the natural goodness in every bite.") The cake was okay, and I could certainly taste the Jack Daniel's in every bite, but the GooGoos were something else.

I confess that I'd never even heard of GooGoos before Kara gave me a box of them. On the packaging, the ingredients are listed as "milk chocolate, pecans, caramel, and marshmallow," which sounds like a hundred other candy bars. But this isn't like a hundred other candy bars. It's round, for a start. Then, tucking in, I find that the GooGoo turns out to be toothsomely sweet and very soft. Melting as they were held and chewed, each one went down effortlessly, even as the next Cluster seemed mysteriously to be unwrapping itself. Read Steve Almond's account of the GooGoo production line in *Candyfreak* and how the GooGoo's *double enrobing* process (the candy goes through two chocolate applicators) accounts for some of its unique flavor.

The GooGoo is a noble and, it turns out, historic candy. It's the world's first ever combination candy bar, invented in 1912 in Nashville. It's hard to believe no one came up with something like this before then. We'd been flying airplanes almost ten years before anyone thought of adding something to chocolate in a candy bar. Perhaps we didn't have the processing technology. It seems 1912 was a big year for candy; Life Savers debuted then, too.

The GooGoo comes in three versions: the pecan Supreme, the peanut Cluster, and the self-explanatory Peanut Butter. GooGoos are famous throughout the South. I was happy to see boxes in a Cracker Barrel we stopped at between Phoenix and Tucson. I was also happy that they reconstituted satisfactorily in our hotel, having melted down in the back of our car. The Standard Candy Company of Nashville anticipates customer bingeing by selling in bulk online. A six-pack is $2.50; 18 six-packs are $40.50, and you can score 288 GooGoos for $103.95.

Buy GooGoo Clusters, Coconut Waves, Cumberland Ridge Nut Rolls at www.googoo.com.

CONTRIBUTION
STEVE ALMOND'S TOP FIVE CANDY BARS

I turned to the candy connoisseur Steve Almond himself for his candy selections.

I spend a lot of my time thinking about candy bars—about half my waking hours, if I'm going to be honest. I also spend a lot of time traveling around the country tasting bars. This is simply part of my job description as a certified Candyfreak. I know, it's a tough gig, but somebody's got to do it.

With the enthusiastic help of a dozen or so friends, I recently came up with the following mouthwatering winners:

BEST INDIVIDUAL PIECE:
THE CANDYFREAK SIGNATURE

Last year, Granny's Chocolates of Gilbert, Arizona, asked me to design a piece of chocolate. I sent along the following specs: a bite-size piece of soft caramel, infused with cocoa, sprinkled with crisped rice, then enrobed in Belgian dark chocolate and dusted with cinnamon. This was an effort to re-create the now-extinct Caravelle bar, my favorite as a kid. The finished piece sent me a total mouthgasm. It tastes like you're licking the brownie bowl.

BEST CHOCOLATE BAR:
THE LAKE CHAMPLAIN FIVE-STAR BAR

Lake Champlain's chocolate engineer, Dave Bolton, has been known to spend a full year perfecting a single recipe. And it shows. The Five-Star Caramel Bar, for instance, is a sublime blend of buttery caramel, Belgian dark chocolate, roasted almonds, and milk chocolate. This Vermont-made confection costs a little more, but delivers a taste and texture that is priceless.

BEST REGIONAL BARS

Thanks to the economic pressure of the Big Three—Hershey's, Mars, and Nestlé—these delicacies are all on the endangered list, so try them now before they're gone forever. All are available for order online:

Sifers' Valomilk (Kansas City, Kansas)

When Russ Sifers took over the family business a decade ago, he vowed to make Valomilks the way his grandpa did. Mission accomplished. These delicate chocolate cups, filled with vanilla syrup, are a delicious mess to eat. Prepared in small batches, they contain only the finest ingredients, including real bourbon vanilla.

GooGoo Cluster (Nashville, Tennessee)

The official candy bar of the South, the GooGoo is reportedly the nation's first multi-ingredient bar. It is also the only bar I know of that is enrobed in chocolate *twice*. The standard Goo contains marshmallow, caramel, and peanuts. The vaunted Supreme boasts a Southern specialty: pecans.

The Twin Bing (Sioux City, Iowa)

The Bing is still made by hand, as it was a hundred years ago. It features a luscious cherry cream surrounded by chopped peanuts and chocolate. Marty Palmer, the fifth generation to produce the Bing, has no plans to tinker with the formula.

The Idaho Spud (Boise, Idaho)

The Spud is debatably the strangest retail candy bar available in America. Contrary to speculation, it does not contain any potato.

It's actually a small loaf of marshmallow infused with cocoa and maple, then covered in chocolate and sprinkled with coconut. It's . . . spudarrific!

BEST NONCHOCOLATE BAR:
THE BIG HUNK (HAYWARD, CALIFORNIA)

There is nothing else in the candy world quite like a Big Hunk: a slab of chewy vanilla nougat shot through with fried peanuts. Thanks to the secret ingredient (honey), the nougat exudes the rich flavor of cake batter. A quick tip: stick them in a microwave for a few seconds to soften them up. Irresistible.

BEST FAIR TRADE CANDY BAR: EQUAL
EXCHANGE DARK MINT BAR

Sadly, much of the world's chocolate comes from economically depressed countries, where abusive labor practices persist. In the Ivory Coast, for instance, children are often used to harvest cocoa for slave wages.

Fair Trade is a movement that stresses economically just and environmentally sound trade partnerships. The bars that Equal Exchange produces come from cooperative farms in Latin America, Africa, and Asia. They are also unbelievably delicious.

The new Dark Mint Bar is a perfect example: the aromatic mint serves as the ideal complement to the chocolate, which has hints of coffee and cherry. It's one of the best bars you're likely to taste, and the kind you can eat in good conscience. If you're concerned about those who grow and harvest your chocolate, make sure to ask your local retailer to stock Fair Trade products.

Following are the candy manufacturers and candies mentioned by Steve. The manufacturers either sell their candy themselves, or will tell you who does:

Granny's: 1-866-362-CHOC (2642) / www.grannyschocolate.com.

Lake Champlain: 1-802-864-1808 / www.lakechamplain chocolates.com.

Valomilk (for list of stocking stores): www.valomilk.com.

Palmer: 1-712-258-7790 / www.palmercandy.com.

Spud: 1-800-8-YUM-YUM / www.idahospud.com.

Big Hunk (for stocking Web sites): www.annabelle-candy.com.

Equal Exchange (chocolate, coffee, and tea): www.equal
exchange.com.

Other online candy retailers include:

Favorites Of: 1-888-451-2848 / www.favoritesof.com.

Victory Seeds (heirloom seeds *and* candy): www.victoryseeds
.com/candystore/.

Candy Direct: 1-619-216-0116 / www.candydirect.com.

Home Town Candy: 1-215-392-4339 / www.hometowncandy.com.

Candy Warehouse: 1-626-480-0899 / www.candywarehouse.com.

I have a weakness for chocolate and chocolate bars. Is there anyone who doesn't? I have a bad habit of picking the Hershey's Kisses out of my kids' Halloween stashes. On a rainy day we visited Hershey's Chocolate World, where a crawl shows you how many tens of millions of Kisses have been made so far that day. There are lots of big numbers at Hershey, like the fact that seventy million people have taken the Great American Chocolate Tour. It felt like half of them were there the day we visited, but the line went very quickly and my son, Sam, wanted to go around twice, partly for the Disneyworld nature of the ride and partly for the free candy (a small **Take Five** bar both times).

The tour disgorges you into the store, of course, where there's more chocolate product than you've ever seen: five-pound bars of Hershey's milk chocolate, **Hershey's Extra Dark Chocolate** (60 percent cacao), which I'd never seen before and bought a bar of and enjoyed, millions of Kisses and Twizzlers and KitKats, and the aristocratic offerings of San Francisco chocolatier Scharffen Berger (now owned by Hershey's), whose chocolate is decidedly moreish (you have some, you want more).

Away from Hershey's, Trader Joe's Belgian **Dark Chocolate,** at $1.29 for three bars, is good, and for that price, there's a lot to like. More luxurious are the products of Recchiuti Confections of San Francisco. Their **Burnt Caramel Almonds,** coated in chocolate and dusted with cocoa powder, are an extravagant indulgence. As is the **Fève Bar,** 85 percent cacao with flakes of roasted cacao nibs (the raw material of chocolate, and "*fève*" in French) embedded in the surface. Extraordinarily good.

Order from www.recchiuti.com.

Chocolate is supposed to contain endorphins that make you feel good. Eating a couple of square inches of Gethsemani Farms **Chocolate Bourbon Fudge with Pecan Pieces,** a box of which we'd received as a gift, made me extremely happy, but perhaps I was just getting ever so slightly loaded on the bourbon. Gethsemani Farms fudge is made by Trappist monks who live and work at an abbey in Kentucky. Monks came to Kentucky from western France in 1848, and their successor brethren support the order with a mail-order food business. The monks make liberal use of the one particular Kentucky specialty in their fudge, and they've created a sensational taste. The bourbon starts working on your nose before the fudge makes it as far as your mouth. It's a two-pronged attack that's difficult to resist. You can also buy **Butter Walnut Bourbon Fudge** from the monks, as well as cheeses, homemade fruitcake, and coffee that originates from a Trappist monastery in Venezuela.

We tried the monks' cheese, too, and that was fine, but the fudge is surprising and delicious and makes a fun gift. Gethsemani Farms is located on Monks Road in a town called Trappist (what a great address!), which is about fifty miles south of Louisville and near Loretto, Kentucky. The Maker's Mark Distillery is located in Loretto, and a visit here and to the abbey would make an interesting and spiritually intoxicating day trip.

Order bourbon fruitcake and fudge and Trappist cheese: 1-800-549-0912 / www.gethsemanifarms.org.

The buckeye is the seed or nut of the buckeye tree (*Aesculus glabra*)—so called, it is said, because it resembles the eye of a male deer, a buck. The buckeye has long been associated with Ohio, at least since the 1840 presidential run of Ohioan William Henry Harrison, who used buckeyes as a prop in his campaign. Ohio is the Buckeye State, and Ohioans are Buckeyes. The buckeye is the official state tree, and teams at Ohio State University are all Buckeyes. But none of these buckeyes can you eat.

Buckeye candy is another matter. The candy, aka **buckeye balls,** comprises globs of peanut butter with a chocolate coating that are made so they look like the nut or the eye of a deer because of a round patch of peanut butter that's left exposed. Popular as an easy homemade treat, buckeye balls are also store-made. The Anthony-Thomas Candy Company in Columbus makes about a hundred thousand pounds of buckeyes a year to sell at its numerous locations, while the punning folk at Haute Chocolate in Cincinnati make special buckeyes for Halloween, Thanksgiving, and the holidays.

I took the kids down to Jacques Torres Chocolate Haven, on Hudson Street in Manhattan, to pick up some birthday chocolate for Mom. It's a return favor for the boxes of the sublime **chocolate-covered ginger** she's bought me from this store. (We've also enjoyed the Jacques Torres chocolate-covered **cornflakes** and Cheerios. If you look into the shop from King Street there are some interesting Roald Dahl-esque Chocolate Factory appliances with twirling silver orbs and drums to admire. Inside the Chocolate Haven, it's impossible to stop kids from behaving like they're in a candy store. We picked out some bars of chocolate (a terrific **Dangerously Dark Haven Bar,** 72 percent cocoa), **a white chocolate bar,** and some decorative chocolates to put in a box: **love potion** (dark chocolate ganache); fresh ginger; almandine; peanut brittle; **cinnamon praline**. I sent Lindsay back with a third bar because we had enough. A kindly man stepped forward and asked me very properly if he might give the kids a lollipop. This was Jacques Torres, the benevolent proprietor.

I complimented Jacques on his store and asked him about people's appetite for fine foods like his. He's been in the luxury chocolate game eighteen years, and he says that food as a whole has been getting better and better, and especially in the last five years. He puts this down to baby boomers, who have two things in common: disposable income and health concerns. The doctor says no chocolate, so they buy just a little of the very best, which definitely includes Jacques Torres chocolate.

Resist Jacques Torres if you can. Order from: www.mrchocolate.com.

• • •

My Los Angeles tour guide, George Motz, suggested I visit the Edelweiss chocolate store in Beverly Hills if I got a chance. The store has been operating since 1942 and was owned for some of that period, up to 2000, by Shirley Jones of *Partridge Family* fame. The store's walls and display cases were packed with chocolates in all forms, colorfully decorated. Much care is taken here to make sure everything's just so. I hemmed and hawed before I picked some small dark chocolate bars, Halloween balls, and a variety of individual chocolates: **with prunes, with dates soaked in rum, with ginger,** and **with arancia (orange peel).** I made sure to get a few chocolate turtles, my wife's favorite.

I got to chatting with the staff and soon was ushered behind the counter and in back to have a look round. A series of rooms form the factory that makes the chocolates. In the first, a woman was dragging cashews one by one through a kettle of liquid milk chocolate. Against the wall were stacked a series of what looked like large shoe boxes but with odd labels: TEDDY BEAR LOLLIES, SITTING BABIES, BABIES' BUGGIES, ASSORTED HEARTS, SAFETY PINS, PREGNANT LADIES. Within each box was a couple of days' inventory of the chocolate representations of the same.

Madlen Zahir, the owner, found me and graciously let me poke further around the store, showing me the old Rube Goldberg machines used in confectionery making. "Savage Bros. Co. Chicago," read one. "Pats. 1914, 1919." In the very back was a great sheet of nougat, with a beautiful pristine surface. I commented how laborious it looked to make all these candies and chocolates manually, and Madlen agreed. The reason the chocolates are as expensive as they are is that they really are handmade. Making chocolates is one of the few activities where it helps if you have cold hands.

I thought I committed a faux pas when I mentioned Mondel Chocolates, in my neighborhood in New York. (I buy Kara's favorite **chocolate turtles** from there, as well as gift boxes of truffles now and then.) Katharine Hepburn used to go there, I said, and Madlen said that Hepburn came to Edelweiss, too. Madlen started to tell me how the store ships chocolates all round the country when the phone rang and an order came through. Sure enough, the surname Madlen wrote down on the order was extremely well known.

The chocolates came back to New York with me in an attractive red Edelweiss box. Kara loved the turtles, the kids liked the Halloween chocolate, and I ate the fruit ones and savored the deep richness of the dark chocolate. The box stuck around the kitchen for a while, and I picked it up the day I was ready to write about Edelweiss. It was not empty! Inside, I found a small dark chocolate bar and two pieces of what turned out to be the dark-chocolate-coated ginger. I put the box back in the fridge and managed to resist for a good half hour.

Mondel: 1-212-864-2111 / www.mondelchocolates.com.

Edelweiss: 1-888-615-8800 / www.edelweisschocolates.com.

ICE CREAM AND CANDY SUMMARY

RUN, DON'T WALK, FOR . . .

- **Chocolate, strawberry,** or **vanilla ice creme** from Carl's in Fredericksburg.
- **Chocolate-covered ginger** from Jacques Torres in New York and Edelweiss in Los Angeles.
- **Lemon ice cream** from the Magic Fountain in Mattituck, New York.
- Nashville's finest **GooGoo Cluster.**

IF YOU HAVEN'T TRIED . . .

- Steve Almond favorite candies, you should. (Nor have I. Yet . . .)

Part II

EATING OUT

10

BURGERS

Hamburger: Minced (ground) beef shaped into a flat round cake and grilled (broiled) or fried. It is one of the main items of a traditional American barbecue. The name is an abbreviation of Hamburger steak, i.e., beef grilled in the Hamburg style, and the hamburger was introduced into the United States by German immigrants.

—Larousse Gastronomique (1988 edition)

Is there any question that the quintessential American dish, the American eating vernacular, is the hamburger? Other items, like the hot dog, might be included in the debate, but none, the dog included, is as popular across the nation as the meaty champion of sandwiches. Across the world, the most recognized commercial symbol of the American way of life is McDonald's and its golden arches, and McDonald's didn't get to be McDonald's selling hot dogs.

The humble burger has so much going for it. A burger is a quick and easy way to use cheap cuts of meat. It delivers protein effectively. It can be dressed up with any number of condiments and add-ons, and most ways you fix it, it tastes pretty good. Chefs endlessly riff on the theme of the shaped beef patty. Today, the burger is enjoying a new period of coolness. Knowing eaters flock to decades-old burger purveyors and also to a new wave of back-to-basics restaurants like the Shake Shack and the burger joint at the Parker Meridien Hotel, both in New York City, which together may represent a modern paradigm for burger eating.

But we'll begin our modest survey at the beginning, at Louis' Lunch in New Haven, Connecticut. The restaurant was established in 1895. In 1900, the story goes, the hamburger *qua* sandwich was invented when a Louis' customer ordered a broiled beef patty to go and left holding the meat between two slices of bread. Today, the burgers are still served on toast rather than a bun. This was cause for concern once we decided to head up to New Haven for a family trip—would our kids eat a hamburger made using toast? And then there was the ketchup issue. The Web site makes it clear—no ketchup allowed. This was even less likely to sit well with them.

The four of us arrived outside the tiny Louis' building just past noon, the appointed opening hour. One family, who had traveled from northern Connecticut, was already waiting. At 12:07 the door opened, and by 12:17 the place was full. For first-timers, there's not a great deal of posted information to go on. I lined up, and Kara, Sam, and Lindsay sat at the one large table that has four cast-iron garden benches set around it. There are a couple of other small tables and a few stools at the bar. I couldn't see a menu as such, but a member of New Haven's finest was being served a hot dog, so I asked for one of those and three sandwiches—two **cheeseburgers** and one plain. I was told the hot dog wasn't on the menu yet (the hot dogs are generally available after six, and you can order a tuna sandwich on Fridays), so I was confined to the burgers.

You wait for your food in close quarters with the other diners. Some, clearly old hands, asked for the "**worksburger**," which comes with lettuce, tomato, and onion. The burgers are made in a corner behind the counter, and the toast is prepared on a venerable Savory Radiant Gas Toaster. There's a no-go sign superimposed on a ketchup bottle: DON'T EVEN ASK. A couple of pieces of baseball memorabilia are among the few decorations— a Red Sox banner and a photograph of the famous play where Alex Rodriguez tried to knock the ball out of pitcher Bronson Arroyo's hands in the 2004 American League Championship series between Boston and New York. To Red Sox fans, this innocuous incident made A-Rod Charles Manson as well as Benedict Arnold. Seeing this, I knew we were in enemy territory.

Our order was soon ready. The burgers come medium-rare, unless you specify differently, and are dished up in a heap on small paper plates. Lindsay, who'd eaten some "dirty" chips as an appetizer, had a tentative bite of her burger. Sam ploughed right in and didn't mention the *k* word once. One of the sandwiches looked less well done than the others, and I took it. The toast was moistened by the meat's juices but it didn't have a chance to become sodden. The burger, gone in two or three bites, hit the spot for me. It was served unadorned like this, the meat flavor is right at the forefront, and the meat was clearly of a good quality. Sam agreed, pronouncing his meal "Burger-licious."

I had some questions I wanted to ask, but the restaurant was busy. Phone orders were coming in, the line of customers was steady, and the gentleman cooking the stuff was all business. I e-mailed Jeff Lassen, the fourth-generation owner of Louis' Lunch. Jeff confirmed that they grind their own meat every day. He told me the restaurant is in its third location. From 1895 to 1917 it stood on Meadow Street, and then from 1917 to 1975 it was on the corner of George and Temple streets. Then, threatened with demolition, the small building was physically removed to its current location. It should be safe now, Jeff says, because the family owns the property.

From Louis' Lunch, it's a short stroll across the Yale campus to the Yankee Doodle Coffee and Sandwich Shop. I'd heard about the Yankee Doodle a number of times when my brother-in-law Doug reminisced about life in the Northeast. There's a place in New Haven, he would say, where they slather the burger bun with butter. It always sounded good, and now I had an opportunity, and an excuse, to try it for myself. The Yankee Doodle has been on Elm Street since 1950. A couple of extra stools were added in 1953, and it has remained unchanged since, always run by the Beckwith family. The restaurant is a long counter with the grill at the front, by the entrance,

QUICK BITE

There are challenges to Louis' Lunch as the originator of the hamburger sandwich. If you're from Athens, Texas, you'll probably support claims for Fletcher Davis of Athens introducing the hamburger to the world at the 1904 World's Fair in St. Louis. In Seymour, Wisconsin, there's a statue in a park downtown that celebrates the efforts of one Charles Nagreen (there used to be a Hamburger Hall of Fame in Seymour, but it is closed). At the Outagamie County Fair in 1885, Nagreen is said to have placed rolled-out meatballs between two pieces of bread and called what he came up with a "hamburger."

unusually, so passersby can watch the cooking from the street. We got four stools together and ordered frugally, having just eaten.

I ordered a **cheeseburger with tomato**. For $2.25, this is a genuine steal. There is butter involved, but it's more of a schmear than the thick layer Doug alluded to. It's enough butter to taste, though, and with the thin patty and the sweet tomato relish that comes on the side, it makes for a distinctive burger. A couple of people in the know in our party said the **milkshake** was excellent, too. There are little aphorisms dotted about the place. This one is right on:

> *The place is small*
> *The food is great*
> *It's worth your while*
> *To stand and wait.*

Unless you're a vegetarian, it's hard to go wrong at Louis' Lunch or the Yankee Doodle. In fact, they complement each other nicely, and I was happy we'd hit on our two-course burger meal with a stroll in between. Don't try it on a Sunday, as neither restaurant is open.

After the Yankee Doodle, we were all full up and happy and had some time to explore before we hit the famous New Haven pizza restaurants. Across the street from the Yankee Doodle is a big Barnes and Noble. I noticed a table display of books by notoriously challenging French philosopher Jacques Derrida. I took myself off to the bathroom, where there was a collection of absolutely the dumbest graffiti I'd ever seen. So much for lofty thoughts.

Just as I was starting to get serious about burgers, eating them with relish, as it were, John T. Edge's book *Hamburgers and Fries* was published. This is one of his series of four books on what he calls America's "iconic foods," the subjects of the others being apple pie, fried chicken, and do-nuts. Reading Edge's extremely engaging book, you appreciate just how adaptable the burger has proved to be. He describes the onion burger of Oklahoma, pimento burgers in South Carolina, and the butter burgers of Wisconsin. Burgers are breaded in North Carolina and extended with soy or flour (as with the slug and dough burgers) in Mississippi, New Orleans has deep-fried burgers, while in Connecticut they're steamed. Patties are cut with Brie, feta, peanut butter, béchamel sauce, and green chile; from Minnesota comes the Juicy Lucy; from San Antonio the bean burger, with its refried beans, Fritos, and Cheez Whiz; and originating in Iowa, the Maid-Rite, a sandwich made with loose hamburger meat.

When I was planning a visit to Los Angeles, eating an In-N-Out burger was at the top of my wish list. By the end of Eric Schlosser's *Fast Food Nation*, the In-N-Out chain was about the only thing left standing with much integrity. In-N-Out's good reputation has spread far beyond its western power base, even if its restaurants haven't. I live exactly 2,527.52 miles from the nearest In-N-Out, 37 hours and 50 minutes' drive away. I know this

QUICK BITE

On my next trip to New Haven, I want to head north to Meriden, Connecticut, for one of the famous and singular **steamed cheeseburgers** ($3.50) at Ted's, a featured stop on the great American burger tour.

QUICK BITE

In Rhode Island the **Dynamite** is a local specialty that sounds like a Maid-Rite. "This is sort of like a Sloppy Joe," says cookbook editor Amy Treadwell. "It's a spicy mix of crumbled hamburger and chili-like sauce, usually on a submarine sandwich roll or, if making them at home, on a hamburger bun. These are often sold at pizza places/sub sandwich places." The Chelo's chain of restaurants sells Dynamites at its nine locations throughout the state.

fact thanks to a great feature on the company's Web site, which builds detours to In-N-Outs into national driving directions. I read John Edge's book on my Jet Blue flight into Burbank and was pleased to see that he writes, "All burger roads lead to the sprawling metropolis of Los Angeles." The next stop on my particular burger road: In-N-Out.

QUICK BITE

Nearer to home, if I want to take a drive for a good burger, is 96th Street Steakburgers, in Indianapolis, where I'm just 718 miles from a **double steakburger with cheese.**

A mere 1,769 miles away, at James Beard Award-winning Robert McGrath's Roaring Fork Restaurant, in Scottsdale, have a **Big-Ass Burger** in the Saloon. (How does this sound? "Twelve ounces of Grilled Love with Roasted Green Chiles, Colby Longhorn Cheese, Smoked Bacon, Grilled Onion & Fries.") These two burgers were among those voted the fifteen best by America Online users. And there's an In-N-Out in Scottsdale for fortunate burger lovers.

I picked up the car I was borrowing and went straight to the Studio City In-N-Out and had a Number 1 meal. On its own, a **Double-Double**— a double cheeseburger, with onion, lettuce, tomato, and Russian dressing—was $2.75. The burgers are made fresh, and customers stand to the side and wait for their orders. (Check out the Web for In-N-Out's not-so-secret menu of supercustomized—"Animal style" and so on—burgers.) I was interested to see that there were wedges of lemon on offer in the drinks dispenser—a nice touch I hadn't seen anywhere before. My burger came wrapped in paper. Undressed, it was slightly irregular, steaming, and demonstrably juicy. (Subsequent Double-Doubles have been even more delightfully sloppy.) It tasted great—the onion gave the burger a serious jolt, and the cheese and sauce jostled for attention with the meat. The fries were pretty bland, but fries usually are. I remembered what Eric Schlosser wrote, how, unlike other organizations, In-N-Out paid decent wages and benefits and offered genuine chances for advancement for its workers. It treats its own people well, in other words. I felt well looked after, too.

I wanted to put at least an hour between one burger and the next, so I stopped off at Book Soup, on Sunset, where I picked up a host of new restaurant tips. I made for the Apple Pan, on West Pico, a famous burger place where one particular dessert had been highly recommended to me. The restaurant is housed in a small white building. Inside, you find a three-sided counter around a serving station. Four or five people were waiting inside the door and one of them helpfully pointed out a single space down to the right. The diners around me were chowing down enthusiastically. I knew right away this was going to be good.

Dotted through the Apple Pan menu are references to the restaurant's heritage. The inception date was April 11, 1947. The burger recipes hark back to 1905 and 1927; some desserts are made using formulas from the nineteenth century. The motto is the slightly Orwellian "Quality Forever." I ordered a **Steakburger with Cheese** (melted natural Tillamook cheddar). Right after I'd eaten, I had some regret that I hadn't had any fries, and that I hadn't tried the **Hickoryburger,** but the burger I did eat was excellent. Served with a wedge of lettuce, pickles, mayo, and "our own sauce," the Apple Pan burger is a substantial handful whose dominant note is its relish.

QUICK BITE

I rectified my neglect of the **French fries** on a later visit. At the Apple Pan they are spectacularly crisp and among the best I can remember. (Double-cooked homemade fries are fantastic. See James Carville's recipe on page 50, these were close.) On closer inspection, I saw that the difference between a Steakburger and a Hickoryburger lay in the sauce slathered onto the patty. The Steakburger is a great burger. On reflection, I saw that it had a lot more lettuce than other burgers, which alters the biting experience considerably. Think twice before taking out the lettuce—the bite's a stretch, but it's worth it.

Like every place worth going, the Apple Pan is quirky. You start with the seating free-for-all. Once you're settled, you notice the room is decorated with dark wood panels and a complementary section of red tartan wallpaper. My coffee came with a little jug of cream, which, for a skim-milk guy, is quite a change. The fries are served on small paper plates and the soda in conical paper cups. Here, the attitude toward ketchup is the reverse of that at Louis' Lunch. I watched as, unbidden, the server asked if anyone wanted ketchup. If someone does, he heaves a healthy dollop onto

a separate plate from a small glass bottle of Heinz. He slings the empty
bottle in the trash and reaches for another. There's no hint of their refilling
Heinz bottles with a lesser-grade ketchup, because under the counter are
boxes and boxes of the real thing.

John Edge documents the arms race in the world of the luxury burger
in the early 2000s. The skirmish was joined in 2001 after Daniel Boulud
introduced his (lowercase) db burger at the DB Bistro Moderne, on Forty-
fourth Street in Manhattan. Boulud's burger, customized with short ribs,
foie gras, and truffles, clocked in at twenty-nine dollars and was soon challenged by other chefs, with ever more ostentatious sandwiches. One was
made with exotic Wagyu beef; another was all foie gras, and a third was
decorated with gold leaf like a fancy gate. Daniel Boulud raised the stakes
further by adding more fresh black truffles to his burger and charging
ninety-nine dollars for it.

A year or so after the DB Bistro opened, my wife and I visited for my
birthday. We're not in the habit of going out for a fancy lunch, but this was
a good way of visiting a restaurant without having to kill yourself getting a
reservation and without paying for a night's babysitting. Looking at it like
that, I could say the meal was practically free. More important, we'd read
about the **db burger,** and it had prompted our interest in the restaurant.

And here it was, called out in all its finery on the menu.

THE ORIGINAL db BURGER
Sirloin Burger Filled
with Braised Short Ribs, Foie Gras
and Black Truffles
Served on a Parmesan Bun
with Pommes Frites
29.

We had to have one, even though I never wholly trust anything that
willfully drops a capital letter. This was a phase of my life when I eschewed
red meat, sort of, so we decided my wife would order the burger and I'd
have a taste. (It was my birthday.) I asked for some fish for myself. We were
served, and I dutifully ate my fish but I only had eyes for the burger. If it
had been a steak, I'd have been much less interested, but this little tower
of food was a New York celebrity, a mini monument to Gothamite excess.
I duly had my taste. Given the ingredients, it's not surprising that the db
burger is at least one step beyond the normal. I remember it as being in-
toxicatingly rich and fabulous, as in a thing of fables. So what if it's ten

QUICK BITE

"Steakburgers since 1940," says the menu at the beloved Winstead's, restaurants found in and around Kansas City and heartily recommended by (my) literary agent and K.C. native Laura Dail. A **Single Winstead** is $1.99, including its mustard, ketchup, pickle, and onion, plus mayo and grilled onion, should you prefer. Have a Double for $3.09, or a Triple for $3.79, old-fashioned prices for sure. Cheese, lettuce, and bacon come extra, but won't break the bank, either. Try one of the classic fountain treats, like shakes and malts or a **Chocolate "Frosty,"** "the exclusive Winstead drink you eat with a spoon."

times more expensive than a fast-food burger? If you're paying, you go to expensive restaurants for the occasion and something to remember, and the db burger was certainly memorable. The fish I ate I don't recall so much about.

The Shooting Star Saloon in Huntsville, Utah, has been in business since 1879 and is the oldest continually operating saloon in the state. It was

QUICK BITE

My friend Bud went to DB Bistro with his wife, Tamar, to celebrate her birthday. Inevitably, Bud had the burger, and described it like this:

Its intense delights could be described as nearly sexual (it was served sliced, so its pleasure layers were exposed), certainly hedonistic, especially in our health-conscious time. Overlooked in the frenzy surrounding the truffled foie gras center is the burger's secret ingredient: that next layer of shredded short ribs. With that nestled in a layer of rare sirloin, like tartare, then fried, the package was a shrine to the good carnivorous life. What's remarkable is that, like The Beatles, the whole manages to be greater than the sum of its parts. This is a burger only nominally, ironically even—like calling Radio City a movie theater, or the Grand Canyon a hole in the desert.

selling beer before Utah even was a state, which came to pass in 1896. The small town of Huntsville once served silver mining towns like La Plata, twenty miles up the mountain. La Plata's a ghost town now. When the miners used to come down for provisions, they'd drink in the saloon and stay the night across the street. During Prohibition, there was a still out back of the saloon and booze was bootlegged out of the basement.

Shooting Star owner Heidi Posnien, who told me these details, points out that the saloon is a tavern, not a restaurant, so no one under twenty-one is allowed in. She sells beer, but no hard liquor because she'd have to operate as a private club to get the license. Although it's primarily a bar, the Shooting Star makes burgers and has developed a reputation for its **Star Burger,** a double cheeseburger with the works, with a knockwurst on top. I ask Heidi if you can eat this with your hands, and she says you'd better, because it would make a royal mess otherwise. The burger is six dollars, which is a deal, but not as good a deal as the jukebox, which plays seven songs for a buck. A lot of the songs are old country 45s that are rotated in and out of the machine.

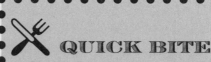

QUICK BITE

In Cincinnati, you can get your chops round a Mettwurst at Zip's Café, which serves what it calls a **Girth Burger,** a burger that comes with a split Mettwurst on top, a cousin, perhaps, to the Utah Star Burger.

People may labor under the misconception that the influence of the Mormon Church, whose members don't drink, means that the whole state of Utah is dry, as in alcohol-free. Not so. You can get a drink in the Beehive State. The state runs the liquor stores, and mandates that three types of licensed establishments can serve alcohol: private clubs; restaurants; and brew pubs, beer bars, and taverns (no hard liquor in these). According to the New York State Liquor Authority, there are approximately 1,900 establishments with full liquor licenses in Manhattan (24 square miles) compared with roughly 800 in Utah (85,000 square miles). So you just have to plan ahead if you want to drink with your meal in Utah.

The Shooting Star Saloon also features a near-three-hundred-pound St. Bernard called Buck, who is stuffed and mounted in the bar. Buck lived in West Yellowstone, and when he died a friend of his owner had the dog mounted. Buck was so big they had to use a stand built to hold a grizzly bear. Buck was put on display in a local bar until the bar was sold and Buck reverted to his original owner. The story is that the man's wife wouldn't let the dog back in the house in his exhibition condition, so Buck stayed in the man's truck. This was until the owner came up to Huntsville and had a drink in the Shooting Star. The man left, but Buck stayed behind. That was thirty years ago.

A QUESTION FOR DANNY MEYER

What do you suggest we eat?

"A Shack Burger from Shake Shack in New York City."

One of the pioneers of the current burger movement is the entrepreneurial restaurateur Danny Meyer. His Shake Shack in Madison Square Park in Manhattan is far more than just a burger place, but his Shack Burger has quickly gained a starry reputation. In 2005, it was *New York* magazine's Editor's Pick for Best Burger in the city.

I have visited the Shake Shack at either end of the summer, and both times the line swelled appreciably at noon. There's consistently a long line, but it is a quick line, really. I came one lovely October day at one thirty and had my food in about twenty-five minutes. Anticipation can be a pleasure in itself. The Shack attracts a big office crowd, and if I worked in the area, I'd find it hard to stay away, too. First time, I went with my son, Sam. He liked his cheeseburger and the crinkle-cut fries but was most taken with the ultracreamy **vanilla shake.** To me, it tasted like liquid ice cream, which I suppose is the point.

I love the **Shack Burger,** which is a works burger with "Special Sauce," that bears some resemblance to Russian dressing but which has its own secret ingredients. I'm not into the "Best of" game, but if there's a better burger than this in New York, give it to me. The burger is a good size but not huge, which allows us to call it exquisite. The meat, sirloin and brisket, which is ground at Meyer's swanky Eleven Madison Park, close by, has always been joyously juicy. The first time I went, if I hadn't been testing the Shake Shack hot dogs, I'd have had two burgers. This is great-value food. Last time I went, a Chicago dog, a Shack Burger and fries, and a Diet Coke was twelve dollars even. And you probably don't have to eat all of that to feel full.

Because you eat at tables set up in the park, you're prey to the vagaries of the New York weather. The restaurant takes no chances with winter and closes before they can get snowed out, which is a shame. The rest of the year, you can take advantage of bad weather, as the Shack itself notes, so come when it's raining to avoid the lines. Dining in this particular park does have one drawback—there's no bathroom. The nearest ones—I guess you could say this is ironic—are in some fast-food chains across the street.

If you haven't been before, the location of the burger joint at the Parker Meridien Hotel on West Fifty-seventh Street in Midtown Manhattan isn't immediately obvious. The hotel pretends the burger place isn't there, so, set just off the main lobby, the entrance is concealed. If you're going at lunchtime, there may well be a line marking the spot, and it's possible to detect the faint whiff of frying food from the lobby. Follow the line to the front and look for the neon burger (with lettuce and tomato) at the end of a passage. Turn right under the neon sign and you're inside. This is an un-dercover venue—over the two exposed sides of the box that houses the restaurant are floor-to-ceiling drapes, and there are no windows.

My lunch companion the first time I visited was my friend Bud. Bud works at Columbia University and always brings an intelligent rigor to the subject at hand. More important, he likes to eat. We arrived right at 12:00 to find a good-size line out the door. It was a quick line, though. We heard that at 11:45 there had been no line, and nor was there one at 12:40, when we left. (I came one day at 12:50 and was in and out in a leisurely 18 min-utes.) Once you penetrate the threshold, you realize there's a second line stretching back from the counter to the door. If you're not eating alone, one of your party should stand in the line to order while the others loiter by the booths or over at the counter that is set to one side so they can grab seats as soon as they're vacated. Advice for eaters: As with the subway, once you're set, don't make eye contact with anyone looking for a seat.

The restaurant looks like a coffee shop with booths and wood panel-ing. On the walls were tacked some recent, not new, movie posters, and the walls and brickwork in the back were adorned with graffiti. On the counter is a tiny menu listing individual items. I asked for a couple of cheeseburgers with fries and sodas.

Eating lunch here could overload your senses. On our visit, the small room was hot and loud, and there was much to look at. This was Election Day, so there was a poster crying VOTE OR DIE. There was a curt sign saying MENU FOR TODAY: CHOICE OF TWO, TAKE IT OR LEAVE IT. Behind us was a wall of decorated napkins. (The one nearest to me said CHIHUAHUA IS A STATE, NOT A DOG.) Above the grill were racks of Arnold burger buns and big cans of Heinz ketchup. Then there were the curious globe lights that seemed out of place. Above the din, we had noted a Bollywood sound-track playing, which was followed in true international style by works from Edith Piaf and Kylie Minogue. Finally, we spotted two Actual French People (Michelin inspectors?).

Our order was ready, the fries in paper bags and the burgers wrapped in butcher's paper. The decent-size **cheeseburger** comes with lettuce, to-mato, mayo, pickle, and a generous slice of red onion (and, once, mustard). By now, I'd come to appreciate certain attributes in a burger—slight loose-ness in the meat and a tendency for the contents to slide away from you once the burger is bitten into. In this case, the "works" worked well. Just delicious. The fries were very good as well. Sitting in the debris of our quickly eaten meal, Bud and I realized we couldn't immediately order an-other burger. This is a flaw in the ordering system because this kind of spur-of-the-moment idea dissipates fast if you have to line up. But now we know, and we'll get two next time.

Bud and I decided that there were two possible explanations for the down-home decor: one, the place was an existing diner reconfigured cheaply into a burger bar; or two, more likely, it was designed to look like it had been there for fifty years, a reverse makeover that would conform to a design style Bud dubbed "neo-retro." When we left, a member of the hotel staff told me the place had been there only a couple of years. As for the look, he figured someone had just gone to Home Depot and thrown it to-gether.

But looking online after I got home, I found a Web site for the designer, McCartan, who took credit for the burger joint, as well as a lot of the ultra-modern elements of the hotel around it. Beneath a couple of pictures, a rubric says of the joint, "It is designed to look like a decades-old family café and is completely hidden, appearing as if the hotel was built around it." Just so.

Meeting at Bud's apartment over home-cooked brats the next day, we agreed that the concept and its execution are utterly brilliant. The burger joint wants to look generic, coyly hiding its not-a-name name in lowercase letters. Its fake-fake décor is so good it belongs in Las Vegas. Setting this seemingly cheap burger bar inside a swanky hotel makes each place hipper. (Though this location can be disorienting. One time, a guy in line behind me commented to his friend, "This place is cool." He waited a beat, and said, "Right?") But it's here that business lunchers and trend-conscious

Europeans both say, "Let's eat at the hotel." The Parker-Meridien has hidden the place behind curtains and pretends it isn't there. Once you're inside the joint, you don't feel like you're in a hotel at all. The experience makes you feel like you're in on something, that you're an insider. To sum up, the burger joint is a brilliantly cultivated, well-kept secret everyone knows about.

George Motz did yeoman work making *Hamburger America*. He reckons he ate five hundred burgers in two years, half of them when he was promoting the film. These would have been more than enough to help him put on the twenty to twenty-five pounds he gained in this period. The idea for the film came about when George and his wife saw a documentary on hot dogs and realized that no one had tackled burgers from a national perspective. For George, a cameraman on TV commercials, this was his first feature. George's wife, Casey, should win some kind of forbearance award—she is a vegetarian.

Every town and city has its well-loved burger joints. The Old Town Bar and Restaurant behind Union Square in New York is such a joint, but it's better known as a saloon. The bar opened in 1892 and is renowned for many things: the tracking shot of the bar at the start of David Letterman's show and the imperious urinals in the men's room, to name just two. My friend Sam and I eat upstairs every time he visits from London. May the creaky booths and the dark, dark wood paneling never be replaced. May they continue to tell diners who is the patron saint of the day with a note on the menu. (The last time we went, it was Saint Albert the Great Day.) The burger with American, with lettuce, onion, and tomato on the side ($8.25), was fine, though lacking the essential juiciness of others I had around the same time.

Go to the Old Town Bar for the history. Even as great cities modernize and rebuild, they have to keep places like this around lest they lose their soul. The Old Town knows its history but doesn't oversell it. On the wall upstairs is a menu from December 1937 with a corned beef sandwich for fifteen cents, a lot of German food, and a special section for rarebits, the Welsh, the Golden Buck (with a poached egg), the Yorkshire Buck (with bacon), and the mysterious **Long Island.** I haven't been able to find out what made the dish specific to this part of the world.

The Corner Bistro in Greenwich Village is famed for its eight-ounce flame-grilled burgers. I met a couple of friends there late one winter Sunday afternoon to watch football and eat a burger. We failed the Darwinian survival-of-the-fastest test for seats at the bar and ended up being shuffled to the dingy back restaurant. It may or may not be true that the word *bistro* entered the French language from the Russian for *quickly*, but it certainly applies at the Corner Bistro: our **Bistro Burgers**, cheeseburgers with the works and curlicued (deep-fried?) bacon, arrived in about a minute. The big sloppy burger took my mind off our barroom experience, as did the two-dollar beers. Nothing in New York costs as little as two dollars except McSorley's ale at the Corner Bistro.

QUICK BITE •

A burger I am very interested in trying is the **Supreme with Olives** from the Halo Burger chain that originated in Flint, Michigan. Flint is a place with a lot of burger history. Halo Burger founder Bill Thomas got his start at a Kewpee restaurant and went on to take over a couple of local Kewpees and rename them Halo Burger. Thomas died in 1973, but his family still runs the chain, which has eleven restaurants in the Flint area. Burgers had been sold out of the Kewpee Hotel (which was not a hotel at all) since 1923, by Sam Blair, who claimed to have originated the flat-bottomed bun and had the idea of putting lettuce, mayo, and tomato on burgers. A few Kewpees remain, including three in Lima, Ohio. There's a comprehensive Web site on vintage Michigan that has a lot more information on all this: www.waterwinterwonderland.com.

By no means are all burgers created equally. Four-ounce burgers might have a lot in common with eight-ounce burgers, but they're not the same. Ditto flame-grilled and skillet-cooked patties. The next two establishments we looked at serve burgers that are more cousins than brothers. Each is grilled, each is a good size, but at Le Tub in Hollywood, Florida, your choice is cheese or no cheese, while Island Burgers and Shakes in New York City lists sixty-four varieties, with further customization available from a raft of extras. They do have the key factor in common: both make fantastic burgers.

For a restaurant with such a big menu, Island Burgers is implausibly small. And far more than burgers are on offer: every hamburger variation is offered as a churrasco, a grilled chicken breast sandwich. There are numerous salads as well. I can vouch for the **Capo San Lucas,** a giant grilled chicken/avocado/salsa feast—but it is the burgers that are truly special. I favor the **South of the Border Burger,** the meat seared on the outside and perfectly medium-rare within, topped with guacamole, jack cheese, salsa, and five or six rounds of raw jalapeño.

The last time I went I was impressed that the gentleman seated next to me had managed to clamp his burger down—I think it was a **Derby** (bacon, blue cheese, and avocado)—and eat it with his hands. If I tried that I'd dislocate my jaw. I always wimp out and use a knife and fork, balancing quantities of the fixings on top of the burger. I can sit back to savor the bursts of flavor and texture that alternate peppery and soft, spicy and crunchy, all underpinned by the crusted yet moist meat. I'll say the same about the burgers at Island Burgers that I said about those at the Shake Shack—if there's anything better than this round here, I want to know about it.

Island Burgers is a narrow room with alternating yellow and red tables and a surfing theme décor (*Endless Summer* poster, surfboard motifs, etc.). There's a Buddha figure looking down from a shelf and a plastic Christmas tree that was either very early for the holidays or is just always there. One of the numerous pleasures of the place is that they play music I like. Among the stacks of CDs by the stereo, I recognized perennial Brit favorites like New Order, Blur, Pulp, Keane, and Oasis. The last time I went, co-owner Mark Calvino was playing the new Stones CD, which took me nicely through my lunch.

Mark Calvino told me Island has been around more than ten years and was started by him and Californian Will Brown, who thought up 90 percent of the burger names. The two met at Joe Allen, the famous Theater District restaurant, where Mark was a waiter and bartender and Will Brown was the office manager. Mark says Will Brown wanted his own place eventually. Mark made some off-hand comment to the effect that he'd be happy to invest in any venture of Will's, and three years later Will called Mark on his promise. Mark ended up working at Island Burgers before it opened and he's been there almost ever since.

Many of the burger and salad names come from beaches and places in California and Mexico (Capo San Lucas is spelled wrong deliberately) or from prominent Island people. **Will's Burger** (bacon, cheddar, sour cream, onion, and scallion on sourdough) is named for Will Brown; **Charlie's Sweet and Sour** (relish, honey, mustard, and Swiss), for a chef named Charlie. **The Clyde** (blackened burger with bleu cheese, salsa, bacon, and avocado) was created by a customer who was on the phone placing an order and asked if she could come up with a name for a burger. Clyde was the name of the woman's dog, who had been named in turn after New York Knicks legend Walt "Clyde" Frazier.

I ambushed Mark with a pop quiz, asking him to list the ingredients of two particularly challenging-looking items: the **Hippo** and **Princess Grace's** burger, and he passed with flying colors. What are they? I'm not going to spoil the surprise. Go and check them out. Mark told me what he thought the top ten best-selling burgers at Island might be. Not in order, they are: The Clyde, Napalm, Bourbon Street, Cowboy, Tijuana, The Derby, Hobie's, Mona Lisa, South of the Border, and Black and Blue. Sounds like a good menu plan to me.

A feature of the restaurant is that they don't serve French fries. The space was previously a check-cashing place, so the kitchen had to be built from scratch. The architect said they couldn't run a gas oven, a grill, and a Frialator (industrial deep-fryer) from the existing gas supply, and the investors couldn't afford to wait for Con Ed to come in and install a new line. So fries they did without. The menu used to say "fries coming" but the restaurant prospered without them. Mark suggested that they make baked potatoes instead, and that idea took hold. Occasionally a customer will get up from the table and walk out when he hears about the fries. Mark always tells fry-deprived patrons that the chicken place two doors down will happily sell them fries in a cup that they're welcome to bring back with no corkage, but few of the fryophiles ever do. Me, I'm happy not to have the temptation. Island Burgers' marvelous offerings show it's all about the burger.

From Eric Schlosser's *Fast Food Nation* I gleaned a couple of world-class bits of trivia:
Q: Which two American institutions were both founded in San Bernardino, California, in 1948?
A: McDonald's and The Hell's Angels.
Along similar lines:

Q: Which two American fast-food institutions were both founded in Wichita, Kansas?

A: White Castle and Pizza Hut.

The first White Castle was opened in Wichita in 1921, selling five-cent burgers. Today, there are no White Castle restaurants in Kansas. Frank and Dan Carney were students at the University of Wichita when they started their pizza restaurant in 1958. It's said that the modest building they used had room for only three more letters on its sign once "Pizza" was spelled, hence "Hut." (One more letter, and we might have had "Pizza Shed.") Both Wichita restaurants were, of course, the first of many to open under the same moniker.

No sooner were we seated at our weather-beaten table at Le Tub, the bar-restaurant that fronts the Intracoastal Waterway in Hollywood, Florida, than the diners next to us turned our way and said, "You know this place's hamburger was voted the best in the country." "I know," I said. In 2000, we learned you can't trust any vote held in the state of Florida, but Le Tub wasn't voted the best as much as crowned such, by food writer Alan Richman in an issue of *GQ* magazine. That was what had drawn us to Le Tub, as it had countless other trophy hunters and carpetbaggers. "So the burger's good, then?" I asked our lunch neighbors. They confirmed it was, though it took a lot longer to get one these days. We'd been told at least twice that we'd have to wait no less than an hour for our food—it got up to three hours right after the *GQ* piece came out. We got the coloring books out for the kids, ordered a couple of beers, and settled in for the duration.

Lining the sidewalk outside Le Tub are the first of many bathroom fixtures, including cast-iron tubs and toilets that decorate the restaurant. Behind our table is a reminder, painted on the flipped-up underside of a toilet seat, to try the Key lime pie. The barroom is hung with fishing gear and lined with license plates. You look up toward the bar from the door, past a pool table, and the effect is of a ship, with a sunken galley from which pours great gusts of pungent smoke. You can sit round the bar, if you don't mind the smoke. Behind you might be an NFL game on one TV; on another, above the bar, Bobby Flay might be soundlessly describing some dish or other on the Food Network.

Most of the tables are outside and everything—tables, railings, flooring—appears to be made from the same naturally distressed wood.

The menu claims that founder Russell T. Kohuth built the restaurant in the seventies, on the site of a Sunoco gas station, wholly out of "flotsam, jetsam and ocean-borne treasures." The water is right in front of you, and big oceangoing yachts ply up and down the waterway. It's very pleasant to sit here and watch them go by and take in the sun.

Our hot dog (boiled rather than grilled, on our waitress's recommendation) and plate of excellent beefsteak fries and mozzarella sticks came quickly enough, as did my bowl of **seafood gumbo.** Our neighbors had told us the gumbo was hot, as in spicy, and so it was, and also full of shrimp and mighty good.

At an hour ten, the **Sirloinburgers with cheese** arrived. The menu advertises "8 oz. ground sirloin," and the burger, a plastic fork jammed into the melted cheese, looked gigantic. I fixed my burger with the thick slice of white onion accompanying it and went at it with the knife and fork. The burger, ground top sirloin, was meaty and then some. Charred around and pink within, it was the medium-rare I had asked for. Juice ran into the bun, and lubricated with a little ketchup, the burger went down fast. Sam ate half of his, which in itself is a lot of food. I asked the waitress whether there was anything in the meat, and she said it was seasoned with that special secret have-to-kill-you-if-I-tell-you ingredient.

We managed a piece of the **Key lime pie,** and it was nicely sour. The bill topped out at a hundred dollars, nice tip included. Le Tub's burger is the business. Who's to say if it's the best or not, but it certainly is superior. I took a bunch of pictures of my burger and I have found myself looking at them fondly from time to time.

Being written up as "the Best" was probably a mixed blessing for Le Tub. It's now "famous." There's a Budweiser advert on the front door commemorating the Best Burger award, and you can buy a T-shirt that fêtes it, too. Le Tub is really a bar that serves food that's restricted by the fact you can't squeeze anyone in the galley besides chef/part-owner Steven to prepare the great burgers. In time, Le Tub will probably revert to being a neighborhood, rather than a national, joint—and be all the happier for it.

Twenty-something blocks east of the famous Versailles restaurant in Miami we found El Rey de Las Fritas, which stood on Calle Ocho and Twelfth Avenue for more than forty years, but which moved after we visited. There are other locations, including one at SW Fortieth (Bird) Avenue. As it originally stood, El Rey de Las Fritas was a small, cafeteria-style restaurant that featured representations of Cuban fast food, like *pan con butifarra,* a hot dog sandwich, pictured round the walls. I was there for a **frita,** the Cuban burger, which I ordered at the take-out window ($2.65) and didn't take it out of its little bag and look at it till we got back to our hotel a half hour later.

These are not optimal conditions under which to eat anything. Bringing take-out trays back to a hotel room isn't one of life's great ideas. It smells, it's messy, and it encourages snacking. Into this particular room I had brought half a Le Tub sirloinburger, two-thirds of a Versailles Cuban sandwich, and another box I never looked inside before throwing away. I ate one piece of the Cuban sandwich and most of the sirloin burger, but I felt like a carrion crow after and vowed to try to swim off a few of the pointless extra calories the next day.

But the *frita* I had brought back to my room with the best of intentions. I took the sandwich out onto the balcony and inspected it. White bun, small, spiced meat patty with onions and shoestring potatoes sprinkled on top. These potatoes did really resemble shoestrings, unlike most similarly named fries, which would only lace the Green Giant's sneakers. I pressed the top half of the bun back down and the fries crackled. They gave a pleasing crunch under the soft and yielding roll, and the meat was thin but tasty. The whole thing taken together was very satisfying. The hot *frita* is something I want to try and perhaps also a **pan con butifarra** with a **guanabana shake**.

The Bobcat Bite sits five miles or so out of Santa Fe, along the Old Las Vegas Highway. Early one summer's evening, I flopped down at a seat at the counter and ordered the **Green Chile Cheeseburger** I'd been looking forward to for weeks, along with potato salad and a side of green chile. (This would be some general advice about eating chile round these parts: if it's offered, get some on the side, too.) My gratification was delayed by the restaurant's quixotic opening hours: Wednesday through Saturday: 11:00 to 7:50.

The best thing about eating on your own is that you can usually get a seat at the bar or the counter. This evening, my companion to the left looked ahead resolutely and didn't seem like a talker. A couple of guys sat to my right and talked to each other. Fine. I didn't feel like saying much anyway. The Bobcat Bite has a wonderful draw you see best from the counter and I was free to concentrate on that. A big drip feeder stocked with sugar water hangs outside and attracts hummingbirds. The hummingbirds flitted in and out to feed, one, sometimes two, at a time. I was mesmerized.

QUICK BITE

Co-owner Bonnie Eckre told me why the Bobcat Bite closes at 7:50. When the place first opened, this was ranch country and, metaphorically at least, Santa Fe was much farther away. There was a de facto curfew in effect, and ranch workers had to be back in their bunks by 8:00 p.m. Closing the restaurant ten minutes before the curfew meant people had a chance to get home in time. Now the time has a distinctive value. (I certainly remembered it.) But don't mess with it. There's nothing ornamental about it: 7:50 means 7:50.

The back of the menu gives you the restaurant's history. Old Las Vegas Highway is part of the old Route 66. First a trading post, then a gun shop, this building was made a restaurant by Rene Clayton, the owner of the Bobcat Ranch next door, in 1953. The Bobcat Bite changed hands a few times and has been operated by John and Bonnie Eckre since 2001. The name came from the bobcats that would come down from the hills behind the place for scraps before I-25 came through. Pictures of the felines decorate the walls.

Bonnie Eckre told me how the area round the restaurant had changed. She said that the last cowboy who used to ride his horse to the restaurant had just made his final visit. If you ride a horse up the mountain out the back, Bonnie says, you might see a bobcat. But the bobcats no longer come right down to the restaurant—years ago the owners would put out food for the foxes and bobcats. Recently, however, she was out by the porch and a bobcat walked across the street just outside. All told, Bonnie has been working at the restaurant for eighteen years, and that's the closest she's ever seen a bobcat to the Bobcat Bite.

Sitting up front, you get to watch the place working. There were just two servers here, and the kitchen was making a lot of food, much of it for takeout. Inside, the restaurant is small. The parking lot had been full, and those people in parties of two and more wrote their names up on a board outside and waited. All of a sudden I was extremely hungry. I knew from the menu that they ground the meat here every day from choice whole boneless chuck. That wasn't helping. When my food came, I did my best not to bolt it. The ten-ounce burger was done medium-rare and just right. The white cheese was melted over the green chile. With the bun, this is a big burger—a knife-and-fork operation. The chile was toward the hot side and it did the job.

By the time I'd forked down the last piece of my burger, my taciturn neighbor had been replaced by an older gentleman the server greeted as the Professor (who is a professor). "No hummingbirds," he said, looking out the window, and for the last couple of minutes there hadn't been. Sure enough, right on cue, one, and then two, maneuvered into view and hovered, each dipping its proboscis in the sugar water. "Wings beat a thousand times a second," the professor said. I sat and watched a little more before leaving. The burger at the Bobcat Bite deserves its reputation. Go for that reason. And—how many places can you say this about?—go for the hummingbirds, too.

BURGERS SUMMARY

RUN, DON'T WALK, FOR . . .

- **Green Chile Cheeseburger** at the Bobcat Bite: sit at the counter and keep an eye out for what's happening out the window.
- **South of the Border Burger** at Island Burgers and Shakes in New York.
- **Shack Burger** at the Shake Shack, and **cheeseburger** at the burger joint, New York.
- A **Double-Double** at In-N-Out.
- A **Sirloinburger with cheese** at Le Tub, in Hollywood.

IF YOU'VE NEVER TRIED . . .

- A *frita* in Miami, it's a genuinely different burger experience.
- Chile on a cheeseburger. See next chapter . . .

11

CHILI, CHILI, CHILE

The chili purist is in love with the romantic notion of the cowboy
on the range—who rustled up a stew made only with water, dried
chilies and meat. This was chili con carne . . . Of course, the meat that
idealized cowboy probably used was pemmican, or preserved bison,
which he had tucked under his saddle near his rifle. I don't hear
the purists clamoring for pemmican.
—David Rosengarten, *It's All American Food* (2003)

At least three distinctive types of dish have emerged in this country based on the spicy power of the chile pepper. Ask for "chili" in different regions and you'll get very different dishes, or you'll be asked to be a lot more specific. In New Mexico, much more information is needed to make a meal, as red and/or green *chile* are accompaniments to huge numbers of other dishes. As is the case with pizza, the hot dog, and all kinds of barbecue (but not so much the more utilitarian burger), there are people who'll tell you how chili *has to be*. Not I. Rather, we'll look at the three main varieties, centered in Texas, Cincinnati, and New Mexico, and enjoy and appreciate them all.

If, as David Rosengarten contends, "authentic" Texas chili needs to be made with bison jerky, then the familiar argument about whether or not you're allowed to add beans is beside the point. Still, the key ingredients in Rosengarten's modern recipe are the dried red chiles and cubed beef chuck. As for the origin of the dish, Root and de Rochemont write that it was created in San Antonio some time after the Civil War and popularized with the 1902 invention, in the town of New Braunfels, Texas, of chili powder by a German immigrant.

When and where this culinary advance occurred is disputed, of course, although Willie Gebhardt of New Braunfels is known to have registered his Eagle Brand Chili Powder in 1896. Gebhardt started by grinding up fresh red chiles using the meat grinder in the restaurant he owned and then dyeing the resulting powder. The extra seasoning—cumin, oregano, black pepper—came later. Gebhardt's powder went on to a long life of healthy sales and his company wound up as part of the giant ConAgra conglomerate, where it remains as one of its brands.

My brother-in-law Doug is involved with the Hard Times Café chain, which operates restaurants, some (known as cue clubs) with pool halls attached, in Maryland and Virginia, with an outpost in North Carolina and one at RFK Stadium for Washington Nationals games. I resisted Doug's lighthearted entreaties about Hard Times chili, the dish for which the restaurants are best known, until *USA Today* named the chain as one of the top ten places to get a bowl of chili in the country. Then I figured I should go and try some.

Doug took me to one of the Virginia stores, where I bought him lunch. As we sat down, we were given a taster with a couple of tablespoonsful of each of the company's four chilis arranged on a plate. They are **Texas Chili, Terlingua Red, Cincinnati Chili,** and Vegetarian Chili. (Terlingua Red is named for the Texas town in Big Bend Country where the first chili cook-off took place.) The restaurant serves its chilis plain in a bowl or over spaghetti for a Chili Mac, along with chili dogs, Coney dogs, and similar fare.

I worked my way round the taster. The Texas is the spiciest of the four chilis, made with coarse ground beef and Texas spices centered on chili powder. The overall texture is dry—some customers ask for their chili "wet," which means it comes with extra "juice," or grease to you and me. Terlingua Red has a tomato-based sauce, hence the name, and is formulated from restaurant co-founder Jim Parker's championship recipe, with which he competes worldwide. This is a recent addition to the Hard Times menu and quickly established itself as the best seller. The Cincinnati uses a finer-ground beef and milder spices, wherein I tasted a pleasant breath of cinnamon. The Vegetarian, made with soy flakes, was pretty good and would make a viable alternative if I weren't having meat. This wasn't one of those days, though, so we ordered a bowl of Texas, a Bowl of Red (Terlingua), and a **Five-Way Chili Mac** (Cincinnati Chili, spaghetti, cheddar cheese, onions, and pink chili beans, for more on which, see page 187.)

I took my chili without beans and with the fixings on the side— some cheddar, sour cream, and diced onion. I had to admit to Doug that he'd got me. The chili was all good: honest, strong, and spicy. I liked the more robust flavor of the original Texas Chili the best, but the Terlingua Red held its own, and we managed to make a good dent in the Chili Mac, too.

Doug also sent me packages of Hard Times chili mixes (for the Texas, Terlingua, and Cincinnati chilis) created by Jim Parker and his brother Fred. I bought two big bone-in chuck steaks from ace New York city delivery merchant Fresh Direct and made pots of Texas Chili and the Terlingua Red using the Hard Times mixes.

At the time I was making the chili, we didn't have a functioning cooking scale in the apartment. (This makes it sound like this was an aberrant situation, but we still don't have one.) To weigh the cubed steak, I hopped on the bathroom scales holding Ziploc bags of meat and then not. Even allowing for the resulting inexactness, and holding back from adding as much chili powder as recommended, the Hard Times recipes make quite blistering, and solidly meaty, chili. The bowl of Red had a lovely color and a big bold taste. Very fine indeed.

Buy Hard Times chili mixes and more: www.hardtimes.com.

When I visited, Hard Times was gearing up for its twenty-sixth annual cook-off, to be held in Rockville, Maryland. The Hard Times event was the Maryland State Championship with competitions in red chili, green chili, salsa, freestyle, and showmanship (which is cooking in fancy dress) categories. The winners in the first three categories advance to the chili world championships, held each October in Omaha, where champions are selected in Red, Chili Verde (green chili), and Salsa categories.

Chili cook-offs are a big deal. So much so that as with professional boxing, there is more than one sanctioning body. The chili organizations raise a lot of money for charity, which is not the case with professional boxing, unless I'm mistaken. The father of cook-offs was Francis X. Tolbert

(1912–1984), newspaper writer, author of a book called *A Bowl of Red,* and chili promoter. Tolbert organized a cook-off in Terlingua in 1967. The Omaha event is run by the International Chili Society (ICS), which was founded as a breakaway organization from Tolbert's in the seventies. ICS can run two hundred cook-offs with a million participants in a year. The original Chili Appreciation Society International (CASI) still holds its International Chili Championship in Terlingua, Texas, each November, and sanctions even more cook-offs all over the country, about five hundred, from Addison, Illinois, to Zuehl, Texas, where contestants earn points to qualify for the big dance.

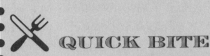

QUICK BITE

The Tolbert chili legacy also lives at Tolbert's restaurant in Grapevine, Texas, ten minutes from the Dallas Fort Worth International Airport, with chili available, naturally, as **A Bowl of Red,** and with pinto beans as **North of the Border.** You can also get **Frank's Frito Chili Pie,** the famous chili dish made with Frito's corn chips.

There is a third group, also founded by Frank Tolbert, called Original Terlingua International Championship Chili Cookoff (OTICCC), or, informally, Tolbert, which also cooks off at Terlingua in the first weekend in November. Check out the chili sites: CASI at www.chili.org, ICS at www .chilicookoff.com, and Tolbert at www.abowlofred.com.

Note also that since 1989, the Lone Star Vegetarian Network has organized a Vegetarian (vegan) Chili Cook-Off. In 2006 it was held in November at the Austin Zoo. Information is available at www.lsvn.org.

BUCKEYE CHILI

I never saw any numbers on menus in Cincinnati, but it is accepted that a customer can walk into any chili parlor—an Empress or a Skyline or any of the independent neighborhood parlors—and say "One three-way" and be assured of getting chili on spaghetti with cheese. Cincinnati eaters take it for granted that the other ways to serve it go up to a five-way (chili, spaghetti, onions, cheese, and beans) and that the people who do the serving are Greeks.

              — *Calvin Trillin,* American Fried *(1974)*

How much do the people of Cincinnati like their chili? The three hundred thousand–odd Cincinnatians and the two million people who live in the metro area must eat a lot of the stuff because they support a very large number of restaurants. The largest chain, the Skyline Chili Company, alone has upward of eighty-five parlors, as chili restaurants are known, in greater Cincinnati. There are other chains: Gold Star, which has more than seventy restaurants in Ohio; and Dixie, which set up its stall over the river in Kentucky. Then there are the independents, and people who make it at home or buy chili from Kroger's, a Cincinnati-based store chain, or from Empress Chili, in whose Vine Street parlor it all started. "Chili is the real thing," Polly Campbell of the *Cincinnati Enquirer* told me. "People eat it all the time, at the chains, at neighborhood places; three, four, five ways. It's great."

The Empress began life as a hot dog joint, opened on Vine Street in 1922 by the brothers Tom and John Kiradjieff. (It got its name because it was situated next to the Empress Theater.) Many accounts say that the Kiradjieffs were Macedonian; others, that they were Greek. Macedonian and Greek aren't coterminous by any means, but the men who followed in opening their own chili parlors were mostly described as Greek. Each cook had his own recipe for what Tom Kiradjieff cooked up at the Empress, which he called chili. Kiradjieff added spices he knew from home, like cinnamon and cloves, to ground meat (some recipes include chocolate). He served his chili over spaghetti, and he had a hit on his hands.

Two of the other Cincinnati chains had their origins at Empress. Nicholas Lambrinides worked at Empress, figured out his own chili, and opened the first Skyline Chili with his family in Price Hill in 1949. And Nicholas Sarakatsannis opened his Dixie parlor in 1929 after learning his trade at the Empress. The Gold Star chain was started by the Daoud brothers, immigrants from Jordan, in 1965. Among the independents are Price Hill Chili, Blue Ash Chili, and Pleasant Ridge Chili.

Polly Campbell says you often get a dish of oyster crackers with your order. Pour a little hot sauce into the open edge of a cracker, if you wish, for a taster before your main course. When the chili comes it will likely have a thinnish con-

QUICK BITE

For a fun twist on your regular beef chili, try a plate of **White Chili** at Kate Mantilini's in Los Angeles: white chicken breast is teamed with white rice, white beans, white cheese, and lime salsa. It's a dish that feels like it just might want to be a curry but which maintains its own deliciously satisfying personality.

sistency. It's heaped on a plate of thick spaghetti. The chili always seems to be served on the smallest possible oval plate so that almost none of the plate is showing. In addition to taking your chili with spaghetti, you can have it served on little wieners, with cheese on top, for a Coney Dog.

When it comes to ordering the chili, it's available **plain** or **two-way,** which is just spaghetti and chili. Then ingredients can be added on a sliding scale:

- **Three-Way**—chili, spaghetti, and cheddar cheese
- **Four-Way**—chili, spaghetti, cheddar cheese, and onions
- **Five-Way**—chili, spaghetti, cheddar cheese, onions, and kidney beans

At Dixie there's a **Six-Way,** which is "chili, spaghetti, beans, onions all topped with fresh chopped garlic and cheese."

GREEN ON RED

Corn is the earth in Santa Fe cooking, and chilies are the fire.
                                    —*Huntley Dent,* The Feast of Santa Fe

Thanks to its remote location and the successive waves of peoples who have moved into the area, Santa Fe, New Mexico, has developed a quite distinctive cuisine. In the first decade of the seventeenth century, some years before the Pilgrims came ashore at Plymouth Rock, the Spanish built a fort here, in the northern reaches of their territory of Nuevo Mexico. They wanted to convert the local Native Americans to Catholicism, and the two groups lived inharmoniously for two hundred years before Santa Fe became part of a Mexican colony. The region was Mexican territory until the United States forced the Mexicans out in the 1840s.

Practically speaking, supplies could come into Santa Fe only along the road from the south, the Camino Real, the route of the present-day I-25. Once a new power controlled the town, its influence on the food in the area would be profound. "The Indians subsisted on corn gruel and chili, the poorer Spanish blended in that fare some pinto beans, tortillas, and little else," Huntley Dent writes in his cookbook/history of Santa Fe. After years of Spanish, and then Mexican, rule, the Americans arrived, cowboys and settlers with their own tastes and preferences. As far as the food of

Santa Fe was concerned, this was like overlaying Mexico City with Kansas City.

Throughout this period, and until relatively recently, the dominant theme of the local cuisine was scarcity. It wasn't until affluent vacationers, many of them Europeans, started coming to Santa Fe and Taos that what we now think of as Santa Fe cooking took full shape. The restaurants in northern New Mexico weren't so much celebrating local food as reinventing it, with more and better ingredients. I, for one, have been very happy to take advantage of the popularity of Santa Fe. I love the place. The air is clear; the country is beautiful; the people are great. Feed your mind at Collected Works, a treasure of an independent bookstore, and then fill your stomach at any number of places around town. This is easy for me: I love chile, red and green—I could happily eat both all day. One particular twenty-four-hour stretch I tried to do just that. It is a day I'll remember with a wonderfully warm greenish, reddish glow for a long while.

All chilies grow fresh on the vine in a green state and proceed to ripen through various stages of yellow, orange, flame red, dark red and brown-red. For commercial purposes, the green chilies are sold to be eaten immediately or else pickled, while the red-ripened fruit is dried to be sold either whole or as a powder.

—*Huntley Dent,* The Feast of Santa Fe

Let's be clear what we are talking about when we talk about chile: *chile* is the fruit; *chili* is the dish (as distinct from the Greek-inspired dish of the same name in Cincinnati, and the Texan dish, also of the same name). Dent prefers the usage for the fruit that renders the Spanish *chile/chiles* into chili/chilies. Brits and former colonies might add an additional *I* and then follow either usage, meaning you might get a *chilli pepper* in Australia but a *chillie* in India. But for our purposes, *chile* is the fruit, separated on menus in New Mexico into green and red varieties, and *chili* is the dish.

And what we're talking about is a fruit, the fruit of the capsicum family that we call a pepper. The fruit includes a substance called capsaicin, or capsaicinoid, that affect the same receptor in our mouth that detects high temperature. Hence the burning sensation when we eat chiles, and also our description of such food as "hot." This heat can be measured by something called the Scoville scale, which ranges from zero units in the thoroughly benign green pepper to hundreds of thousands of units in some habañeros and various other dangerous Indian varieties.

According to the Chile Pepper Institute at New Mexico State University, peppers evolved their heat to prevent their being eaten by mammals, who digest the seeds—which is of no use to the propagating pepper. The seeds of the fruit are spread by birds, who lack the capacity to break them down, and so disseminate them in their droppings. This idea may have worked on most mammals but not on the ever-perverse human, who decided he liked the taste and went out of his way in certain parts of the world to actively seek it. So in New Mexico you'll see *ristras,* garlands of red chiles, drying in the hot sun. The state is also the location, between Las Cruces and Truth or Consequences, of Hatch, "Chile Capital of the World," where a chile festival is held each Labor Day, swamping the small town with chile fans.

Order fresh Hatch chiles: 1-888-336-4228 / www.nmchili.com.

Before my visit to Santa Fe, I consulted Joline Glenn of the *Albuquerque Tribune.* I asked her about chile. In New Mexico, she tells me, chile is a matter "of great pride and seriousness and specialty." She goes on to say, "The official state question is 'red or green?' referring to what type of chile you prefer on your food." She happens to say green. In her opinion, nowhere else pays such homage to the green chile. Not in Arizona, and not in the parts of the country that think of the jalapeño, which is not the same thing at all. "In the early fall, the smell of green chile roasting is definitive New Mexico."

Joline tells me that locals get a year's supply and freeze it. What do they eat it with? "**Green chile** goes on *everything,* but for sure cheeseburgers, enchiladas (especially chicken), green chile stew, stuffed sopaipillas, eggs." (The sopaipilla is the divine fried dough dish that puffs up into a little pillow. You can eat it savory with chile or sweet with powdered sugar and/or honey.)

I asked Joline for restaurant recommendations in Santa Fe and Albuquerque, and she gave me the names of a lot of places. When I reached Santa Fe, everyone I asked gave me at least one new name. Santa Fe is a small town, with only a certain number of restaurants. Perhaps they're all good. I certainly wasn't disappointed. I went to four places Joline recommended, and to Katherine Kagel's Cafe Pasqual's, whose reputation preceded it.

I got into Santa Fe in the evening, checked into my hotel, and walked a short way across town to Tomasita's, on the promise of what Joline had described as "some of the hottest green chile." I was girded up for it, so I was very happy to see on the wall as I entered the restaurant, a not-so-serious health warning:

A MESSAGE TO OUR OUT-OF-TOWN GUESTS
"THE CHILE IS HOT"

Please ask you waitperson for a sample or order it on the side. We are not responsible for too hot chile! Please let you waitperson know if you are a vegetarian.

Thanx, Georgia

Tomasita's is housed in a handsome-looking building that was once the station house for the Denver and Rio Grande rail line, whose "Chile Line" ran the seven-hour trip between Antonito and Santa Fe. Literature at the restaurant says the line "connected villages, pueblos, towns, and cultures. The D&RG was the timekeeper, the newspaper, the friend of children, and the transporter of local goods—lumber, piñon, wool, chile and fruit." The station house was built in 1904, before New Mexico became a state, and the last run of the line was September 1, 1941.

Now, Tomasita's is a temple to northern New Mexico cuisine. I sat at the bar, ordered a margarita, and pored over the menu. I had a tough time choosing from among the enchiladas, burritos, stuffed sopaipillas, chalupas, and taco plates. All of the combinations were alluring, but on the recommendation of the bartender, and because it included both red and green chile, I chose the **Mexican Steak Platter:** "A five-ounce choice sirloin served with a red chile cheese enchilada, chile relleno with green chile, Spanish rice and pinto beans," a ridiculous bargain at $12.95. When it came, the plate resembled the scale model of a small volcanic nation: mountain ranges of enchilada and the stuffed pepper; lurid rivers of red and green chile feeding into lakes of cheese with hillocks of rice and beans, and a steak mesa presiding over it all.

This was a boyish joy I was feeling. I tried to hold back, but the food went down quickly. I managed to relish it nonetheless. The **sopaipilla** on the side was flaky and crisp and perfect for dipping and mopping up. I love steak, but find large steaks monotonous. The eighteenth bite is much like the first. A five-ounce steak, therefore, is a perfect size, and surrounded by such riches so as to be an accompaniment, not the centerpiece. The red chile was indeed hot but not overpowering. It felt warm and sweet and complemented the green perfectly. The slightly smoky green chile had a broader and more complex flavor. It popped with every other taste: pieces of chicken, the hot cheese, rice, pepper, spice.

Two men were sitting a couple of stools down from me at the bar. They'd finished eating and were chatting. This was the end of the evening. I asked the nearer of the two something anodyne, along the lines of "Do you come here often?" and he said, "I should, I'm the owner." Iggy Palacios waited while I paid up, then kindly, and proudly, showed me round the kitchen. Here was the fryer where they made the sopaipillas during the day. They're little more than flour, baking powder, and salt water. When fried at 400°F, the envelope of dough billows out. At each table is a small bottle of honey to eat with your sopaipilla.

Iggy showed me a rain barrel full of whole dried red chiles. To make them into the **red chile sauce** I'd just eaten, the restaurant purées the chiles using a meat grinder. They can get through a hundred gallons a week. The barrel, packed with spice, gave off a lovely sweet scent. As for the green chiles, after being gathered in the September harvest, they are steamed and then double roasted. I asked Iggy whether he's a green guy or a red guy. "I like my chile Christmas style," he said, meaning he likes green *and* red. For Iggy, the red is smoother, the green is chunkier, and each has its place.

Iggy was born, and grew up, in Brooklyn and he's taken to northern New Mexico with a flourish. I asked him to name some restaurants he liked other than his own, and he reeled off a list: Tia Sophia, Diego's, Tortilla Flats, the Pantry, Cafe Pasqual's, the Shed. More and more names.

Half an hour later, and I was floating, satiated and perfectly content, in

QUICK BITE

At the church suppers of Teresa Nielsen Hayden's youth there would be **Sloppy Joes, tamale pie,** a green salad, rolls, and root beer made from root beer extract, water, and sugar cooled with a piece of dry ice right in the glass. Theresa's mother's parents were farmers who became schoolteachers in central Arizona. I asked what else one would eat there, and Teresa said that her grandparents would get up and have scrambled eggs with canned jalapeños. Lunch might be a grilled cheese sandwich with jalapeños. For dinner, they might go out and have Mexican food with green chile or stay home and make something—with green chile.

the small pool on the roof of the El Dorado Hotel, looking at the stars on a perfect, clear Santa Fe night.

It would have taken ten days to eat everywhere I wanted to, but I had only one, the day following my dinner at Tomasita's. The challenge on a day of eating like this is to find meaningful ways to kill the time between meals. After a breakfast at Cafe Pasqual's, my next stop was in Albuquerque, an hour away, so I looked at my e-mail and pottered around the hotel before driving down the interstate. As far as I could tell, everyone drives between eighty and ninety miles per hour in New Mexico. If you go any slower than seventy-five (the limit), someone is likely to drive right up your tailpipe until you either speed up or get out the way. So it was not a leisurely trip to Albuquerque.

I found the Duran Central Pharmacy, which sits along the old Route 66. The restaurant is tucked in the back of a medium-sized pharmacy, which is something I was unused to seeing. Taking on the personality of the store, it is scrubbed and functional, like a canteen. I ordered the special of the day, **Chicken Enchiladas,** which came in their own sea of green chile. As I ate, I watched the staff come and go. I'd never seen so many people work such a small restaurant. The food was good. I liked the chile a lot, but it was lying third after Tomasita's and Pasqual's. I knew that I was spoiled, because these enchiladas were so much better than any I had eaten back east. This was also without a doubt the best meal I'd ever eaten in a drugstore.

The Duran Pharmacy is very close to Albuquerque's grand old square, which is a lovely place to sit and watch the world pass by. I had numerous eating options in the city, but I needed to put some time between my enchiladas and the next meal. I was very interested in the famous green chile cheeseburger at the Owl Cafe. There's an Owl Cafe in Albuquerque and another way to the south, in the small town of San Antonio. I'd asked about San Antonio at the hotel that morning, and the agent asked what I wanted to go down there for. When I said, for a cheeseburger, she commented that it must be good if I was going to drive 140 miles to try it. Sitting in the square in Albuquerque, I decided I should go and check it out.

From Albuquerque going south, I was driving into the sun. Soon the outside temperature was over 100°F. For a while, I rode alongside a thundercloud, and a couple of times in the distance, I watched trails of rain fall and quickly evaporate. A few miles north of San Antonio, I read a road sign announcing VERY LARGE ARRAY TELESCOPE. On a whim, I took the exit and looked on the map to see how far it was. It looked to be another fifty miles or so. Why not?

QUICK BITE

In Santa Fe, Siritrang Khalsa said I should check out Leona's, a restaurant/ stand in Chimayo, on the grounds of the sanctuary, a church sometimes called the American Lourdes. She and I never made it up there (the restaurant is closed Tuesdays and Wednesdays), but I'll make a point of it next time. Siritrang told me people come from a hundred miles away for the tamales and **Chocolate Tortillas.** Leona Medina-Tiede started the restaurant as a stand beside Highway 76 in 1977. On the Web, Leona talks up her homemade posole and **Carne Adovada** (a pork-and-red-chile dish)—yet more things I have to try in this town.

Leona's ships fresh tamales (vegetable, pork, chicken), chile sauces and salsa, and *ristras,* the lovely strings of red chiles: 1-888-561-5569.

As I suspected, the National Radio Astronomy Observatory Very Large Array Telescope, a collection of dishes spread across the Plains of San Augustin, is featured in the movie *Contact*, a personal favorite. I watch it every time it's on HBO, which is a lot. This is the place where Jodie Foster picks up the extraterrestrial signal. (A couple of years before, in Puerto Rico, I'd dragged my friend Ivan away from his family to come with me to the Arecibo dish, which is also in the film.) Out in the New Mexico desert, I wandered around, looked at the jackrabbits, and marveled at what we can do when we put our minds to it.

San Antonio, New Mexico, is a very small town set just off I-25. Conrad Hilton, as in the Hilton Hotel chain, was born here. When I showed up in the early afternoon, the Owl Bar and Cafe was pretty quiet. In New Mexico terms, San Antonio isn't far from the Trinity Site, where the first atomic bomb was exploded in 1945. On the wall of the bar there are clipped newspaper stories about workers from the Manhattan Project stopping by. I ordered the **Green Chile Cheeseburger** ($4.35), which came with lettuce, tomato, onion, pickle, and mayo. The hamburger patty was pounded quite flat and protruded unevenly out from the border of the hamburger bun. That day's chile wasn't quite hot enough for my taste, but the burger was quirky and satisfying. And gone in three bites.

I made the straight shot back, 140 miles, to Santa Fe in less than two hours, which was a joy in itself. I rested up a while in the hotel—I'd driven four hundred miles—and consulted the food oracle. I wanted to walk somewhere for dinner, and the Shed is an agreeable stroll through the Plaza from the El Dorado. I'm happy to say I made a great choice. The restaurant has been at its present location, lodged in a seventeenth-century building, since 1960. It's an attractive and welcoming spot. At the bar that evening was a bunch of locals and out-of-towners, all of whom happened to be charming and a pleasure to spend time with.

I ordered the **Taco Plate:** soft blue-corn tortillas filled with cheddar cheese, avocado, tomato, lettuce, and blackened chicken, with red and green chile and a side of salsa, pinto beans, and posole. **Posole** is made from nixtamal (hominy-like corn), which, here, was stirred in with lean pork, garlic, and oregano. I was looking for some heat so I took some extra red chile on the side. The blue-corn tortillas were a delight and made a perfect vehicle for the hot red (if not red-hot) chile. It was another terrific meal, each dish carefully put together and bursting with thrilling flavors and tastes.

In five meals over a twenty-five-hour period I ate a lot of chile, green and red, separately and together. Which do I prefer? I'm with Iggy Palacios and the Christmas approach to chile. Why choose one over the other when you can have both?

QUICK BITE

To start my dinner at the Shed, I had a bowl of **Cold Red Raspberry Soup.** It was described on the menu as "Fresh red raspberries with rosé wine, lime, and a hint of sour cream." The raspberry flavor was lip-smackingly sour, cut with wine and softened with cream. Just wonderful.

CHILI, CHILI, CHILE SUMMARY

RUN, DON'T WALK, FOR . . .

A dish with green and red chile at Tomasita's in Santa Fe. Make sure you get both, and have some more on the side.

▦ On second thought, any dish with green or red chile in New Mexico.

▦ Try the chili sampler at **Hard Times Café** and take your pick.

IF YOU'VE NEVER TRIED . . .

▦ Chili over spaghetti, Cincinnati style. It works.

▦ Adding some heat. Exercise those taste buds.

12

STEWS, GUMBO, SOUPS, AND CHOWDER

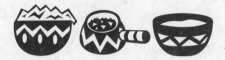

> *When Dr. Creed Haskins and several of his friends returned from a*
> *day's hunting in the woods of Brunswick County, Virginia, in 1828 or*
> *thereabouts, they found their loyal black retainer, Uncle Jimmy Matthews,*
> *stirring a stew he had concocted in their absence. They ate it, hesitantly*
> *at first, then smacked their lips and called for more. By then, it did not*
> *dampen their appetites to learn that Matthews's thick and flavorful ragout*
> *was made from nothing more than butter, onions, stale bread, seasoning*
> *and a passel of squirrels the same slave had shot that morning.*
>
> —Raymond Sokolov, *Fading Feast* (1981)

In his fascinating catalogue of endangered American food, first published in 1981, Raymond Sokolov recounts the legend of the origin of Brunswick stew. There are competing legends (Georgia and North Carolina also have their Brunswick counties and their stews), but no mind.

Sokolov details how the original recipe for this hunter's stew has changed over time. Dr. Haskins himself threw in brandy or Madeira; people added vegetables and removed the squirrels (at which point it evolved into a hunter-gatherer stew).

In his book, Sokolov eats **Brunswick stew** (with chicken, lima beans, tomatoes, and potatoes) at Larry's Lunch in Lawrenceville, Virginia, at the time the sole restaurant in the Brunswick County seat. The restaurant owner, Larry, had eaten Brunswick stew with squirrel in his youth, but he couldn't put squirrel in his stew if he wanted to because of the prohibition on serving wild game to the public. (I'd never thought of squirrel as a game animal before.) Sokolov lamented that he couldn't find real Brunswick stew.

Is there anywhere in Lawrenceville where you can get Brunswick stew today? I called Cook's BBQ and Sandwich Shop in Lawrenceville and heard that Larry's Lunch has been gone for several years. But Anne Burke at the Brunswick County/Lake Gaston Tourism Association in Lawrenceville tells me that the Cinnamon Cafe in town does indeed have Brunswick stew on the menu. You can also get some homemade stew most weekends because civic groups, churches, and the like sell it at fund-raisers. Sure enough, I found that the volunteer fire department in nearby Gasburg was selling it that week for five dollars a quart.

Anne Burke is from Victoria, in neighboring Lunenburg County, where they have their own stew, so she knows all about it. Anne said that on the second Saturday of October each year, since 1996, Lawrenceville has

 QUICK BITE

Bigos is another hunter's stew, this one based on kielbasa and sauerkraut. It's popular in Poland and also sits on the menu at New York City Ukrainian restaurant Veselka (the Ukrainian word for "rainbow"). An East Village veteran, Veselka started as a candy store opened by a wartime refugee and has been a restaurant since 1954. It's a great source of winter-beating soups and stews like meaty beety **borscht** and a rich **Hungarian lamb stew** over noodles I enjoyed there recently. Kara's **beef Stroganoff** would have done the job almost as well. On the side I had a small dish of sinus-clearing **beet salad with horseradish** that I should have bought a barrel of to stave off winter agues.

hosted a Brunswick stew cook-off with two competitions: one for people from in-county and one open to anyone. While the basic ingredients are now well established—chicken, corn, lima beans, etc.—you can taste subtle variations in the entries, Anne says. And the last Wednesday in January is Brunswick Stew Day in Virginia, a day when locals go up to Richmond to serve stew to the legislators on the grounds of the state capitol. Anne said there had even been cook-offs with folks from Brunswick County, Georgia. Of that state's version of Brunswick stew, she says it's spicier and more like chili.

QUICK BITE

I don't need to travel very far from my Manhattan home to get Brunswick stew: they sell it at Brother Jimmy's BBQ, over on Second Avenue and at other locations in New York City. It's a tasty and pleasingly spicy stew with chunks of chicken rather than the shredded meat I remember eating in North Carolina. These hunter's stews—a big mess of ingredients thrown in a pot—seem to be universal. What's the best local or international version where you live?

I ate a good Brunswick stew at Parker's restaurant in Wilson, North Carolina. It was thick and full of meat in a tomato sauce, with corn and beans and other good stuff. I called down to the restaurant later for the recipe: tomato purée, corn, lima beans, string beans, and chicken. Not a hint of any game meat, squirrel or otherwise. All this obviously needs more exploration. I notice that Lawrenceville is less than half an hour from Emporia, Virginia. Next time I'm down that way, I'll try to sneak off and find some more Brunswick stew.

In the same chapter in *Fading Feast* that recounts the story of Brunswick stew, Sokolov looks at the origin of **Burgoo,** another hunter's stew that used to include squirrel. In Kentucky, it is associated with James T. Looney, who would cook it for up to ten thousand people at a time. (One of his recipes calls for eight hundred pounds of beef.) Looney was known as the Burgoo King, and a horse with that name won the Kentucky Derby in 1932. Sokolov writes that burgoo is available in Louisville and its surrounds, and is good made with mutton around Owensboro, where that particular type of lamb rules.

QUICK BITE

How We Cook in Tennessee, published by the Silver Thimble Society of the First Baptist Church of Jackson, Tennessee, in 1906, includes recipes for stewed and broiled squirrel. Here is the bare-bones recipe for Squirrel Stew for Twenty Gallons. The ingredients are twenty squirrels, five pounds of pork, half a bushel of tomatoes, half a bushel of potatoes, three quarts of okra, six onions, eight red peppers, three packages of cornstarch, ten dozen ears of corn, three pounds of butter, and salt and pepper. "Boil for five hours," the instructions say, "stirring often."

The Moonlite Bar-B-Q Inn, in Owensboro, Kentucky, is today well known for its **hickory-smoked barbecued mutton** and also for its burgoo. There is a barbecue festival in the town each April that features smoked mutton and burgoo. The restaurant itself acknowledges various and competing burgoo traditions. Theirs is a soup, and mutton, they say, gives the burgoo the oomph that squirrel used to provide both to burgoo and to Brunswick stew. The Moonlite burgoo includes mutton, chicken, vegetables (including corn and potatoes), and seasonings, including cayenne pepper. You can make it for yourself because the restaurant generously posts the exact recipe on its Web site.

Shop for barbecue mutton, Kentucky country ham, and burgoo at Moonlite: 1-800-322-8989 / www.moonlite.com.

Burgoo has gotten around. There's been a burgoo festival in Arenzville, Illinois, for a hundred years, for example. The festival is held the first Friday and Saturday after Labor Day, and the burgoo (which is described variously as a soup and as a stew) is cooked over wood fires in fifty-gallon kettles. The recipe is a secret, but is chicken- and beef-based. Other towns in west and central Illinois—Franklin, Bluffs, Chandlerville, and Winchester—hold burgoo festivals.

Since the mid-nineties there has been a burgoo cook-off in the small town of Webster Springs, West Virginia, on the Saturday of Columbus Day weekend. Merle Moore organized the first event under the auspices of the Main Street Project of the National Trust for Historic Preservation. Merle had been to chili cook-offs, and she wanted to adapt these events to a local West Virginia tradition. Near Webster Springs is the community of Bergoo (note the spelling), which was named, together with a creek, after a logging camp where the bosses up from Charleston served Kentucky burgoo three times a day.

When Merle makes burgoo herself, with a nod to the Kentucky version, she likes to put lamb chops in it. But the first winner of the Webster Springs contest used a recipe whose first line was "Take a live rattlesnake . . ." Webster Springs is in hilly, wooded country. It's also lumber and coal country, both boom and bust businesses. Right now, lumber is in a boom, and trees are being cut down all over the county. There is a salt sulfur spring in town, with a public spring in the town square. There used to be a fancy resort hotel, but it burned down in 1924. A long time ago, the town was known as Elk Lick, because the animals used to come and take the salt in the spring. There's still a lot of edible wildlife in the woods around town, not just rattlesnake. Merle says that people do hunt squirrel round there, and she ate it growing up. I ask, "What's it like?" "Like any meat you fry too long," says Merle.

Whatever else has been imprinted on me by the Irish side of the family, some axioms of food have stayed with me. As I mentioned before, porridge (oatmeal) should be taken with milk and salt. (It's an option.) Food should be boiled. (Not true.) Guinness tastes best in Ireland. (True.) There is no place in Irish stew for carrots. (We'll see.)

In weak moments in the restaurants of Irish-themed bars in this country, I have ordered **Irish stew** and it has always, for want of a better word, sucked. To make matters worse, the undifferentiated pool of heated-up ground meat (what we called "mince" in the United Kingdom) would always include what appeared to be predigested pieces of carrot. I would invariably point them out and say pompously, "It's not supposed to have carrots," as if that were the worst of the dish's indignities.

My mother's Irish stew included cheap cuts of mutton—scrag end or neck—slices of onion and potato, and half a teacup of water slow cooked for hours over an open fire in a cast-iron pot. Okay, she actually used the gas oven, but she might as well have used a fire for this ancient dish. Same with the vast ox tongues I remember her boiling up on a couple of occasions (**fresh tongue** is delicious). In my youth, Irish stew was what my mother made best. Meat hung off the mutton bones, and we sucked out the marrow before piling the stripped bones on a plate. The onions were stringy (in a good way), and the potatoes had just the right flouriness to soak up the plentiful gravy.

When I call my mother for positive reinforcement of my memories, to my horror she says, "Some people put carrots in, which is fair enough." As English footballers put it, I'm gutted. Later, she calls back and makes amends with news from a 1956 Irish cookbook that says, "The pure flavour is spoilt if carrots, turnips or pearl barley are added." So there.

The cookbook that salvaged my image of Irish stew is *A Taste of Ireland,* by Theodora Fitzgibbon, which is, according to Amazon.com, still in print in a new edition. My mother talked to me about **Brotchan Foltchep,** an Irish soup that unites two of my mother's (and my) favorite foods: leeks and oatmeal. Essentially, you boil up flaked oatmeal and leeks in milk or stock and add parsley.

Leek and oatmeal soup sounds somewhat medicinal. The only soup that gets much of a run out in our house is **chicken soup,** a dish that has legendary, if doubtful, healing properties. If we roast a chicken, and I'm feeling sufficiently motivated after cleaning up, I'll boil up the carcass and make soup. It's extremely easy to make good soup. Pull off the meat, crack the bones some, and boil it up. (I keep it going until just before I need to go to bed.) Skim off some of the material that accumulates on the surface and drain into a pot. Add some vegetables you've been softening in the meantime: onion, carrot, celery. Salt and pepper the mix (add a bay leaf if

QUICK BITE

My friend Deborah recommends the **oxtail soup** specialty at New York City Korean favorite Gahm Mi Oak, called *sul lung tang,* a good remedy for hangovers, it is said. Like Gahm Mi Oak, nearby Han Bat Restaurant is open twenty-four hours. Korean food is great late-night eating. Bud and I feasted on delicious pickles and **kimchi.** There are more than a hundred kinds of this traditional Korean dish—in America, it usually refers to the red-peppery pickled cabbage version. If you want to try one Korean dish, have **bibimbab.** At Han Bat it came super hot in a stone dish—rice, vegetables, meat, red pepper, with an egg broken over the top. Stir it up and get eating. The rice crisped to a shell against the stone pot, and it was fun scraping away every last morsel with chopsticks.

you like). Throw in a handful of rice for a thicker soup. Which begs the question: At what point does a thick soup become a stew?

The title of this book is *Eat This!*, but the rubric for this next item might read *Be Thankful You Don't Have To*. This is **Son-of-a-Gun Stew,** which Huntley Dent describes in his *Feast of Santa Fe*.

> One recipe I have seen instructs the cook to slaughter a beef—in fact, the most usual animal was a calf—and cut only its liver, brains, sweetbreads, kidney and marrow gut (a tube connecting two of the cow's stomachs) into ½-inch dice. The meat itself went for another purpose. Salt and chili were tossed in for savor, along with a chunk of fresh suet, and then the pot was stirred for several hours to reach the final result.

Which presumably was then eaten. In reality, as Dent writes, this dish was more often called "son-of-a-bitch stew." It went by other names: "boss's," or "foreman's," stew, because these, presumably, were the sons of bitches who'd made off with the best parts of the slaughtered cow.

[A] warm savory steam from the kitchen served to belie the apparently cheerless prospect before us. But when that smoking chowder came in, the mystery was delightfully explained. Oh, sweet friends! hearken to me. It was made of small juicy clams, scarcely bigger than hazel nuts, mixed with pounded ship biscuit, and salted pork cut up into little flakes; the whole enriched with butter, and plentifully seasoned with pepper and salt. Our appetites being sharpened by the frosty voyage, and in particular, Queequeg seeing his favorite fishing food before him, and the chowder being surpassingly excellent, we despatched it with great expedition . . .

—Herman Melville, Moby-Dick *(1851)*

Given chowder's fierce regional association, it's fascinating to read food historian Raymond Sokolov's exploration of its origin:

Our chowder descends from a fish soup of France's Atlantic coast. In name, at least. Long ago it must have happened that French fishermen crossed the Atlantic and took their favorite fish soup with them. Then, in the mouths of neighboring English speakers, chaudrée *turned into chowder.*

(Why We Eat What We Eat [1991])

It is either from *chaudrée* or *chaudière,* a Breton fish stew, that chowder gets its name, Sokolov says.

The chowder enjoyed by Ishmael and Queequeg at a Nantucket Inn is the iconic New England dish. I will always take it over Manhattan clam chowder, the red, tomato-based version that, to me, is much less distinctive. Amy Treadwell is a native New Englander who now lives in San Francisco, where she is a cookbook editor for Chronicle Books. First on her list of things to eat in New England is this selfsame clam chowder.

"**Clam Chowder** (of course) and only the white kind, not the tomato-based Manhattan clam chowder. If you even mention that red clam chowder is worth eating anywhere in New England, you'll be run out of town by an angry mob. When I fly from Logan Airport in Boston back to San Francisco, I always pick up a quart or two of Legal Seafood's clam chowder, which you can buy frozen in little freezer packs, specifically to survive the plane trip. You can find literally hundreds of chowder festivals around New England, each one claiming to crown the best chowder in New England."

In addition to two locations at Logan Airport (in Terminals B and C) there are Legal Sea Food restaurants up and down the East Coast, many in shopping areas, from the Town Place Mall in Boca Raton to the Garden State Plaza in Paramus, New Jersey, the Walt Whitman Mall on Long Island, and the Burlington Mall in Massachusetts.

In the next chapter, we'll meet Chef Bobo, executive chef of the Cal-

QUICK BITE

For me the best New England Clam Chowda is located in Menemsha [on Martha's Vineyard]. It's served at a little shack called "The Bite." This isn't the gloppy, creamy style that most attribute to New England. It's a true milky, briny broth-type of New England Clam Chowder made with butter, clams, and potatoes. It's the best.

—David Remillard

houn School in Manhattan and an expert on the food of New Orleans. As a taster, Bobo tells us about **gumbo,** the famous New Orleans stew. I made a gumbo once, and it was far too thick and floury and could have been watered down to feed my family for months. Recipes differ wildly, including which fish and shellfish you want to use, though most will have some kind of white fish, crabmeat, and shrimp. Chef Bobo says, "Gumbo comes from Africa and uses French techniques. The whole success of a gumbo is in the roux, and that's French. If you screw up the roux, you screw up the gumbo. It's the real taste of New Orleans. The fat in the roux is what cooks the flour and what gives it the depth and the smoky flavor. You have to make it as dark as you can without burning it. Chef Paul Prudhomme in New Orleans makes it a reddish black. The key is that reddish black—when it turns black, it's over. It's the most incredible flavor in the world." In New Orleans, they'll use peanut oil or lard, while cooking at the school Bobo has to use a blended oil because they can't use any nut oils. Still, they get their gumbo dark: darker than peanut butter.

QUICK BITE

On a visit to the Reading Terminal Market in Philadelphia, my friend Bud talked about looking for a can of **Bookbinder's Pepper Pot Soup,** a famous dish from a famous old Philly restaurant that has tripe as its main ingredient. Bud mentioned the **Campbell's Pepper Pot** he ate frequently as a kid, which was, he added, one of the Campbell's varieties Andy Warhol painted in the early sixties. I recalled a quote I wrote down from a funny little book from 1949 that I found in the New York Public Library called *Greenwich Village Gourmet,* in which New York artists wrote up their favorite recipes. The painter, Stuart Davis, made as a contribution his recipe for Philadelphia Devilled Crabs: "Philadelphia," Davis wrote, "as a center of Colonial artistic culture, produced alleys, artists, cats, Pepper Pot, and a crab mixture that really knocked people out." Campbell's Pepper Pot may be more famous as an artwork than as a dish, but it's hanging on better than the deviled crabs seem to have done.

If you can't find Campbell's Pepper Pot near you, you can buy it online. Amazon.com sells it by the case, for example.

I found an interesting recipe for gumbo in *La Cuisine Creole*, which was written around 1885 by a fascinating individual named Lafcadio Hearn (1850–1904). (Half Greek, half Irish, Hearn was born in Greece, grew up in Ireland, and worked as a newspaperman in New Orleans, where his interests included the local food. He later moved to Japan, married a local woman, and, as Koizumi Yakumo, took Japanese citizenship and worked as a teacher and lecturer.)

QUICK BITE

Another cookbook from recent antiquity, *Gourmet's Guide to New Orleans*, by Natalie Scott and Caroline Merrick Jones, published in 1933, has an interesting take on the origin of the name of bouillabaisse, the famous Provençal stew. It's taken to come from a combination of the two French verbs *bouillir* and *abaisser*, "to boil" and "to reduce." But according to Scott and Jones, "As for the name, the story is that in the first days of its glory, as the chefs hovered over it, when one saw that the rich brew was bubbling too rapidly, he shrieked a warning: 'boullit: baisses!' It's boiling: lower the fire."

As well as a recipe for "Crayfish Broth for Purifying the Blood," Lafcadio Hearn's book includes one for "Maigre Oyster Gombo," *maigre* food being that which can be eaten on a day of fasting.

> *Take 100 oysters with their juice, and one large onion; slice the onion into hot lard and fry it brown, adding when brown a tablespoonful of flour and red pepper. When thick enough, pour in the oysters. Boil together twenty minutes. Stir in large spoonfuls of butter and one or two tablespoonfuls of filee, then take the soup from the fire and serve with rice.*

(Filee, or filé, is made of dried and pounded sassafras leaves.) Note here the hundred oysters and figure out how much that might cost you. Also note the extremely sparse directions typical of old-time cookbooks. The soup/stew conundrum raises itself again. How thick, would you say, is "thick enough"?

STEWS, GUMBO, SOUPS, AND CHOWDER SUMMARY

RUN, DON'T WALK, FOR . . .

- **Brunswick stew.** Parker's in Wilson, North Carolina, was a good place to start for me.
- New England, not Manhattan, clam chowder.

IF YOU'VE NEVER TRIED . . .

- Proper **Irish stew** made from mutton, onions, potatoes, and no other vegetable.
- Making gumbo. Easy to make, hard to make well.

13

SEASIDE FOOD AND SUSHI

*One of the primal pleasures of Maine is to sit at an outdoor picnic table
on a deck over the water with a messy toasted lobster roll dribbling on
your fingers, or with a bowl of lobster stew clearing your sinuses,
or with the ancient crustacean itself set boiling and steaming before you,
ready to be hand-wrestled for its claws and tail.*

—Charles Kuralt, *Charles Kuralt's America* (1995)

Charles Kuralt spent years "on the road," crisscrossing the country for *CBS News*, adventures he was eloquent about before the camera and on the page alike. In his 1995 book, he suggests you follow your instincts when you want to find a lobster. In Rockport, Ogunquit, Southwest Harbor, Deer Isle, or wherever you happen to find yourself at lunchtime, he says, "just go along to the water to where you think a lobster wharf ought to be—and there is."

The **lobster roll** is to seafood what *Dubliners* is to *Ulysses*. Each is an easy way to dip a toe into a whole universe of flavor and texture. Some of us will venture this far and no farther. We know there's more to Joyce than the short stories; we're told how bounteous and rewarding the Great Novel is, but we just can't bring ourselves to do it. But even if we're in the don't-eat-fish camp, or have never relished grappling with a red sea-bug using a nutcracker and a miniature fork, we should all eat a lobster roll—a *good* lobster roll—if only once.

In New England and on Long Island, the lobster roll is a regional signature dish. This means that practically every eating establishment—including the local McDonald's, in some places—serves one. Its obligatory presence on menus ensures that many lobster rolls are perfunctory and worthless. The key is the ratio of mayonnaise to lobster meat. Too many rolls are filled out with a sickly paste of mayo and chopped vegetable sundries with little actual lobster. I had one such in a bar/restaurant in New York City recently that should have come with its own sluice to wash off the mayonnaise. What you're looking for is large chunks of meat, a little mayo and paprika, perhaps, and a bun playing its supporting role—and that's all.

The first couple of lobster rolls I ate may as well have been made with tuna salad, or chicken salad, for that matter. Then, at my friends' oceanfront home in Kennebunkport, Maine, I had a real lobster roll that my friend Seana brought home from Bartley's Dockside. Before I turned the roll on its side and bit into it, I admired the aesthetics—big pieces of lobster set on the square-sided toasted roll and dusted generously with paprika. I couldn't see it, but when I started in, I could taste the light coating of mayonnaise on the roll. As lunch, with a cold beer, it was fantastic. Now I see the point of this, I said to myself.

Up the coast from Boston is the old town of Ipswich, founded in 1633. More than one person has recommended the Clam Box, built in Ipswich in 1938. I was sitting eating barbecue at the Block Party in New York City and got chatting with a guy who said the lobster roll at the Clam Box was the best he'd tasted. Definitely worth a visit, he said.

David Remillard recommends another Kennebunkport establishment for lobster roll. "The perfect **Lobster Roll from Cape Porpoise Lobster Company** in Cape Porpoise, Maine (in the village of Kennebunkport). Delicious entire lobster with just a touch of mayo in a great white bread bun."

The Cape Porpoise Lobster Company offers a fantastic range of seafood for sale, starting with live lobsters up to five pounds each shipped next-day UPS, as well as local shrimp, crab, clams, lobster tails, haddock, scallops, and Alaskan king crab legs to boot. 1-207-967-4268 / 1-800-967-4268 / www.cape porpoiselobster.com.

Since my first great one, I've had other lobster rolls that come from the lobster salad school. There's nothing inherently wrong with decent lobster salad, and you're more likely to get away with spending about twelve to fifteen dollars, when a sandwich made with chunks of lobster may well cost a lot more. Anyone who's driven to Montauk, out on the eastern end of Long Island, will be familiar with the restaurant called The Lobster Roll (aka Lunch), alongside the Montauk Highway on the slender isthmus that makes up the community of Napeague. This is one of the few restaurants in this part of the world where you don't have to pay the bill in gold bars. The Lobster Roll's eponymous sandwich is more salad than chunk: good, but not extraordinary. I'd say the same about the roll at Claudio's in Greenport, out near the tip of the North Fork of Long Island. Claudio's has great people-watching when the bikers come in, and the ferries plying the short sound over to Shelter Island are soothing to watch.

Lobster rolls can get very fancy. West of Lunch, on the (main street) in Southampton, is Silver's Famous Restaurant, where a lobster roll on a baguette would set you back thirty-two dollars the last time I checked, which was in the fall. The lobster roll at the Oyster Bar in Grand Central Station in New York City is up there in the twenties, and it sounds like a compli-

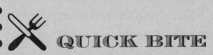

QUICK BITE

From Boston, Chris Lyons points out that there are essentially two kinds of lobster roll, each served on a buttered and grilled hot dog roll: the cold, with a little mayo on the meat; and the hot, with the lobster sautéed in butter. The lobster salad roll has no place here. Chris says these babies can cost up to twenty-five dollars (and more). Bargain hunting for lobster rolls is not advised: "Beware of the under-ten-dollar lobster roll," says Chris.

QUICK BITE

For **whole lobster,** I have fond memories of Duryea's Lobster Deck on Fort Pond in Montauk, where you'd sit outside and watch the sunset with disposable plates of great seafood, lobsters included.

There's more than one way to eat a lobster. At the famous Locke-Ober restaurant in Boston, a fixture since 1879, you can try a **lobster bisque, JFK's Lobster Stew** (as enjoyed by you-know-who), and the decidedly decadent **Lobster Savannah,** in which the lobster meat is removed, sautéed with sherry, and replaced in the shell for serving. (**Lobster Newburg** is also made with sherry but includes butter, egg yolks, and heavy cream.)

Lobster Savannah, by the way, sounds a lot like the oddly named Irish dish **Dublin Lawyer,** which sounds more like the start of a joke than a recipe. The lobster meat is temporarily removed from the shell, cooked in butter, flambéed in whiskey, and then doused in cream, which sounds to me like a good way to go.

cated cousin of your New England relations: Maine lobster and jumbo crabmeat in a toasted potato bun with sweet potato chips and jicama slaw.

The **lobster roll** I really covet is one that's always in this particular conversation, that from Red's Eats, the roadside establishment on Water Street (Route 1) in Wiscasset, Maine. It's an incredible bargain. For your fourteen dollars, you get the whole pound-plus lobster, claws and tail, and all heaped into a buttered bun. And there's butter and mayo available on the side. This, ladies and gentlemen, is a lobster roll.

A treat I'll allow myself every now and again is a plate of **linguine with white clam sauce.** I'm sparing because *sauce* seems to mean "gallon of butter with clams and shaved garlic," and every now and again, there's nothing wrong with that—if you let the sauce pool and eat toward the other side of the plate, that is. From broadly this family of foods, Amy Treadwell also includes:

> *Clam Cakes. These balls of dough are deep-fried and the best ones have bits of clams in them that you can actually see, though many greasy-spoon restaurants seem to make them without any discernible clams. They are greasy, and yet, somehow irresistible. This is one of*

those strange foods that people crave, compulsively eat, regret it, then eat them again two days later.

When she's feeling nostalgic for her childhood foods, Amy says, she might head out to the Yankee Pier, a "lovely restaurant in Marin County that calls itself a clam shack (but it's really too nice for that). They fly in their clams from Woodman's in Essex Massachusetts." On the menu is a **Fried Ipswich (Whole Belly) Clam Platter,** six ounces of East Coast clams served with coleslaw and Kennebec fries ($18.95). (Kennebec is a variety of white potato. In-N-Out Burger uses 'em, too.)

QUICK BITE

I made some long-distance selections from the menu at Caprial's Bistro in Portland. They offer, for an appetizer, **Northwest clams** steamed in coconut milk, lemon grass, ginger, kaffir lime, chilies, and basil, garnished with curry-dusted fried wontons. Then, a **smoked salmon salad,** with crispy romaine lettuce and Bistro-smoked salmon, tossed with horseradish-buttermilk dressing, fried capers, and cornichons.

In Rhode Island, at restaurants like George's and the Harborside, in East Greenwich, the local specialty is **Stuffies,** which are baked stuffed

QUICK BITE

Golf writer and editor Robin McMillan told me about a place in Guilford, Connecticut. Its name is easy enough to remember. "The place in Guilford, Connecticut, is called 'The Place.' It's right on the Post Road, has a huge wood-burning grill, and you all sit on tree stumps; hence the T-shirts that say PUT YOUR RUMP ON A STUMP. There's no liquor license, but a lot of people make it a big family/group thing and bring coolers. The signature dish is the **Roast Clam Special.** They grill the clams, then, when they open up, they pull them off and stick in a dab of margarine and a squirt of cocktail sauce. Then they put them back on the grill. Seriously good."

quahogs. The clam is chopped up with breadcrumbs and onions (and butter) and put back in the shell and baked. These might be baked clams or stuffed clams somewhere else, but in Rhode Island, they're Stuffies. (Rhode Island has a couple of popular drinks peculiar unto itself—summertime favorite **Del's frozen lemonade,** made from fresh lemon and sold from trucks all over the state, and **Coffee Milk,** made from coffee syrup and milk, and which beat out Del's lemonade to become the state drink in 1993.)

THE CUISINE OF NEW ORLEANS

I went to talk to Chef Bobo, executive chef of the Calhoun School in Manhattan about his fabulous lunch program (see pages 349–52) and also about the food of New Orleans, of which he is a knowledgeable and passionate advocate. Chef Bobo was born and raised in Texas but lived ten years in New Orleans. Bobo found New Orleans cuisine a step up from the Tex-Mex and southern staples he was familiar with. "You go to New Orleans and you learn how to *taste* food because they know how to cook it," he says. "There is a very strong French influence in the way they bring out the flavors in food."

In the years before Chef Bobo was Chef Bobo, he lived in New York and worked in corporate America before taking on a second career. He attended and then taught at the French Culinary Institute, set up a catering business focused on Louisiana cuisine, and found a measure of celebrity cooking for kids in Manhattan and campaigning for better food for youngsters. (He was too modest to mention his other sideline: cooking for Yankees shortstop Derek Jeter.)

New Orleans is the major inspiration for Chef Bobo. As we're talking, we never stray too far from the ocean and its treasures. This is after Katrina, so we know, too, that the waters give and they take away. The cuisine is an essential mix of Creole, based on African cooking, and Cajun, the feisty, saucy, country food of the French who were evicted from Acadia in Nova Scotia by the British in the eighteenth century and ended up in the Delta. These two influences are seasoned with a bit of classical French influence, some Italian, some Spanish.

And by and by we reached the West End, a collection of hotels of the usual light summer-resort pattern, with broad verandas all around; and the waves of the wide and blue Lake Pontchartrain lapping the thresholds. We had dinner on a ground veranda over the water—the chief dish the renowned fish called the pompano, delicious as the less criminal forms of sin . . .

We had opportunities on other days and in other establishments to test the pompano. Notably at an editorial dinner at one of the clubs in the city. He was in his last possible perfection there, and justified his fame. In his suite was a tall pyramid of scarlet cray-fish—large ones; as large as one's thumb; delicate, palatable, appetizing. Also devilled whitebait; also shrimps of choice quality; and a platter of small soft-shell crabs of a most superior breed. The other dishes were what one might get at Delmonico's, or Buckingham Palace; those I have spoken of can be had in similar perfection in New Orleans only, I suppose.

—Mark Twain, *Life on the Mississippi* (1883)

The pompano, Chef Bobo tells me, you're not going to find so much in New Orleans anymore. You're much more likely to see **redfish,** and the great cornerstones of New Orleans cooking: shrimp, oysters, and crawfish. To cook them, you need to figure out how to make a good roux, the basis of the essential gumbo that we've just looked at. One roux-based dish is **crawfish étouffée.** *Etouffée* doesn't mean stuffed—Bobo said he'd been into a New York gourmet food store and found a readymade "étouffée" dish stuffed with breadcrumbs. It means smothered. To the roux you add the New Orleans "holy trinity": onions, celery, and green pepper. A crawfish étouffée will include fish stock and maybe sausage. At Calhoun, Bobo makes a chicken étouffée and takes any leftovers home to freeze for anticipated summer cravings.

Chef Bobo prefers his crawfish cooked another way: "I like 'em **steamed** or boiled. In New Orleans, you go to a crawfish bar. They put a big sheet of brown paper out, or newspapers, and pour a whole pot of them out on the table. It's got **andouille sausage,** which is the Cajun sausage, it's got whole boiled potatoes and corn, like a lobster boil. You get pitchers of ice-cold beer. You pop the heads and pinch the tails and they can go so fast you can't believe it. If you overcook them, they won't pop; if you undercook them, they won't pop; you have to cook them just right." Chef Bobo had visited the city for Mardi Gras. (He was also too modest to mention he's the chef of the Krewe of Orpheus, a festival parade organization set up by New Orleans native Harry Connick, Jr.) This was the first February after Hurricane Katrina, and the oysters were just coming back. "They were better than I could ever remember them being, which is maybe because I wanted them to be. **Gulf oysters** are beautiful. They are large oysters, a mouthful literally. They have that wonderful taste of the sea in them which all oysters have, but these are just a little bit sweet. All you need is a little Tabasco sauce on them." I asked Chef Bobo to recommend some restaurants in New Orleans. I have visited the city just once, on a deliriously exciting Halloween trip numerous years ago, when fine food, or even food at all, was way down on my list of priorities. I stayed a few nights at the youth hostel and made Rice-a-Roni to conserve funds. I ate **red beans and rice** someplace, listened to some blues in an out-of-the-way bar, and finished off Halloween with a sunup serving of beignets (the powdered sugar-coated donuts) and the delicious **coffee and chicory** at the famous Café du Monde.

CHEF BOBO'S
NEW ORLEANS RESTAURANTS

BAYONA

"Bayona's chef is a woman named Susan Spicer, who's avoided any notion of becoming a rock star. She's a great, great chef. She has two restaurants, Bayona in the French Quarter and Herbsaint in the Warehouse District."

DOMILISE'S

"Domilise's is a po'boy [the New Orleans French bread sandwich] shop in the Garden District that has been there ever since I can remember . . . You have to stand in line, as you do at a lot of restaurants in New Orleans. That's just a way of life. Here, they don't take reservations. You're just lucky if you get a seat. There are two sizes of sandwich, and the cutting board has two notches on it according to the size. **Oyster po'boy,** shrimp, roast beef, andouille sausage—it's all they sell. You can have **Zaps Chips** if you want them, and the local Barg's root beer, Dixie beer, or Budweiser."

CAMELLIA GRILL*

"The Camellia Grill isn't open yet after Katrina. It's situated right where the river bends—where uptown meets Carrollton. Carrollton was pretty heavily damaged in the floods. It's like a diner with stools next to the counter. Once you get inside, you sit on couches to wait to get a seat.

"Half of it is the guys who are cooking. They are hysterically funny and are having fun doing what they're doing, which is to make gigantic omelets on the griddle. They make incredible **pecan waffles.** I just hope it comes back."

We talked about restaurants Bobo liked in other parts of the country: Mike Fennelly's restaurant Santacafé in Santa Fe, and Cafe Pasqual's, also in Santa Fe, where he ate his breakfast, lunch, and dinner when he was there. Chef Bobo was planning a trip to Austin to talk about a healthy lunch program and was looking forward to getting some good barbecue at Mesquite and then heading up to Dallas to Sonny Bryan's. As for good New Orleans food in New York, Bobo said the only time he'd found that was many years before, when Paul Prudhomme used to take his restaurant on the road for the month of August, which is oppressive in New Orleans. He brought his whole staff from the dishwashers to the cooks up north and cooked for the month. This reminded Bobo of two New Orleans restaurants he'd cooked in himself:

DOOKY CHASE*

"It's owned by Leah Chase, who is a wonderful woman. It's closed right now, but I think she's coming back. She makes the best fried chicken in the universe. If that restaurant doesn't come back, I don't even want to go back to New Orleans."

K-PAUL'S

"The temple of Cajun cuisine is K-Paul's. Paul Prudhomme's whole goal in life was to put Cajun cooking on the map, and he

---

* As of 2007, these restaurants were working toward reopening.

succeeded very well. He's not cooking anymore but he's still there at the restaurant. The food is incredible. It's not an inexpensive restaurant, but the food is exceptional. His cookbooks are outrageous they're so good, and every recipe in them works. I worked there twice. He would let me come in during vacations and work helping and what we call trailing. Chef Paul is a generous wonderful man.

"I was showing a friend of mine the French Quarter over Mardi Gras. We stopped when we saw K-Paul's was open and we looked at the menu. All he saw was **fried chicken, black-eyed peas,** and **hot biscuits,** and he said, 'Let's come here for dinner.' We came back for dinner but they were closed evenings over the weekend, and this was Friday. I don't think I've ever seen anybody so disappointed in all my life."

This same friend is a New York restaurateur. Chef Bobo took the friend to the Acme Oyster House in the French Quarter. It's another place that gets a line, but it's fast moving, especially if you're willing to sit at the bar. The friend called up Chef Bobo when they were back in New York.

"He asked me to tell his chef how they cook the **oysters at the Acme Bar and Grill.** Simplest thing in the world—they take the oyster and put it on the grill, and it opens. Then they put cheese on it, put it in a salamander, and serve it. They're outrageous."

―――――――――――
―――――――――――

Nathalie Dupree is the author of, among numerous other books, *Nathalie Dupree's Southern Memories* and *New Southern Cooking.* Nathalie told me about a couple of Charleston/Low-Country specialties: **she-crab soup** and **shrimp and grits,** the last of which she was in the process of writing an entire book about. "The best place for she-crab soup is Tristan in Charleston, and the best place for shrimp and grits is my house. Barring that, try Slightly North of Broad, a restaurant in Charleston. Do not under any circumstances think that the shrimp and grits flavored with andouille and tasso, from New Orleans, are Charleston shrimp and grits. Charleston shrimp and grits are shrimp (preferably small 'breakfast' shrimp, caught early in the morning), butter, salt, pepper, and grits. Both original recipes are in the 1930 edition of *Charleston Receipts*." I looked in *200 Years of Charleston Cooking,* recipes gathered by Blanche S. Rhett, and found a nice description of what makes she-crab soup so special:

> *The Crabman charges ten cents a dozen extra for "she" crabs with the eggs in. The crab eggs are picked and put with the crab meat and give a delicious, glutinous quality to the soup which makes it very different from regular crab soup.*

JOE'S STONE CRAB

The take-away section of Joe's Stone Crab restaurant is a highly attractive store at the very southern tip of Miami Beach, where it would be very easy to drop a couple of hundred dollars. Even as I tried to focus on my take-out order, I picked up a jumbo chocolate chip cookie that turned out to be a huge hit on the plane ride home the next day. Joe's is also hyperefficient. We'd placed our large order from Kara's friend Jessica's house in mid-Beach and were told it would be ready in fifteen minutes, which meant we had to leave right away for the ride south.

The traffic snailed its way up Collins Avenue on our way back. We had three bags of food in the trunk of the car, and I could picture Sam's cheese-burger hardening into a hockey puck and the seafood bisque turning to cement. The cars idled along at four or five miles per hour in a procession of drivers who seemed to be choosing to go along at this speed. Some aborted shortcuts later we were seated at the kitchen table with a substantial spread of take-out food that was not so much one meal, as parts of three different ones.

Along with the burger and fried chicken we had the seafood bisque, my stone crab claws, two chopped salads, a blackened mahi-mahi sandwich, and a random order of creamed spinach. The couple of bites of Jessica's **seafood bisque** I tried were great—thick and mushroomy—and left me wanting more. The **stone crab claws** (eight mediums for $19.95), full of meat, came ready-cracked and complete with butter and **mustard sauce.** Fresh seafood like this really needs an oceanfront setting and a cold beer, but I closed my eyes and made it halfway there.

We were eating when Jessica's husband, Michael, got home. He is a big fan of the rolls from Joe's (a great **pumpernickel roll with onions** among them) and also the chopped salad (dressing on the side), but not, alas, of much of the seafood. I was a little sorry that it would be he who was going to Joe's Restaurant for a business dinner the next day and not me. Reporting back later, I heard that Michael had salmon, the fish of choice for people who don't like fish.

 Joe's will ship stone crabs, mustard sauce, implements with which to open the crabs, *and* Key lime pie: 1-800-780-CRAB (2722) / www.joesstonecrab.com.

My friend Rick works in television. He lives in New York but he's frequently in Los Angeles on business. Years ago Rick told me about his favorite L.A. restaurant—a sushi place in a strip mall in Studio City. He tells me the only way to experience the place is to sit at the counter and eat *omakase*—chef's choice. Rick reported that some say the chef can get a little cranky. When I heard that Rick was traveling to L.A. and staying the weekend, I planned a trip. We agreed that he and I would go around and eat at some places I picked out and then I'd visit this sushi joint he liked for dinner.

I know next to nothing about sushi, but I do know I like it—it's my favorite way of eating seafood (just ahead of the prosaic English favorite, fish-and-chips). Sushi Nozawa, the name of this particular restaurant,

QUICK BITE

From publisher Cynthia Frank of Cypress House: "Here's a treat from the Mendocino Coast in California. A local fisherman taught me this recipe years ago when I ran a small restaurant in Mendocino."

ALBACORE AND BACON

- Cut fresh albacore into thick strips about 1½-inch thick.
- Wrap spiral fashion with thin-cut bacon held in place with toothpicks.
- Marinate for ½ hour in white wine with a little crushed garlic and a dash of tamari [a thicker type of soy sauce].
- Barbecue and cut into serving pieces.

didn't mean anything to me. But as soon as I looked into it a little, I found that it is a semi-legendary establishment in Southern California. Its unassuming lodgings notwithstanding, the food is consistently rated among the best available in the city. I wondered without consequence if this was going to fit in with the remit I was using for my book.

When I headed to pick up Rick at his hotel, I idiotically failed to make allowances for L.A.'s notorious traffic. Setting out to drive from West Hollywood to Burbank at 5:15 on a Friday evening is a terrible idea, especially if you're going to misplace yourself a couple of times. What took about an hour and three-quarters at rush hour took twenty-seven minutes in reverse four hours later. I've said it before (but never just as I'm about to go anywhere)—planning is everything.

After eating a piece of sushi, eat a slice of pickled ginger to clean your palate, have a sip of tea, then eat the next piece of sushi. Japanese green tea removes oiliness after eating fish and prepares the palate for the next piece. Sushi bars serve tea that has a slightly bitter flavor—sweet tea should be avoided, as it diminishes the flavor of the sushi.

—Hideo Dekura, Brigid Treloar, and Ryuichi Yoshii,
The Complete Book of Sushi *(2004)*

Sushi has penetrated the American eating universe to an extraordinary extent. One of the most extravagant eating experiences in the country is offered by sushi superstar chef Masa Takayama, at the restaurant Masa in the Time Warner Building in New York City. A *New York* magazine critic reported he spent exactly $834.31 for each of two meals (for two) there, and this was in 2004. Spending that kind of money, I'd be worried about committing some terrible sushi faux pas. There's no menu at Masa, so at least I wouldn't have to worry about what to order.

A few words about eating sushi and some of the terms involved. In Japan, the word *sushi* refers to the rice cooked with vinegar that forms the basis of the food. *Sashimi* is the raw fish that can be eaten on its own. When a piece of rice is topped, usually with a piece of fish, often with a dab of wasabi between the two, this is *Nigiri-zushi,* or hand-rolled sushi. *Wasabi* is Japanese horseradish and is very expensive: most wasabi is ersatz, regular horseradish dyed green. The sushi can be dipped in soy sauce, but you might be advised to dip the topping, not the rice, so as not to overwhelm the flavor.

Makizushi, or just *maki,* are filled rice rolls encased in *nori,* seaweed. The rolls are cut into pieces before serving. *Temaki* are rolls that are shaped by hand rather than rolled on a mat. They're looser and can be cone-shaped. *Uramaki* are inside-out rolls that have the rice on the outside and might be covered with sesame seeds. *Gunkan-zushi* are filled cups of rice and seaweed. The Web site Japundit.com has a section on sushi where there's a link to bayosphere.com and a fascinating series by Noriko Takiguchi on sushi eating. Sushi developed relatively late in Japan, in the early nineteenth century, and it's meant to be a fast food.

As for the sushi toppings and fillings, if you order *omakase,* the chef will orchestrate your meal like a musical conductor, probably starting with lighter tastes and heading toward more intense flavors, just as Chef Nozawa did for Rick and me. As well as cleaning the palate with ginger, diners can select an omelet for the same effect. Traditional or not, I love to finish off my sushi meal with a bowl of **red bean ice cream.**

SASHIMI/SUSHI TOPPINGS

- **Aji**   horse mackerel
- **Ebi**   cooked shrimp
- **Engawa**   fluke fin
- **Hamachi**   yellowtail
- **Hirame**   fluke
- **Hotate**   sea scallop
- **Ika**   squid
- **Ikura**   salmon caviar
- **Kani**   mock crabmeat
- **Maguro**   tuna
- **Mirugai**   giant clam
- **Saba**   mackerel
- **Sake**   salmon

◆ **Sawara**   Spanish mackerel

◆ **Suzuki**   sea or striped bass

◆ **Tai**   snapper

◆ **Tako**   octopus

◆ **Tamago *or* tamagoyaki**   fried egg or omelet

◆ **Tarabagani**   king crab

◆ **Tobiko**   flying fish roe

◆ **Toro**   fatty tuna (belly)

◆ **Unagi**   eel (freshwater)/*Anago* eel (seawater)

◆ **Uni**   sea urchin

───────────

Rick and I pulled into Sushi Nozawa's strip-mall lot a little after seven. My traffic-induced irritability faded when we lucked into the last parking space. Rick had not overstated the humdrummery of the location. The restaurant sits between a shipping center and a nail salon and looks like nothing much outside, or, indeed, in. There are a few glass-topped tables and nine seats at the counter. I was thankful there was space for us in front, where Rick said the action is. Our hostess said we could sit there, but "chef's choice—okay?" Okay. In case you miss the point somehow, there are helpful signs up on the walls. TRUST ME, says one. And TODAY'S SPECIAL: TRUST ME. And DON'T THINK: JUST EAT. The signs are arranged on painted cinder block walls otherwise adorned with little more than strips of red neon. A bright blue picture of tuna running in the ocean hangs front and center. The other diners were eating almost soundlessly. The message is clear. Here it's all about the food.

The assistant takes our drink order and Kazunori Nozawa gets to work. The glass case holding the fish is opaque in back, so from where you sit, you can't see Nozawa's hands, and that's a shame. But you can see his face, which wore a perfectly benign expression that evening. He may even have offered a hint of a smile when we said our thanks and left barely more than half an hour after we had arrived.

Very soon, the first dish came. The rest followed quickly, one after another, with the assistant enunciating quietly what was on the plate, but so quietly I wasn't sure I got what each one was. The meal was extraordinarily simple. Generous pieces of fish—**yellowtail** and **toro, red snapper** and

king mackerel, eel and **abalone,** set on top of warmish, and quite loose, blocks of rice. **Crabmeat** and **lobster** hand rolls made of squares of crunchy seaweed, which was folded rather than rolled tight. The food kept coming until the assistant asked, "Enough?" We had one more plate and that was indeed enough.

Rick insisted on paying. Of course, we hadn't seen anything written down during the process, so I was concerned at the damage we had done. But $132.77 before tip seemed eminently reasonable, despite the extremely breezy nature of the meal. I lack the gustatory vocabulary to properly describe sushi, but the fish was clearly fresh as can be. Also, each offering was subtly different from the previous one, and the flavors crescendoed up to the last plate, what I am calling **hot eel,** which was strong and meaty. I'd never eaten an assemblage like this, and it was wonderful.

Perhaps more than any reviewed restaurant I have visited, Sushi Nozawa is a place that is focused on the food to the exclusion of everything else. There's almost nothing to look at. There's little point starting a conversation, because the dishes are presented so rapidly and the place is so quiet it doesn't seem appropriate to chat. The bright room is not particularly comfortable or inviting to sit in. When we visited, Sushi Nozawa scored a full twenty points higher in Zagat's for food over décor (on a scale of thirty, twenty-six to six), a heroic discrepancy.

If you visit Sushi Nozawa, and you should, just follow the signs and trust Nozawa-san. He surely knows more about sushi than you do. I hope to place myself in his care again. Sushi Nozawa exists to provide fabulous food, not to give you a good time and not for chitchat, whether between dinner companions or with the chef. I'm extremely grateful to my friend for his recommendation, and for the dinner. As much as any place I know, Sushi Nozawa proves that if you put food quality first, second, and last, and you know what you're doing, your customers are going to win out bigtime.

SEASIDE FOOD AND SUSHI SUMMARY
RUN, DON'T WALK, FOR . . .

- A seaside **lobster roll** from some place by the cold Atlantic in New England.
- Clams!

- **Crab claws** from Joe's Stone Crabs in Miami Beach. Clean your plate and then you can have some Key lime pie.
- Sushi Nozawa.

IF YOU'VE NEVER TRIED . . .

- **Sushi** omakase style. Put yourself in some capable hands.
- The palate-cleansing properties of red bean ice cream.
- New Orleans. This great city deserves our support and won't disappoint.

14

HOT DOGS

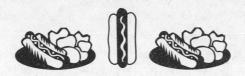

> Dunbar sat up like a shot. "That's it," he cried excitedly.
> "There was something missing—all the time I knew there was
> something missing—and now I know what it is." He banged
> his fist down into his palm. "No patriotism," he declared.
>
> "You're right," Yossarian shouted back. "You're right, you're right,
> you're right. The hot dog, the Brooklyn Dodgers. Mom's apple pie. That's
> what everyone's fighting for. But who's fighting for the decent folk?"
>
> —Joseph Heller, *Catch-22*

In *Eating in America*, Waverly Root and Richard de Rochemont detail the various stories of how the frankfurter made it to the United States. One version has it entering the country as a German exhibit at the Chicago World's Fair. Another has a man named Antoine Feuchtwanger selling franks in St. Louis. Third, Charles Feltman is said to have introduced the frankfurter at Coney Island, New York, where it became known as "Coney Island chicken." (Feltman, incidentally, is one of more than 560,000 people buried at the Green-Wood Cemetery in Brooklyn, a giant necropolis-within-a-city. Also at rest here is Reuben Kulakofsky, who may or may not have been the inspiration for the sandwich that bears his [first] name.)

Along the way, the frankfurter became part of the hot dog (another event wrapped in mystery and conjecture). As the frank was assimilated, an American institution came into being. The hot dog has worked its way into the essential fabric of America. Its genius is its simplicity. You couldn't get two more basic words. *Hot. Dog.* Whether frankfurters were first popularized in Coney Island or not, Coney Island and hot dogs have become synonymous. In Coney Island itself, the biggest name in hot dogs is Nathan's, named for Nathan Handwerker, who left the employ of Charles Feltman and in 1916 opened his own stand, where he sold hot dogs for a nickel.

Today, Nathan's Famous is a sizeable operation that runs a number of franchises, and sells a lot more than hot dogs. The flagship is a large boxy building on Surf Avenue in Brooklyn, a block from the famous boardwalk. It is a giant stand designed to accommodate heavy summer traffic. The sides are open to the street, and the stand boasts stretches of counter space and multiple serving stations. Seating is provided at heavyset concrete tables and benches outside.

My son, Sam, and I found ourselves in the Coney Island neighborhood when we were paying a visit to Totonno's Pizzeria, which is just round the corner from Nathan's. After a long trip on the subway, Sam was hungry. We showed up at Nathan's just after eleven o'clock on what was an unseasonably cool June morning. Even though the schools had got out the day before, there were few people around. It would need someone with a better imagination than mine to sit at a concrete table at an almost deserted restaurant and conjure the old Coney Island. The teeming masses of fairground goers and bathers from yesteryear forever define the place, and they live on in the work of photographers like Diane Arbus. Today, a couple of men were asking if anyone could help them out with something to eat. One of the men had a quarter inserted face-out in his ear.

Sam and I both had an order of **Nathan's hot dogs and fries.** My dog, with onions, was fine but felt like it had been on the grill too long. The fries, skin-on, thick, and crinkle-cut, were excellent, fried hard and crispy on the outside, soft and pillowy within. I thought back to the Nathan's dogs we'd had a few weeks before at Shea Stadium. Boiled rather than grilled, they were plumper and, to me, more satisfying. On a fine day in the upper deck with Flushing set before you, the planes coming and going from LaGuardia, and the Mets having a good afternoon against the Giants, a good dog is the perfect complement. This dog at Coney Island more resembled one you'd find at Yankee Stadium, where the only notable feature of the food is the sticker shock. Two hot dogs and two beers cost twenty-four dollars. You feel like you should get a hot dog at the ball game, but those prices make you think at least twice.

So what constitutes a great hot dog? To me, it's a grilled, kosher-style frank served on a lightly toasted bun with slightly spicy mustard and a homemade onion or pickle relish that is neither too sweet nor too hot.

—Ed Levine, New York Times *(May 25, 2005)*

In his *Times* article, Ed Levine describes *kosher* and *kosher-style* dogs. The former is all-beef, encased in collagen, and rabbinically supervised. The latter has a natural casing, which isn't allowed by kosher rules, and is usually made from sheep intestines. "It is the natural casing that gives the best hot dogs their wondrous snap and bite," says Levine.

The hot dog is best when it stays close to these utilitarian origins. Foot-longs and other gimmicks just seem wrong. Take the gourmet hot dog. The Old Homestead Restaurant in New York City, which is best known as a steakhouse, sells a Kobe Beef Frankfurter for nineteen dollars. It comes with white-truffle mustard. It seems as if, in all the fuss, they made a hamburger out of a hot dog. (Old Homestead does a Kobe Beef Burger, too, for forty-one dollars.) My wife was at Da Silvano in the Village with someone who ordered the restaurant's **Kobe Beef Hot Dog**, which is a foot-long that comes sans bun and is $21.50. She tried a piece and said it tasted like a "very, very, very good hot dog," so perhaps I should be more tolerant.

No, I won't condemn anyone for putting ketchup on a hot dog. This is the land of the free. And if someone wants to put ketchup on a hot dog and actually eat the

awful thing, that is their right. It is also their right to put mayo or chocolate syrup or toenail clippings or cat hair on a hot dog. Sure, it would be disgusting and perverted, and they would be shaming themselves and their loved ones. But under our system of government, it is their right to be barbarians.
— *Mike Royko,* Chicago Tribune *(November 21, 1995)*

In 1995, columnist Mike Royko wrote a scathing piece in the *Chicago Tribune* defending what he saw as the impinged honor of the **Chicago hot dog.** No, *scathing* isn't the right word. *Scalding* is better. The recipient of the piece was Senator Carol Moseley-Braun, who had submitted, no doubt with the best of intentions, a recipe for a "Chicago hot dog" for a cookbook. Alas, there were sins of omission, of such key components as sliced tomatoes, chopped onions, and celery salt. The senator went on to commit the worst no-no of all by including ketchup. Royko clearly couldn't believe that someone representing the city of Chicago (as part of the state of Illinois) in the United States Senate could do such a thing. "It is said that power corrupts," Royko wrote. "I didn't know that it brings on utter madness."

Doug Moe, who wrote *The World of Mike Royko,* recounted this story to me. What's so bad about putting ketchup on a hot dog? people wrote to Royko to ask. To them Royko replied, "It is wrong because it is not right." Moe says that Royko, who died in 1997, wrote a lot about Chicago food: about pierogis on the North Side of the city, about his own Chicago Ribfest, and about hot dogs. If the tradition of being, er, dogmatic about food lives on in the Second City, I'll have to tread carefully.

I'll start on relatively safe ground: New York. I had a **Chicago Dog** at the Shake Shack in Madison Square Park in New York City, to go with my Shack Burger. The dog's lengthy list of ingredients leaves out nothing that should be there and includes nothing that shouldn't. Take a "Vienna all-beef dog in a poppy seed bun," say the instructions, and "Drag it through the garden," meaning pile on lettuce, tomato, sport peppers, green peppers, pickles, onions, neon relish, cucumber, celery salt, and mustard. I enjoyed it immensely, though it seemed like I was getting a hot dog with a side salad piled on top. Sport peppers, by the way, might also be called serrano sport peppers, which are pickled.

In Chicago itself there are numerous well-known and respected hot dog places that were recommended to me. Many of them would make my all-name team for their punning ways. So we have Hot Doug's, which calls itself "The Sausage Superstore and Encased Meat Emporium." "The Dog," their Web site says. "Chicago-Style Hot Dog with all the trimmings: 'nuff said" ($1.50). Hot Doug's features a couple of named dishes: "The Jennifer

Garner (formerly the Britney Spears) Fire Dog: Mighty hot! $2.25"; and "The Madonna (formerly the Raquel Welch and the Ann-Margret) Andouille Sausage: Mighty, mighty, mighty hot! $3.50." I wonder which is worse: to have a hot dog named after you, or to formerly have had a hot dog named after you?

Also making the all-name team is the Wiener's Circle on North Clark, where the self-explanatory, grilled-up **Char Dog** has been highly recommended to me.

━━━━━━

CONTRIBUTION

Adam Langer is a journalist, playwright, and filmmaker and the author of the much-praised novels *Crossing California* and *The Washington Story*. Adam is a native of Chicago and the neighborhood of West Rogers Park, which feature prominently in his two books, both set in the period between the late seventies and 1987.

> *Larry didn't find anyone so he drove back north to Peterson to get a hot dog at Wolfy's instead. Wolfy's hot dogs weren't kosher, especially when slathered with cheese, but the temptation of a double cheese dog with everything and a large fries was too great to let Jewish doctrine interfere.*
> (Crossing California)

Adam gave me a few ideas for foodstuffs to sample in Chicago, starting with "the classic Chicago-style hot dog, of course—mustard, relish, onions, jalapeños (one doesn't eat them whole; one squeezes the jalapeño juice onto the frankfurter), celery salt, no ketchup. The best varieties of these can be found at Wolfy's, a long-standing West Rogers Park establishment. Others opt for the **cheese dogs** at The Wiener's Circle."

━━━━━━

Coney Island is so deeply associated with the hot dog that in many parts of the country, certain types of hot dogs are known as "Coneys," and the restaurants that sell them, as "Coney Islands." This phenomenon is rampant in Michigan: Detroit has numerous Coney Islands, including the

QUICK BITE

If there's more than one way to skin a cat, there are hundreds of ways to serve a dog. Walter's Hot Dog Stand in Mamaroneck, in Westchester County, New York, has been operating since 1919 and has served its hot dogs out of a roadside Chinese pagoda since 1928. **Walter's own-brand dogs** are split in half, spread with butter, grilled in secret sauce, and served with homemade mustard.

And at yet another Greek hot dog joint, venerable Pete's Famous Hot Dogs of Birmingham, Alabama, the signature dog is served **"All the way,"** with mustard, kraut, and the local, secret special sauce. Wash it down with Grapico, a local soda. What's your local dog favorite?

famous Lafayette and American Coney Island Restaurants, which are right next to each other. Something else many of the restaurants have in common is that they were founded by Greek immigrants, in the case of American Coney Island, by Constantine "Gust" Keros, who came from Greece in 1903 and started the restaurant in 1917, just a year, note, after Nathan's was established in Coney Island.

The chili served in parlors in Cincinnati originated in a recipe created by a Greek American in 1922. When this chili is spooned over a hot dog, you get what they call a Coney. This is how the Skyline chain describes the dish: "Our classic **Cheese Coney** is a specially made hot dog in a steamed bun, with mustard, covered with our original, secret-recipe Skyline Chili, diced onions and a mound of cheddar cheese."

QUICK BITE

In some parts—eastern Pennsylvania, for example—a Cincinnati-chili-like meat sauce designed for spooning over hot dogs or burgers is known as **Greek Sauce.**

I was guided through some of Michigan's meaty morass by chef Eric Villegas of the Restaurant Villegas in Okemos, Michigan. Eric hails from Saginaw and his wife is from Flint, Michigan, outside of Detroit. Round here the key is in the kind of sauce that goes on the hot dog that creates, along with mustard and chopped onions, the Coney Dog. "The Detroit sauce, or the 'wet' sauce, is actually a midwestern version of chili," says Eric. "So it does contain ground beef, beans, onions, et cetera. The Flint style, or 'dry,' sauce is more akin to a midwestern taco filling: finely ground beef (some of the older versions use beef heart) and highly spiced." One of the manufacturers of wet sauce for Detroit Coneys ("Hot Dog Chili Sauce"), who also distributes Abbott's dry sauce for Flint-style dogs, is Koegel's, located just outside Flint. (Both their sauces, which are available online [see page 84], contain beef heart.)

Eric Villegas told me not to forget about Todoroff's, in Jackson, Michigan, who say that they, in the person of founder George Todoroff, invented the Coney dog back in 1914. George made up his chili (ground beef, onions, and secret spices), first put it on a dog in 1914, and went on to sell seventeen million Coneys at his restaurant before he retired in 1945. Todoroff's, like Nathan's, is a franchised operation today.

So the Coney dog is centered in, but by no means confined to, the Midwest in general and Michigan in particular. There are also Coney Islands in Texas, like the James Coney Island chain, with locations all over the Houston area where you can pick up a classic Coney as well as various kinds of Texas chili. James Coney Island was started by Greek immigrants Tom and James Papadakis in 1923. And a **chili dog** is eighty-nine cents at one of the Coney Islands in La Crosse, Wisconsin, which was started by Jim Kapellas and Tom Sideras in 1922.

———

"In Toledo there is quite a famous place called Tony Packo's," says Eric Villegas. "It's interesting for a number of reasons but one thing they do is have visiting celebs sign a Coney bun, which then gets encased in a plastic frame for all eternity for everyone to gawk at." Tony Packo was a Hungarian-American who started a restaurant in 1932. In those tough times, Packo would sell a half-a-dog for a nickel, rather than a whole one for a dime, which many people couldn't afford. Packo put his own chili sauce on his "Hungarian Hot Dog."

In 1976, actor Jamie Farr, who is from Toledo, mentioned Tony Packo's Hungarian hot dogs on television. Luckily for Packo's, Farr was playing Corporal Klinger on *M*A*S*H* at the time. Farr gave the restaurant a number of shout-outs. Getting a name check on the most watched program in American television history, the *M*A*S*H* finale in 1983, cannot have hurt sales.

Burt Reynolds, in 1972, was the first well-known visitor to sign a
hot dog bun to be fossilized and displayed round the restaurant
as Eric describes. The idea was Reynolds's own, apparently. On
the menu are **Tony Packo's World-Famous Hot Dog** (smoked
sausage, mustard, onions, special sauce); stuffed cabbage
(stuffed with rice, pork, and beef and simmered in sour cream);
and Midwest specialty Chili Mac (in this case, chili over dumplings with cheese and onions).

In some parts of Pennsylvania, hot dog joints have "Texas" in their
name—Altoona's Original Texas Hot Dogs and Texas Hot Wieners, for
example. The Coney Island-Texas-Pennsylvania circle is squared at Coney
Island Lunch, a restaurant in Scranton, Pennsylvania. Coney Island Lunch
was started by a Greek immigrant, Steve Karampilas, in 1923. Now they
serve what they call a **Texas wiener,** which is a grilled beef wiener with
mustard, chopped onions, and their homemade chili sauce.

In and around Paterson, New Jersey, also in restaurants operated in the
main by Greek Americans, is served what are known locally as **Hot Texas
wieners.** The distinction here is that the dog is deep-fried before being
entombed in onions and chili sauce. (On the side, you can take fries with
gravy known in northern New Jersey, when with cheese, as **Disco Fries.**)
Rutt's Hut, in neighboring Clifton, is well known for its deep-fried dogs,
which are known as **Rippers.**

In Rhode Island, the local version, once again a Greek American
creation, is the **New York System Hot Wiener.** (Perhaps you'd
call it a gagger. What you wouldn't call it is a hot dog.) In a story
in the *New York Times* on the gastronomic oddities of Rhode Island, Paul Lukas writes that the System was propagated among
the Greek hot dog sellers in Providence in the 1940s and then
became customary throughout the state. This is what the System does to the hot dog:

> *The wieners are cut short, usually about four inches. They*
> *cook slowly on a low-heat griddle all day and are served in*
> *a soft steamed bun. Counter clerks apply mustard, chopped*

*raw onions, celery salt and the true hallmark of hot wieners:
a greasy ground-beef sauce that's not quite chili, not quite
gravy, distinct unto itself.*

Places that serve wieners this way advertise it in their name:
Sam's New York System or Riverside Kitchen New York System
or Olneyville New York System, all in Providence. To cement the
New York connection, some places call the chili-like stuff they
put on the wiener "Coney Island Sauce."

———————

Proliferation of hot dog styles stretches way beyond Texas wieners and
Coneys. Around Plattsburgh, in the North Country region of New York
State, there is the **Michigan,** a chili dog variant that has its own secret
meat sauce. This name appears to be a reference to the Coney dog's popularity in Michigan that made its way back to the home state of New York.
Gordie Little writes a column called "Small Talk" for the *Press-Republican*
in Plattsburgh, and he looked into the history of the Michigan. "The
Coney is not the Michigan, and the Michigan is not the chili dog," he told
me. "Each region of the country has its own sauce for hot dogs, but for the
most part, they are not directly related."

So to sum up, we have Michigans in New York and Texas Hots in Pennsylvania and New Jersey; New York Systems in Rhode Island and Coneys
all over the place: Cincinnati, Houston, Detroit. I checked with a spokes-
woman for Nathan's, and she confirmed what I thought: Nathan's of Coney
Island doesn't sell anything called a Coney, although you can get chili on
your dog (for a chili dog). So we can tentatively say, the one place where
you're not going to see a Coney called a Coney is Coney Island.

Many restaurants feature signed pictures of celebrities on the wall. If you
look at the faces, some you'll know and some you won't. But at Pink's, near
the corner of Melrose and La Brea in Los Angeles, they have a better class
of celebrity—real stars like Steve Martin and Nicole Kidman, rather than
the local weatherman. Pink's has graduated from a pushcart in 1939 to the
landmark it is today.

On a warm day in October, my L.A. eating buddy, Rick, and I stood in
line at Pink's and debated what we were going to have. We were early
enough that we could line up in the shaded section of the cordon, but

before long, and still before most people would consider having lunch, there was a good-size line heading up the street. We decided that one of us at least had to have a chili dog, which Pink's is renowned for, but what else? We watched quietly as orders of **chili fries with cheese** were put together. Onto a pile of the fries is ladled chili. Onto the chili is squeezed some cheese product, and onto the cheese is ladled more chili.

Rendered speechless by this spectacle, Rick and I looked over our pink menus. Among Pink's super specials are a bunch of goofy names, dogs named for Martha Stewart and Rosie O'Donnell, another commemorating Harry Potter (Polish sausage, onions, mushrooms, bacon, and cheese) and one for the Lord of the Rings (BBQ sauce and onion rings). My favorite name was the **Three Dog Night,** which, joy to the world, is three dogs in a tortilla with cheese, bacon, chili, and onions, for $5.95.

Rick decided to be cute by asking for a **New York Dog,** hold the onions. (A New York Dog is simply a dog with onions.) "You want a hot dog, then," our phlegmatic server said, and went about his work with efficiency and economy. I took a **Chili Cheese Dog,** $2.75, and a **Guacamole Dog,** $2.95, and we shared some fries (no chili, no cheese) for $1.95. Pink's is a hot dog stand with a place you can sit out back so you don't have to worry about spilling chili gunk on your car's upholstery. To my taste, the chili was a little greasy and the guacamole wasn't anything to shout about, but the experience of eating here was a hoot.

QUICK BITE

Mark Calvino of Island Burger in New York City has fond childhood memories of trips up to the Poconos, when he was nine or ten. The family would stop at Hot Dog Johnny's, on Route 46. (A great feature of the Internet is going online to see if your favorite childhood place is still around. Mine, Billy's Baked Potato, by the Tower of London, isn't.) Hot Dog Johnny's was opened by John Kovalsky, whose daughter Pat has worked at the restaurant since 1944. What Mark Calvino remembers is an oval-shaped building and chest-high tables. As a New York kid, Mark was used to having sauerkraut on his hot dog. But Hot Dog Johnny's didn't serve kraut, which was a shame as far as Mark was concerned. Mark now operates a burger restaurant that doesn't sell fries, so he's more understanding.

The best hot dog I ever ate was served up by El Guero Canelo of South Tucson, a popular Mexican fast-food joint. If you're thinking about visiting Tucson but wavering, let this dog put you over the top. El Guero Canelo is made up of a couple of cinder block structures, a separate hot dog preparation trailer, and a shaded patio where you eat your food. There is a giant menu posted above the cash windows that includes every Mexican dish I've ever heard of and many I haven't. Fortunately, Kristen Cook of the *Arizona Daily Star* said I should get a **Sonoran Hot Dog** and a **Chicken Torta** (a grilled chicken sandwich with avocado and mayo) here, so I didn't have to think too hard. I threw in a taco made with **carne asada,** for luck. I picked up a chit after paying and sat for a while with the family on the enclosed restaurant patio, munching on the delicious roasted peppers and giant spring onions you can pick up at a serving station.

I'd already delivered the sandwich and taco and waited while someone's take-out order for dogs was being filled. Here, at a cart the size of small trailer, the dogs were frying in their jackets of bacon. The smell of fried bacon fat was making me hungry, and I tried to wait patiently as hot dog after hot dog was assembled before I got mine. When I got the dogs back to the table, they lasted a hundredth of the time I'd waited for them. The bacon-wrapped dog sits in a large, soft bun and is buried under a mess of beans, jalapeño relish, onions, and tomatoes finished off with a mayo flourish. Divinely wicked and wickedly divine, and just two dollars each. "I don't like hot dogs," says Kristen Cook, "but I love these."

HOT DOGS SUMMARY
RUN, DON'T WALK, FOR . . .

- A **Sonoran hot dog** from El Guero Canelo in Tucson. My favorite hot dog isn't even served in a hot dog roll.
- A **Dodger dog** at Dodger Stadium. Don't leave the game before the end.

- A **Chicago dog** with everything. A handful, but practically a balanced meal.

IF YOU'VE NEVER TRIED . . .

- A chili dog. Not for the faint of heart, and keep a napkin handy, but it's sometimes worth going the extra step and adding some meat to your sausage.

- Try this, or any other signature dog. Any joint that thrives long-term selling its own dog creation has got to have something going for it.

15

BARBECUE

The strongest memory from my childhood is waking up to the smell of smoke. I'd lie in my bed with my eyes still closed, take a deep breath, and smile. That aroma meant that we'd be having a good supper that night.
—Mike Mills and Amy Mills Tunnicliffe, *Peace, Love, and Barbecue* (2005)

What are this country's great cultural contributions to the world? Three come immediately to mind: baseball, jazz, and barbecue. In this bounteous nation, you can find meat prepared every way possible, but across a great swath of the country, barbecue has been honed and polished into an art form. Who first cooked meat indirectly by means of smoke isn't known, but like baseball and jazz, the contemporary versions of barbecue are American variations on a multinational theme. Pork, the meat on which so much barbecue cuisine relies, was introduced to the Americas by the Spaniards. They found Native Americans cooking meat over fire on grills that the Arawak Indians called "barbacoa," which may be where the modern word comes from.

However it came to be, barbecue is now a huge business and is close to a spiritual movement. Millions of Americans perform their own rites and rituals in yards across the country, although most people grill over an open flame rather than barbecue in the strict sense of the term. There are barbecue restaurants everywhere, with pits and smokers catering to the faithful. Barbecue traditions run deep. If you so desired, you could draw maps of the southern United States across to Texas and up into the Midwest based on the dominant meat and serving style. If you're in South Carolina, for example, you might find mustard sauce on your pork; if you're in the western parts of North Carolina, the sauce on your meat will quite possibly be vinegary. Utilizing the more prominent pitmasters from across the barbecue nation, a barbecue circuit has been assembled that travels round the country cooking for crowds of appreciative acolytes in underserved outposts like New York City.

Danny Meyer has operated Blue Smoke, a well-regarded barbecue restaurant in New York City, since 2002. Meyer was prompted to organize the Big Apple Barbecue Block Party in 2003, and it has been a roaring success each year since. It's a noncompetition event where top pitmasters come to New York to show off their craft. Tens of thousands of 'cue-hungry fans hang out in Madison Square Park and along a closed-off section of Madison Avenue. Billows of fragrant smoke and sundry incongruous scents fill the air as, for one weekend, some of the glorious dishes of the American South are fixed right in Manhattan.

At first glance, the world of big-time barbecue looked intimidating to this outsider. Many barbecue followers are very knowledgeable. Some of them are as bad as the more zealous oenophiles. Fact is, there's always going to be someone who knows more about barbecue than you. It's certainly not hard to find someone who knows more about barbecue than me. Visiting the Block Party, I was concerned that I'd be wading in over my head with the pitmasters, but they were all extremely solicitous, even of the most basic, dumb questions. Kathleen Purvis, the *Charlotte Observer*'s food editor, helped

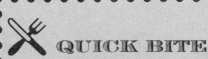

QUICK BITE

Kathleen Purvis says that the best version of South Carolina's elusive **mustard sauce** is to be found at Sweatman's Barbecue, in St. George, South Carolina. "If you're really lucky," Kathleen says, "they'll have a big pan of **pork skin** on the buffet."

me with some suggestions for barbecue in the Carolinas. Kathleen has been writing about barbecue for fifteen years and she uses qualifiers like *usually, mostly,* and *maybe* when describing local specialties, differences, and distinctions. So it's not an exact science. There's nothing to be afraid of. Dig in.

At the Barbecue Block Party, the first person I spoke with was Carolyn McLemore, from Big Bob Gibson Barbecue, in Decatur, Alabama. Big Bob Gibson's is among the barbecue elite, and I talked to Carolyn through a throng of people eager to get their hands on the paper trays of barbecue. Carolyn reeled off some of the prizes the restaurant has been awarded on the cook-off circuit. Its **pork shoulder** has been six-time world champion at Memphis in May, the barbecue Olympics. National magazines had decreed its ribs the best in America; it won Best Ribs at the Houston Livestock Show; and so on. Carolyn said that the newest dish the restaurant was trying was **brisket,** and that had already won a prize at an event in Kansas City. The brisket had been on the menu only four weeks, and already out-of-towners were making return trips for it.

I asked Carolyn what was distinctive about the meat at Big Bob's. "If you come to our place and you order pulled pork, it will stand alone, although we have championship sauces that a lot of customers put on it. What we do to the pork enhances the flavor of the pork; it doesn't cover anything that would change it to apple or cinnamon or something." I can vouch for **Big Bob Gibson's Championship Barbecue Sauce.** It's a fantastic red color, tangy and slightly sweet, textured with pieces of onion, and light-years removed from any store-bought sickly brown sludge. It was in 1996, and with this sauce, that the restaurant started competing. It won first place at the Memphis in May competition that year and the next, and

QUICK BITE

Barbecue sauce can be the stuff of legend. At McClard's, in Hot Springs, Arkansas, the story is that a guy who had stayed two months at Alex and Gladys McClard's hotel couldn't pay his ten-dollar bill, so gave up the recipe for **"the world's best bar-b-q sauce."** And the McClard's went into the barbecue business. The recipe, the story goes, is in a safe-deposit box downtown, where it's earned the ten dollars back a few times over. **Ribs and fry** are on the menu here—that is, ribs covered with fries—together with barbecued beef and pork and tamale plates.

McClard's ships the debtor's sauce: 1-866-622-5273 / www .mcclards.com.

has won all kinds of other awards. The championship sauce has spawned other sauces, Carolyn tells me. "From that sauce we developed a mustard sauce and a **habañero sauce** using the same basic ingredients."

I must have been distracted by the thought of habañero sauce because Carolyn was the lucky recipient of my first stupid question of the day. I indicated a gentleman tending some meat and asked if this was Big Bob himself. No, this was Carolyn's husband, Don McLemore, the restaurant's owner. Big Bob Gibson was Don McLemore's maternal grandfather, who started the business in 1925. Carolyn is part of the third generation—barbecue is often a dynastic affair—and there's a fourth in Don and Carolyn's son-in-law, Chris Lilly, who married their daughter, Amy. With this, Chris married into the barbecue profession. Carolyn told me he was busy preparing his own barbecue show for television. (You may have noticed, these barbecue guys are on TV a lot.)

As for Carolyn herself, she likes **fried catfish** and **hush puppies.** Carolyn wanted to make sure I knew about as much of the restaurant's menu as possible. Big Bob's was well known for its coleslaw, which is vinegar-based, with a little bit of sugar in it. "It goes real well with pulled pork. Some people who come in don't like it by itself but they put it on their sandwich and they love it."

And I shouldn't forget their **barbecue chicken,** which is served with a vinegar-based white sauce. It's not a ranch dressing or a tartar sauce, Carolyn says, but rather is made with mayonnaise, vinegar, and "some other things I'm not allowed to tell you." (Those secret ingredients again.) Apparently Big Bob didn't keep his recipes to himself, and a lot of people in Alabama copied his sauces. The mistake has not been repeated. "Our sauces and rubs that we've added—nobody but us has the recipes for."

Carolyn sent me on my way with some **pulled pork.** She said this was her third time in New York and "you've been very gracious to us up here." I dunked the pulled pork and its potato bun into the red sauce and took a bite. I think it's a misconception that people in New York aren't friendly and accommodating, but perhaps it takes fantastic barbecue like this to make them gracious, which isn't a word you hear bandied about the five boroughs very often. When I looked at the meat, the steaming fibers were surprisingly pale. To the tongue, the meat was succulent and moist and sweet. This was promising to be the hottest day of the year so far, and I was going to pace myself, but, oh my, I was going to eat everything I was given. Not to do so would have violated some fundamental law.

For gift baskets and sauces: 1-800-783-9640 / www.bigbob gibsonbbq.com.

Next I talked to Jake Scherrer, from the Salt Lick Barbecue in Driftwood, Texas, which is just outside Austin. ("The last bit of Texas left in Austin," the restaurant likes to say.) Jake describes the Salt Lick, which has been operating since 1969, as "very, very old school." It's all you can eat, a selection of brisket, sausage, ribs, chicken, turkey. It's also BYOB, because Driftwood is situated in a dry county. All-you-can-eat can be a dangerous game, for any restaurant, especially one in Longhorns football country. "Sometimes we get big offensive linemen who eat eight or nine pounds of brisket, sausage, or ribs, or whatever they eat," says Jake.

Jake does public relations for the Salt Lick but likes to wait tables when he can, to keep his hand in. At the restaurant, his personal favorites are brisket and ribs, but he eats chicken about three times a week, too. "I like it all," Jake says convincingly. I say, "And what do you eat when you don't eat barbecue?" And he says, "I eat steak."

The Texas specialty, Jake tells me, is brisket. Everyone in Texas does it a little differently. "There's eight hundred fifty-four barbecue places in Texas, and I bet you nobody does it the same." Of these 854 restaurants, Jake reckons he's visited about 250.

"There's seventeen million people in the state of Texas, and we have a little bit of everything. In Austin, there's thirty-five hundred restaurants. I can go and eat sushi one day, Chinese food the next day. There's a

QUICK BITE

A QUESTION FOR DANNY MEYER

What do you suggest we eat?

"Great 'cue from any of these six barbecue joints in the Hill Country around Austin, Texas. My favorites are Opie's, in Spicewood; Salt Lick, in Driftwood; Vencil Mares's Taylor Café, in Taylor; Cooper's, in Llano; Crosstown and Southside Market, in Elgin."

Mongolian barbecue there mixed in with Texas barbecue, and your normal hamburger joints and pizza joints."

Jake reckons New York is becoming a great barbecue town. "This is an introduction to barbecue here. They didn't come in wagon trains here and have to cook meat on the back . . . That's what we've got going on right now."

I took a piece of the Salt Lick **barbecue link sausage,** half beef, half pork. The restaurant has it made to their specs. It was good and spicy, and went down well with the piece of Salt Lick barbecue **brisket** I tried. It's meat that often has a good amount of fat, and this was very moist and flavorful. To heck with pacing myself.

Glory! The Salt Lick ships four- to five-pound smoked beef briskets, pork ribs, sauce, and dry rubs: www.saltlickbbq.com.

I grabbed a couple of minutes with Otis Walker of Smoki O's, from St. Louis, before he had to go and fix some meat. Often a barbecue style will feature one predominant sauce. Otis said his sauce is a sweeter, tomato-based sauce that's very tangy. "We cook everything. We cook ribs, pulled pork, chicken, chicken wings snoot— it's the snout of the hog. It's a meal, usually with the tips— **snoot-and-tips combo**—and it brings a crunch to the meaty taste of the tips. People enjoy it. The recipe is a secret." Not that I was going to ask, but with that he had to go off and cook.

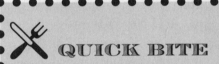

QUICK BITE

Cookbook editor Michael Flamini provides four suggested meals in four locations: brisket at Arthur Bryant's, in Kansas City; **smoked turkey** at Big Bob Gibson's; sausage at Kreuz Market, in Lockhart, Texas; and **fried chicken** at Scott Peacock's restaurant (Watershed), in Decatur, Georgia.

I tried some **snoot.** I liked the taste of pork rind growing up when my mother used to make a Sunday roast with the skin on, which my father was extremely partial to. This reminded me of that. I was told that the recipes used at the restaurant Mr. Walker learned from his mother, who made them in her backyard.

While he was in New York, Ron Blasingame, the owner of the Whole Hog Café, in Little Rock, Arkansas, was looking forward to eating some good Italian food every chance he got. The Whole Hog makes pulled pork and beef brisket, but Ron says people like the ribs the best, the **St. Louis–style ribs** (pork spareribs). The sauce is tomato-based. "We doctor it up with some other ingredients. It's not a secret; we put in citrus juices—lemon-lime juice—some sweet-sour type in there, and balsamic vinegar."

Cooking for Ron Blasingame was Mike Davis. After putting in twenty years' service in the army, Mike Davis started cooking, first in competition barbecue and then in the restaurant business. The Whole Hog Café opened in 2000. "I like to eat fish," says Mike. "Any kind of fish. We got catfish. I like any kind of seafood, cooked any way you want to cook it pretty much. I don't eat it raw. That's fish bait."

QUICK BITE

Thanks to Beverly Lancaster-Hyde of Vanguard Communications for these Washington, D.C., favorites: **short ribs** from the "World's Famous" Florida Avenue Grill, on Florida Avenue, NW (and **coconut cake** when they have it); **pork ribs** from Big Daddy's Ribs, on Twelfth Street (in the Brookland section of D.C.); and the **chili dog** from Ben's Chili Bowl, on U Street, NW.

Gary Roark has been cooking barbecue seriously since about 1989. Gary was representing Ubon's restaurant in Yazoo City, Mississippi, which was then but a year old. There was a second Ubon's, opened more recently in Madison, near the state capital, Jackson. Gary told me that his restaurant uses a dry rub, a marinade, and a sauce that sets their meat apart. The recipe for the sauce has been in Gary's family for generations.

> *The sauce goes back to my daddy's mother and daddy. The story that my daddy used to say was that every Fourth of July my grandfather would cook a whole hog or a side of beef on a spit in the back. He was a farmer in southeast Missouri. He would invite all the neighbors and friends over. The sauce was made in a big Number Three washtub and stirred with a boat paddle he probably fished with the day before. This is how the family cooking started. With us today, we have my wife, my daughter, my son-in-law, my brother-in-law. It's a family gathering for us, too. We don't make it in the washtub anymore. We have to use a stainless-steel vat, all Health Department–approved. That part has changed since my granddaddy's day.*

Gary described himself as a Mississippi boy transplanted from the Blue Hills of Missouri as a young boy. I asked him the same question I asked everyone, whether he thought New York was a good barbecue town. "Well, look at this crowd," he said, indicating the swelling multitudes. "It's a bit overwhelming to a southern boy from a small town. Yazoo City's population's naught but about thirteen thousand. Just a little better than thirteen thousand, and I saw that many vehicles yesterday."

Like everyone else here, Gary enjoys the fruits of his own labors. He works with pork all day, but he still has a craving for it. He said he was watching a program about Memphis in May on the Food Channel recently, and they showed the ribs in competition. "When it went off I was craving a barbecue rib, and I have ribs all the time. I guess it's just in my blood."

The city of Memphis is renowned for its **dry-rub ribs,** which are cooked without sauce. The spices in the dry rub, which is applied before cooking, give the meat its flavor. A couple of years ago I spent some time working in Memphis and stayed in a motel on Poplar, right across the street from Corky's, one of the city's great barbecue places. More than a couple of times, I found myself at Corky's accompanied by a plate of their ribs. Corky's has nine locations in Tennessee and has spread across the center of the country, to cities like Metairie, Louisiana; Duluth, Georgia; Springfield, Illinois; and Evansville, Indiana. And they'll also send you their ribs, using their handy local delivery service, Federal Express. We ordered up a big box of ribs for my daughter's birthday one year and heated the meat up on a grill. Extensive sampling confirmed that air travel didn't do the ribs (or the rubs and barbecue sauce) any damage whatsoever.

Order from www.corkysbbq.com / 1-800-9-CORKYS (926-7597).

In Memphis, I also had the dry-rub ribs at the Cozy Corner, a storefront place that has been around since the time Elvis died. Here they barbecue all sorts of stuff: Cornish hens and baloney, even spaghetti, but I ate a plate of ribs with coleslaw and beans and relished every mouthful.

They'll give you sauce in Memphis, and Corky's sells it with their ribs, along with shakers of dry-rub spices. It's between you and your conscience whether you want to use it or not.

———

On a barbecue pit, ribs pass through the perfect state of doneness for only fifteen minutes. If the bones slip right out of the slab, the ribs are mushy; if the meat refuses to separate from the bones, it is tough . . . With perfectly cooked ribs, the meat between the bones should separate down the center and not from the bones.
     —*Jeffrey Steingarten,* The Man Who Ate Everything *(1997)*

It was hard to talk to Mike Mills without being distracted by the racks of ribs lined up on every flat surface behind and to the side of him at his stand. In front, a small army of helpers was working, each of them wearing orange T-shirts advertising Mike's book *Peace, Love, and Barbecue* (which comes with great credentials: foreword by Danny Meyer and introduction by Jeffrey Steingarten). Mike Mills is a true barbecue star, winner with the Apple City Barbecue of Memphis in May titles in the early nineties and now a major 'cue entrepreneur. Mike's first restaurant was the 17th Street Bar and Grill, in Murphysboro, Illinois, which he took over in 1985. He kept his day job for ten years but eventually concentrated on barbecue full-time. His interests now spread from southern Illinois to Las Vegas and New York.

Mike Mills is a great enthusiast. This day, he was having a fine time, getting a big kick out of cooking barbecue for thousands of people in the street in New York City.

"New York is an awesome barbecue town. Look at this crowd out here today, doing something they don't normally do. This is what this is all about. They're not hustling and bustling; they're waiting their turn. In the Big Apple that's a little bit of an oddity. I was born in Murphysboro, on the southern tip of Illinois. I was sitting here last night drinking a Diet Coke in a lawn chair on Madison Avenue. I was saying, who would ever have thunk it, that this would have been possible? It's gotta be a first."

Like a number of pitmasters, Mike turned to barbecue as a second career, revisiting a family skill and making a business out of it. "I was raised in a barbecue family," he says. "My father was a great barbecuer. But I'm actually a dental technician by trade. I made prosthetic appliances for dentists up until about 1994, and then I decided I was going to get in the barbecue business. I used to just do it to raise funds for different organizations—churches, family organizations—just for the fun of it. I didn't do it to make a living but I changed my mind. Since 1994, I've been at it just hard and heavy."

I commented to Mike that there seemed to be a camaraderie among the pitmasters. They've cooked against one another a lot, says Mike. They all want to beat one another, but they'll help all the way round, other than that period when they're in competition, the time when "you're doing your thing." But right after the contest, they're all friends again. "We'll be happy for the other one," he says. "Maybe we'll take them a bottle of champagne. On any given day it can be anybody's ball game, like a NASCAR race. You never know who's going to win."

Mike divides his time between Las Vegas, where he has three Memphis Championship Barbecue restaurants, and southern Illinois. He's in one of the restaurants every day and he spends time in the pit. His staff is great, he says, and today he's enlisted the help of his friend Ed Wilson, who has his own barbecue place in Fairfield, Connecticut. Ed is tending a mobile smoker while Mike talks. I'm almost impossibly distracted by the shuttle of ribs I can see over Mike's shoulder and by the wafting smoke filling the air. So I ask Mike what he likes to eat.

"**Barbecue pie.** If you've got corn bread with it. I love steak. I'm a red meat person. With potatoes. I've got a strong weakness for desserts. I don't think there's anything that I don't like. If there is, I haven't come across it."

At an undisclosed location in New York City, Mike ate barbecue the night before because he likes to see how other places do it. New York might not be somewhere you'd associate with great barbecue, but neither is Illinois. Murphysboro has always been a barbecue town, Mike says. It's not right in the South, but it's like the South.

Now, about those ribs . . .

"We have a Memphis style of barbecue. I do what we call a wet-dry—a little bit of sauce, but it's not drenched. We have a little bit of vinegar flavor, a little bit of sweetness, a little bit of spice, but not that'll burn you up. I don't want to burn you up. I want you to be able to eat it and taste the meat, the flavor of the meat, and be able to see what it's all about. Not a heavy smoke, not a heavy spice, not a heavy sauce; they all come into your mouth at one time."

I ask about Mike's rub and whether it's a secret. "It was, until I just came out with a new cookbook," he said. I enjoyed listening to Mike immensely. I told him he talks about his cooking so well. "I love it," he said. "It's my life. I'm the luckiest man in the world."

WATCH OUT FOR . . .

When we're grilling for ourselves, it's important to follow safe-cooking guidelines like these from the FDA:

Cook Thoroughly

Cook food to a safe minimum internal temperature to destroy harmful bacteria. Meat and poultry cooked on a grill often browns very fast on the outside. Use a food thermometer to be sure the food has reached a safe minimum internal temperature. Beef, veal, and lamb steaks, roasts and chops can be cooked to 145°F. Hamburgers made of ground beef should reach 160°F. All cuts of pork should reach 160°F. All poultry should reach a minimum of 165°F.

Never partially grill meat or poultry and finish cooking it later.

Reheat Sufficiently

When reheating fully cooked meats like hot dogs, grill to 165°F or until steaming hot.

Keep Hot Food Hot

After cooking meat and poultry on the grill, keep it hot until served—at 140°F or warmer.

Keep cooked meats hot by setting them to the side of the grill rack, not directly over the coals, where they could overcook. At home, cooked meat can be kept hot in a warm oven (at approximately 200°F), in a chafing dish or slow cooker, or on a warming tray.

Serve the Food Correctly

When taking food off the grill, use a clean platter. Don't put cooked food on the same platter that held raw meat or poultry. Any harmful bacteria present in the raw meat juices could contaminate safely cooked food.

In hot weather (above 90°F), food should never sit out for more than one hour.

(*continued on next page*)

Handle Leftovers Properly

Refrigerate any leftovers promptly in shallow containers. Discard any food left out more than two hours (one hour if temperatures are above 90°F).

Safe Minimum Internal Temperatures
◆ Whole poultry: 165°F
◆ Poultry breasts: 165°F
◆ Ground poultry: 165°F
◆ Hamburgers, beef: 160°F
◆ Beef, veal, and lamb (steaks, roasts, and chops): 145°F (for medium-rare); 160°F (for medium)
◆ All cuts of pork: 160°F

For the complete guidelines: www.fsis.usda.gov/Fact_Sheets/Barbecue_Food_Safety/index.asp.

Now it was my turn to get lucky. **Mike's ribs** were fashioned pretty much like the ideal, as described by Jeffrey Steingarten. The meat had a reddish hue and broke apart effortlessly and in the right places. Then the taste was, as Mike said, a little bit of this, a little bit of that, and not too much of anything that would swamp the meat. Just perfect. You've got to get your hands on some of Mike's ribs.

Mike Mills was right: these barbecue stands and the crowds around them did make quite a sight. Nothing was quite as striking as Ed Mitchell's ten big smokers laid out in a row along Madison Avenue. I watched as Mitchell hauled open the top of one and tended to the beast inside. Lying in state on the rack was half a hog minus its head. I grabbed a moment with Mr. Mitchell and commented on the scale of this operation. He said he had an eighteen-wheeler parked round the corner. "That's what I do," he said.

I asked if he traveled round the country.

"Yep."

"How do you find New York as a barbecue town?"

"They found me."

I asked for that.

Ed said he'd been cooking since he was fourteen. He uses recipes that have long been in his family, passed down from his grandfather and his grandfather's grandfather.

For Ed, it's all about the pork. He likes fried chicken fine, but starting with eggs and bacon for breakfast, he prefers pork. His interest in this subject runs broad and deep: Ed said he was involved with North Carolina A&T University in a project trying to raise the perfect pig.

I said that I'd seen the hog in the smoker. This is your specialty, the whole hog?

"That's all it is. This is real barbecue . . . You have a chance to blend all of the meat together to get the original taste of all the different types of flavors hitting the taste buds: from the bacon, from the ham, from the different parts like the pork shoulder. Until you blend it all together . . . that's when you really get the thrill of what it all tastes like. The whole hog."

I tried some of this whole hog, which was presented in a roll as a **pulled-pork sandwich.** Indeed it was a richer, more complex taste than other pork I remembered. I was approaching a level of satiety, but I wanted to finish my assignment. There were two stands I hadn't visited, but I had eaten at the Dinosaur Barbecue and at Blue Smoke in New York City, and I could get to their food readily. But the guys from the Southside Market had come up all the way from Elgin, Texas. Mike Mills told me he'd traded with Southside to get some of their sausage, and he said it was unbelievable.

I talked to Bryan Bracewell from the Southside Market. Bryan was the third generation of his family specializing in the sausage business. In 1968, his grandfather, Ernest Bracewell, Sr., bought a firm that had been making sausage since 1882. Bryan's father, Ernest Jr., joined the firm, and then Bryan. His wife was at home carrying twins, Bryan said, working on the fourth generation.

Bryan said the company was using much the same recipe that the original owners used in the nineteenth century. Southside Market includes a processing plant, a restaurant, and a butcher's shop. Here, they make two million pounds of sausage a year and ship it round the world. Bryan says the Elgin hot sausage is an all-beef sausage with a natural pork casing. The sausage is hot, but not as hot as it used to be. Southside makes a vinegar-based hot sauce for customers to heat up the sausage if they so desire.

Bryan eats a lot of barbecue himself. "Sometimes when you smell like it, it's hard to eat it," he says. Nonetheless, "I eat it every day, just about."

QUICK BITE

It's quite true that the fajita plate, with its dramatic sizzle and forest of condiments, was cooked up in Texas. But fajitas did not become outrageously popular until 1973—when Ninfa's opened in Houston and began selling tacos al carbón—and that was after the classic Tex-Mex era.

—Patricia Sharpe, *Texas Monthly* (August 2003)

Read Patricia Sharpe's *Texas Monthly* piece on "Tex-Mex 101," a fine serving of food history. Sharpe details the three cornerstones of Tex-Mex: yellow cheese, chili. con carne, and tortillas, and why she thinks the cuisine came and has peaked. **Fajitas,** like chimichangas, are more American than apple pie. The fajita is thought to have originated in the *tacos al carbón* at Ninfa's, who have many locations in Houston today.

"When I'm not eating barbecue, it's probably good Mexican food. Central and South Texas—we have great Mexican food. Great Mexican culture. Tex-Mex is Mexican food, Texas style, with an extra kick, I guess. It's not dummied down for—anybody—it comes hot and it's real good."

This was Bryan's first time in New York professionally. People had welcomed them with open arms, he said. Bryan had driven up from Elgin with his father in their custom-built mobile smoker, which looked like a small gas tanker. They'd driven for 32 hours, a total of 1,783 miles. This will sound familiar to plenty of people: Bryan said that he and his father hadn't had a cross word till they got to within the New York City limits.

I tried some Southside sausage, which was fantastic. It was very rich and meaty, and with a real bite. By this stage, I couldn't really do it justice, so when I got home, I ordered a bunch of sausage that UPS delivered next-day from Texas. I got two pounds each of **Smoked Elgin Hot Sausage,** Regular Summer Sausage, and **Jalapeño Summer Sausage** along with bottles of hot sauce and barbecue sauce. I couldn't exactly replicate the flavor Bryan achieved in his smoker, but I didn't expect to. Over the summer, I grilled some of each of the hot sausage links and the larger summer sausages. My favorite was the jalapeño, which came out best when cut into slices, about three to an inch, and cooked quickly right over the heat of the coals. Rich and spicy, it tasted great dunked in French mustard and eaten as hot as tolerable, with a cold Rolling Rock to wash it down.

From Southside Market, sausage and more, right to your door: www.southsidemarket.com.

CONTRIBUTION

Louise Owens is a food, wine, and spirits writer and a regular contributor to the *Dallas Morning News*. She recommends Sonny Bryan's original barbecue place on Inwood Road in Dallas. Sonny Bryan's is "most famous for their **Barbecued Brisket**, moist and filled with the smoke of sixty years of wood-burning fires. Then you add the barbecue sauce, which is kept in Corona beer bottles in a warmer—two styles, regular and spicy. The spicy is the joint."

The other place is Cooper's Old Time Pit Bar-B-Q in Llano, Texas, in the Hill Country. A dozen or so massive cast iron pits are filled with brisket, sausages, chicken, pork, ribs. . . . The heat in the middle of summer is almost unbearable, so you figure out what you want way before you get there. You tell the pit guy what you want, he slaps it on a tray, then it gets weighed up inside where you order your sides. You must have the **fried okra**. *Then, dine in air-conditioned comfort.*

For Cooper's mail order, call 1-325-247-5995 or 1-877-533-5553, or visit www.coopersbbq.com and browse the pictures of brisket, smoked sausage, and barbecued pork chops.

Sometimes, you see a place and you just know by looking at it the food's got to be good. It has a lot to do with age: an independent restaurant that has been operating since 1950 must be doing something right, even if it's not stayed in the same family the whole time. The feeling also has to do with style. You want the people running a place to make an effort but not to overdo it—if they're trying too hard, the food must be deficient. In the spirit of this book, next time you see some little side-of-the-road eatery that looks good, stop and find out if it is.

I was driving with my brother-in-law Doug round Fredericksburg, Virginia, when we had two such moments in one day. We were driving along Route 1—the Jefferson Davis Highway—looking for Carl's ice cream place (see page 139), when we passed a small redbrick building. The red sign on the roof, decorated with the outline of a pig, said PIT COOKED BAR-B-Q, and the name on the side was Allman's. I said to Doug, "I bet that place is good," and promised myself to make a trip back to make sure I wasn't wrong. A few minutes later we saw the old-fashioned frontage of Carl's ice cream stand, which is somewhere you *know* right away is going to be good.

Next day, the family piled into Doug's truck and went for lunch at Allman's. We showed up early and took seats at one of the small array of tables. There are chrome stools in front of the counter, over which the head of a boar presides thoughtfully. The walls are decorated with prints of old diners from round the country, so this is somewhere that is aware of its heritage. Allman's does pork barbecue, available minced or sliced, in a sandwich or as a Bar-B-Q Plate, together with burgers and hot dogs. I wanted some of the seasonal **Pork Stew,** but it was out of season. I decided on a **Bar-B-Q Deluxe Sandwich** with fries and coleslaw, and we ordered some onion rings to share.

When the two servers called in their orders to the kitchen, they addressed them to "Mom," as in, "Cheeseburger, medium-rare, Mom," or "Mom, can I get an order of fries?" Knowing what the answer was going to be, I asked the young man serving us if it was really his mom back there, and he said no. Allman's has been in business since 1954, and Mary Brown, universally known as Mom, has been there for more than forty years making the barbecue.

The **onion rings** were devilishly good—thick battered and steaming hot. The fries were also good and crisp. The pork was unadorned, so I added the house's sweet-and-sour barbecue sauce, which was sweeter than I like. But the pork was aromatic and tender and, with some of the wet, thick-cut slaw, made a good hearty lunchtime sandwich. The platter was $5.62, and you can order the pork, the rolls, the sauces, slaw, and beans in bulk from a handy portion guide on the back of the take-out menu. (For five people: one pound of meat, half a dozen rolls, six ounces of sauce, a quart each of slaw and beans.)

As we left, we poked our heads in the kitchen to say hello to Mom. "Thanks for the food," said Lindsay, who'd gnawed her way happily round the outside of a good-size cheeseburger. Then we headed for Carl's ice cream stand and our dessert.

• • •

Kenny Callaghan is the pitmaster at Blue Smoke, in New York City. The day was clearly going fantastically well for the hosts of the Big Apple Barbecue event. Kenny looked at the thousands of people enjoying the food. At that moment, Danny Meyer was holding a "wine and swine" tasting at Eleven Madison, his restaurant nearby. There were other 'cue-related events and symposia going on, and each was presumably as packed as the next. Kenny said he'd worked for Danny Meyer for twelve years, including four as executive sous-chef at the Union Square Café, before Blue Smoke opened. I'd eaten the Memphis-style ribs at Blue Smoke soon after it opened, which was a mistake, because I was eating a lot of ribs in Memphis around the same time. The Blue Smoke ribs I ate at the Block Party were lovely, with a light, smoky flavor. I made a note that there was a little hot and a little sweet in the sauce, and it was a fine mix.

Kenny had been going around the stands, sampling everyone's barbecue. "Today, I like the whole hog from Ed Mitchell down there," he said, pointing south toward Ed Mitchell's impressive lineup of smokers. "That's what the whole barbecue community's about. People coming together and sharing good food and a friendly atmosphere."

Having grown up in New York, Kenny Callaghan is a fan of the city's fabled thin-crust pizza. But Blue Smoke led a modest barbecue charge in the city that's seen a number of restaurants opening up in recent times, despite the number of city regulations you have to deal with. Kenny mentions John Stage's Dinosaur Bar-B-Que, in West Harlem, a hundred-and-something blocks to the north of where we were standing. "He's a great guy, and I love going up there. He's got a nice friendly atmosphere."

Dinosaur Bar-B-Que was opened at the end of 2004 on Twelfth Avenue at 131st Street, out in Manhattanville, a thinly populated part of the city where Columbia University is planning a massive expansion over the next few years. There are two elevated streets, Riverside Drive and the West Side Highway, that run along here, and also the fabulous uptown Fairway Market. I drove past Dinosaur Bar-B-Que, which opened very quietly, a few times before I realized there was a restaurant here.

Dinosaur is often described as an upstate New York institution, having started in Syracuse in 1987 and expanded to Rochester in 1997. The place is a real assortment: it's a biker-themed place with a lot of graffiti in the bathrooms that's at the same time very friendly and accommodating to kids, even gaggles of messy toddlers. And you can't say this about everywhere in New York City, but there's always a lively conjoining of folk in the

QUICK BITE

Also in New York City, check out Righteous Urban Barbecue (or RUB) hard by the landmark Chelsea Hotel on 23rd Street. In addition to standard barbecue fare like pulled pork and ribs (which are great) you can check out **Szechwan Smoked Duck,** which I intend to do next time I am in the neighborhood and picking up my own lunch tab. For dinner, if someone else is paying, **the Empire** takes the eye. It consists in part of a dish called "The Taste of the Baron," after co-owner and Kansas City Baron of Barbecue Paul Kirk, consisting of a tasting of beef, pork, ham, pastrami, turkey, chicken, sausage, ribs, and sides for $45.75. Throw in a bottle of Dom Pérignon, and $275.00, and you have your Empire.

place: students, business types, Harlemites, Upper West Siders, out-of-towners, tourists, and people who are two and three of these things at once.

The Dinosaur has a huge menu, and I've eaten most if not all of the items. I like the **fried green tomatoes,** all the ribs, the **Syracuse Style Salt Potatoes** (a boiled potato bathed in a salty lake of butter), the mac and cheese, all the vegetable sides, the **Tres Hombre Plate** (barbecue pork, beef brisket, and ribs), and the **barbecue pork sandwich.** My son, Sam, goes straight for the **Bar-B-Que chicken wings** with blue cheese sauce, ordered mild, and he always saves room for the **Chocolate Icebox Pie.** Or, rather, he doesn't, but he orders it anyway.

I'll always think fondly of Dinosaur because my kids like it so much. Lindsay, who gnawed on her first turkey leg at age two, ate her first rib here at five. Is it the best barbecue in the world? Who knows and who cares? It certainly tastes very good to me. Barbecue is so much less uptight than other cuisines. You eat with your hands, mostly, and make a big mess. Everyone shares and hands round food with abandon while bones and other debris pile up. Forget the décor. What's the atmosphere like? Barbecue is about good food *and* good times, and at the Dinosaur, they're both in happy abundance. Look around for a reliable kick-back place like Dinosaur where you live.

• • •

Before I left the Barbecue Block Party, I listened to guitarist Chris Bergson and his band playing the blues on a stage in Madison Square Park. It started to rain quite hard, but most people who rolled up to listen stuck around to catch the whole set. I picked up a copy of his CD *Another Day*, along with a couple of bottles of barbecue sauce, at the concession stand. I read up a little about Bergson later. He's from New York. I thought later that the day—what a blast; you have to spend some time at a Big Apple Block Party if you can came to a fitting end, watching a guy from New York playing blues for a crowd feasting on barbecue from Texas, Alabama, and North Carolina, all cooked up on Madison Avenue. Proof once again, for this friendliest and most welcoming of foods, it ain't where you're from, it's where you're at.

BARBECUE SUMMARY

RUN, DON'T WALK, FOR . . .

- Mike Mills's ribs—if you're lucky, prepared by Mike Mills himself.
- **Southside Market hot link sausage**—hot and juicy. Jalapeño Summer Sausage, likewise.
- **Memphis-style ribs** with almost no sauce at all, from Corky's.
- A Carolina pulled-pork sandwich with slaw. Lip-smacking and vinegary.

IF YOU'VE NEVER TRIED . . .

- Barbecue brisket like the Salt Lick's or Big Bob Gibson's. Move beyond the chicken and the ribs now and then.
- Snoot.

16

SANDWICHES AND PIES

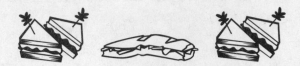

*"You know, a lunch truck. Sold soda, egg sandwiches, and hoagies to the
guys fishing off the docks. That's how hoagies got its name, you know."
Jackmann went to the front of the boat and pulled a fishing rod from
a chrome holder . . . "Guys sold them to the longshoremen and sailors
down the old Navy Yard, off Hog Island. So they called 'em hoagies."*

—Lisa Scottoline, *Killer Smile* (2004)

It's in the relatively mundane worlds of sandwiches and pies that we find
some of the most interesting regional food variations. Many of these
items are made with ingredients that are available throughout the country
but they've taken root in a particular area and flourished to the extent that
they now help define the region. Take the cheese-steak and hoagie, each of
which is inextricably linked with the richly sandwich-laden city of Philadelphia. (Here, Philadelphia thriller writer Lisa Scottoline spices some
hoagie lore into her novel.) Then there is the spiedie and the beef on weck,
both from upstate New York. Throw in a runza, from Nebraska, and a
pasty, from Michigan by way of Cornwall, in the southeast of England.

• • •

My friend Bud hails from Philadelphia. For years we'd talked about making the short trip down from New York to visit the Marcel Duchamp collection at the Philadelphia Museum of Art, but for one reason and another, we'd never made it. Great art alone hadn't been enough incentive for us to go, but as soon as we decided to study the local cheese-steaks, hoagies, and scrapple, we made a plan. Pedro Martinez was pitching for the Mets at the Phillies' that night, too, in case we got bored with eating and wanted to catch some baseball.

After a breakfast of scrapple and chipped beef at the Reading Terminal Market, I took a turn round the market while Bud waited for a friend of his who was meeting us for coffee. There was a small display of other good American markets, and to represent the Los Angeles Grand Central Market there was a photograph of Roast to Go (see page 336). I passed by the produce corner, a place advertising hoagies and salads, a cookbook stall, and Pearl's Oyster Bar. Alas Dutch Corner, the Pennsylvania Dutch section of stands and stalls, is open only Wednesday to Saturday, and this was Tuesday. Dutch Country Meats was open, though, with its **ham hocks** and **landjaegers**—hard, dry "hunter's" sausage—prominently on display.

Bud's friend, Chuck Stokes, a self-described Philadelphia lawyer, showed up and we bought our coffee. On a day when I'd already knocked back a plate of scrapple and was planning to eat a few cheese-steaks and other sandwiches, I was perversely concerned about my intake of caffeine. I chose decaf green tea. Like old friends do, Chuck and Bud picked up a conversation as they if they had last seen each other the day before, rather than three months ago.

The coffee stand was selling **Jewish Apple Cake,** which set off a brief debate between Bud and Chuck. Chuck said the adjective is a key descriptive. He's seen the dish described as "Jewish Apple Cake" in kosher delis, where you'd think the adjective might be redundant. Chuck also filled us in on the Down Home Diner, where we had eaten our breakfast (see page 300). The owner, Jack McDavid, is from southern Virginia, Chuck said, which might explain the grits on the breakfast menu, as well as the **black-eyed pea and hog jowl soup,** pulled pork, catfish, ribs, and so on.

I lamented the fact that the Dutch section of the market was closed and asked Chuck if he shopped there. He said he liked the rotisserie chicken lunches, which wasn't what I expected to hear. From where we were sitting, we could see Tommy DiNic's famous pork-and-beef stand,

and Bud and I figured we'd come back for a roast pork Italian sandwich for lunch.

Bud and Chuck talked over our eating plan. I wanted to make sure we were going to be using our time efficiently and effectively. For sure we'd be trying the quintessential Philly staple, the hoagie. Chuck described it for me. Essentially, it's an Italian submarine sandwich made with capacola (or capicola, an Italian processed meat, pronounced by some as *gabagool*) and Genoa ham, provolone, lettuce, hashed hot peppers, tomato, oil, vinegar, salt, pepper, and oregano. And numerous variations thereof, with different meats, vegetables, and seasonings added and subtracted.

Chuck said we probably knew there were various explanations for the name. I didn't, and was happy to be told. The most common legend (per Lisa Scottoline) is that many years ago, a local purveyor of cured meats put together the sandwich to sell to Italian shipyard workers on Hog Island, in the Delaware River, hence the name "hoggies," or "hoagies." (Sounds good, but tell it to residents of Chester, Pennsylvania, where it's claimed the sandwich originated. Hoagy Carmichael was born Hoagland Howard Carmichael, by the way, in case that name just popped into your head.)

Bud and I mentioned Pedro Martinez and the Mets, which prompted Chuck to tell us about the "Schmitter," a sandwich available at the Phillies' new ballpark, where he said you can get great sausage. (Can you get anything edible at the ballpark near you? Best ballpark food I remember: Candlestick Park, in San Francisco [no longer a ballpark], and Autozone Park, in Memphis.)

Prematurely pleased with myself, I asked if the Schmitter sandwich had anything to do with former Phillies great Mike Schmidt. Bursting my little bubble, Chuck said no, it had something to do with a bar on Germantown Avenue. On the Phillies Web site later, I find that **the Schmitter** you can buy at the ballpark is in fact a registered trademark of H&J McNally's Tavern, Inc. McNally's is a Chestnut Hill bar that serves a cheese-steak on a Kaiser roll with fried salami, fried onions, tomato, and a special sauce. It's apparently named for the favorite beer of a regular who customized his sandwiches this way. Fried salami, wow.

Over coffee at the market, Chuck was proving himself to be a fine resource. I asked him what he thought the essential Philadelphia dishes were. He said he thought if you asked 1,000 Philadelphians that question, 990 of them would answer: (1) cheese-steak, (2) hoagie, and (3) scrapple. So this is sandwich city. I was pleased we seemed to be on the right track.

When we were finished talking about sandwiches, Bud walked his

QUICK BITE

Bud told me that as a general principle, Philadelphia can take something unhealthy and make it more unhealthy. I'm talking about this idea at my son's school with Joe Surak, who in addition to having a career in education is also a professional chef well versed in Philly ways. Joe says he remembers a dish from a street cart that illustrates this perfectly, a concoction featuring the exciting twin bill of bacon and mayonnaise. Joe promises to check with a relative in the city and he e-mails me. "I received confirmation from my cousin yesterday. The breakfast of champions in Philly is, in fact, called **'Bacon, bacon, mayo, mayo.'** It's a hoagie roll slathered with mayo and stuffed with three cups of chopped bacon. Enjoy with black coffee and a cigarette." For a ex-smoker like me, this sounds like what I'd have for my last meal.

friend back through the spruced-up City Hall to his office building. After a dull start, it was now a beautiful spring day, so we changed plans, deciding to keep walking rather than return to the garage to pick up the car. We wound our way around to South Eighteenth Street, to Tony Jr.'s, a small branch of the well-known Tony Luke's. I'd been to the Tony Luke's operation in New York City, and I knew exactly what I wanted—**a pork and greens sandwich** with broccoli rabe, not the spinach option. Because of the punishing nature of our eating timetable, we ordered one sandwich ($5.70) to share and took it to the nearby garden in Rittenhouse Square to eat.

Bud commented that the Rittenhouse Square garden is scaled and laid out like a park in London, and he's right. It's a lovely spot for lunch. We sat on the grass, and I cleft the roll in two. Thinking back, this half sandwich was the best thing I ate all day. The sliced pork is served in what the menu describes as "seasoned pork juice." This flavorsome liquid ran into the seam of the roll and on into the bread. You have to eat it soon after you leave the store because it gets soggy as it cools. The meat was thin cut as advertised and laid over strands of sharp, tart broccoli rabe that was cooked full of garlic. What made the sandwich so great for me were the texture and the delayed afterburn. First, the supremely moist and tender meat and soft roll piqued by the greens. Then—and this all took place in just a second or two—the red pepper flakes crescendoed over the strong garlicky baseline. Once the half sandwich was gone, I was left with a wonderful garlic glow and red pepper burn. Fantastic.

Bud and I left the sun-drenched park and made our way to the Mütter Museum of the Philadelphia College of Physicians. In 1858, surgeon Thomas Mütter donated his collection of anatomical specimens and medical materials to the college. The museum was originally intended as a doctor's resource, but now they'll let anyone in. Aside from the macabre and downright unnerving objects, there were a couple that will live long with me. One is the small jar that shares a display case with cancerous growth removed from President Grover Cleveland. The jar is labeled PIECE OF JOHN WILKES BOOTH. ("You want a piece of me?")

The museum owns a plaster cast of the torso of Siamese twins Chang and Eng. The brothers' livers were connected by a slender piece of tissue, and the conjoined liver is at the museum, too. It's kept below the twins in a modest container with a clear lid that I could see was heavily beaded with condensation. It was not the twins, or the livers themselves, but rather, for some reason, the moisture collecting over the top of the organ that got me.

From one mind-expanding experience, we made our way to another, the Duchamp exhibit. I was especially excited to see *Etant donnés,* a vivid panoramic installation set up behind an old wooden door since 1969, ready

---

QUICK BITE

You like a beef sandwich? In Los Angeles, on your way to the Grand Central Market or the Disney Theater, check out Philippe the Original, where, it is claimed, the **French Dip Sandwich** was invented. Philippe has the feel of a place where good, serious eating takes place. Sawdust on the floor, counter service, big plates of food.

Chicago's Al's #1 Italian Beef was originally a street stand, which opened in 1938. Now it has sixteen restaurants, and in 2002, *Chicago Magazine* named it one of Chicago's seven food legends. Their **Italian beef sandwiches** are sized Little Al, Regular Al, and Big Al, "Actually good, as well as touristy," says chef and publicist Ellen Malloy in Chicago.

And in the North Shore area above Boston, a regional favorite is the **roast beef sandwich,** available from places like Kelly's in Revere and Mike's in Saugus.

QUICK BITE

Some months before going to Philadelphia, I'd visited the Tony Luke's fran-chise in New York with my friend Ivan. When it first opened, the place, lo-cated on Ninth Avenue just north of the Port Authority bus station and across from the entrance to the Lincoln Tunnel, was a take-out location but tables and chairs were added. Ivan and I selected a **cheese-steak with sharp provolone and fried onions** ($6.75) and a **roast pork with greens** (broccoli rabe; $7.25). These sandwiches are great whether you eat one in Philly or New York. I took a picture of Ivan with his cheese-steak, and in it, he's taking a giant chunk out of his sandwich and looks like he could down the whole thing in three bites.

Then, in March 2007, I heard that Tony Luke's in New York was no more. I called and asked what was up. The place was now called Shorty's. "Same food?" I asked. "I'm watching the guy cook the broccoli rabe right now," said Evan Stein, the new owner. Evan said I should stop by and say hi. He'd taken over no more than ten days ago and was living in the restaurant. "So you'll be the tired-looking guy?" I asked. "Yup, the tired-looking guy covered in Cheez Whiz." Evan said.

to trap the unwary. I put my eyes to the tiny holes in the door to see the model of a naked woman lying spread-eagled graphically in front of me. She's lying on a bier of branches and holds a lit gas lamp, and behind her is a Christmas-card landscape with a twinkly little waterfall. "The strangest work of art in any museum," Jasper Johns said. After two or three last looks, it was high time for some cheese-steaks.

As with other regional dishes, there are rivalries and controversies over the cheese-steak. The main competition is between Pat's King of Steaks and Geno's Steaks, both in South Philadelphia. These two establishments are natural rivals because of their proximity. Pat's sits on East Passyunk Avenue, which crosses South Ninth Avenue at an angle. And right across the street, staring into Pat's gunwales, is Geno's. Because of the sharp fronts of each store on the facing lots, they look just like two ships on the ocean, bearing down inexorably on each other. Each is a large stand with a serving window and plastic seats on a triangular section of sidewalk. Geno's is larger and brighter—it's bright orange, in fact—while Pat's is smaller and of quieter aspect.

Bud and I parked and walked up to Pat's window. We chose Pat's first in part because we had parked nearer but also because it had been here first. Pat Olivieri started the stand in 1930. Olivieri had cooked up some sliced steak on his hot dog grill and served it with onions in an Italian roll, which means Pat's is the first name in steak sandwiches. Whose idea it was to add the cheese is the subject of debate we don't need to go into here. Before you order your sandwich at Pat's, you need to decide what you want on it. Pat's helps out with a slightly self-mocking guide: "Step 1. Specify if you want your steak with (wit) or without (wit-out) onions." Then you have to specify the cheese: plain (none) or provolone, American, or Cheez Whiz. A Pizza Steak, with pizza sauce, is also available. So an order for a cheese-steak with Cheez Whiz and onions could theoretically be rendered as "One, wit, Whiz."

At Pat's, you order, and receive, your sandwich at one window and then pass by the mound of steak (ribeye, sliced thin) being cooked on a counter-top griddle to a second window, where you order fries and drinks. We took one **cheesesteak with onions and provolone** (seven dollars) plus giant cups of birch beer soda and a couple of hot cherry peppers you pick up gratis from a condiment station. We ate and sat and looked at the scenery. Mets and Phillies fans were eating here before the game. Together even. We took in a large mural of Philadelphia music celebrities on the back of a building: Frankie Avalon, Chubby Checker, Bobby Rydell, Fabian, Al Martino, Eddie Fisher.

QUICK BITE

In Lizzie Kander's famous *Settlement Cookbook* is a recipe for a "Milwaukee Sandwich." Lizzie Black (Mrs. Simon) Kander helped establish the settlement, which was a charitable institution in Milwaukee designed to assist Jewish immigrants with assimilation into American life. The first edition of the cookbook was published in 1900. The edition of *The Settlement Cookbook* I looked at in the library was from 1921, and the book is still in print. A **Milwaukee Sandwich** is made with two slices of buttered white bread with the crusts cut off. Slice some cold chicken, add grated Roquefort and paprika, toast, and serve hot. It sounds good (the grilled cheese-and-chicken/turkey combo will become a theme later), but does it shout "Milwaukee" to you?

The cheese-steak itself lasted less time than it takes to say those names.

Pat's is soaked in its city. On the pavement in front of the soda and fries window is a brick plaque commemorating the filming of the first *Rocky* movie: SYLVESTER STALLONE STOOD HERE NOVEMBER 21, 1976. As we prepared to move across the street, Bud pointed out a message painted on the side of Pat's: DON'T MAKE A MISTEAK.

Pat's is a mix of aluminum fixtures, red plastic seats, and off-white siding. Geno's is Day-Glo orange all over. Prominently displayed on Geno's prow is a memorial to Philadelphia police officer Daniel Faulkner, who was murdered in 1981. Geno's has been around since 1966, opened by Joe Vento, whose father was already in the cheese-steak game. Vento's son Geno works in the family firm—Geno was named after the restaurant, not the other way round.

After Geno's, Bud and I got lost, then drove toward South Street and Jim's, where we completed our triumvirate of South Philly cheese-steaks. We had split a **cheese-steak with provolone** at Geno's, as we had at Pat's. Standing in the line at Jim's, we decided to go our separate ways. I wasn't feeling gut-wrenchingly full by any means, and I was holding out against the Whiz, to Bud's mild consternation. So I had another **With, with provolone**; Bud, a With, with Whiz. Here, the catering-size can of Kraft Cheez Whiz sat on a corner of the griddle surface so it could be spread when it settled at the appropriate viscosity. With deliberation, our chef put the Whiz right on the Italian roll and chopped the strips of meat with a spatula before overturning the roll and pressing it down on top of the meat. The onions went on last. I took a sprinkling of hot peppers on my hitherto more prosaic sandwich. Jim's, which doesn't sell fries, does sell another Philly product, the Tastykake (see page 128), and cans of Rolling Rock, Pennsylvania's finest and one of my very favorite brews. I took a beer and left the cakes on the counter.

As soon as I entered Jim's, I realized, from seeing the distinctive black-

> ## ✕ QUICK BITE
>
> I read around a little online and found that the last year for which records were available at the time, *Philadelphia* magazine voted the cheese-steak at Tony Luke's Beef and Beer Sports Bar the best in the city. So Bud and I have the first stop on our next trip down the turnpike lined up for us.

and-white floor tile, that I'd been here before, in another lifetime fourteen years before or so. This location on South Street has been in business since 1976; the original Jim's, in West Philadelphia, opened in 1939. Jim's has a couple of other area locations, and Geno's, a place at the Phillies ballpark, while Rick Olivieri, a relative of the original Pat, operates Rick's Philly Steaks in the Reading Terminal Market.

Bud and I sat upstairs at Jim's and compared the cheese-steaks we'd tried. At $6.15, Jim's cheese-steaks were the cheapest. They were also the fullest, which made the feat celebrated on a sign downstairs, of a gentleman who ate twelve in one sitting, more unfeasible still. Jim's sand-wich was slightly drier than either Pat's or Geno's, but Geno's roll was too thick for the amount of meat, I felt. You pays your money, but I enjoyed Pat's for the flavor, and also Jim's steak for the heft. And at Jim's you can sit inside and watch the people go by on South Street.

It was now past seven in the evening and our last task was to pick up a couple of hoagies to take back to New York. We went back to Tony Jr.'s and took a couple of **Italians**—capicola,

QUICK BITE

A lot of chili parlors in Cincinnati sell **double-decker sandwiches,** the local variant of a club sandwich. Double-deckers are made up of three pieces of toasted white bread with various fillings. They go: bread, one filling, bread, a different filling, bread. So you have turkey and ham; egg salad and ham; and so on. A **hippo** is a roast beef and ham double-decker sandwich.

coteghino, Genoa salami, mild provolone, lettuce, tomato, oil, and vinegar ($5.85). We stuck the hoagies in the cooler and drove out of town, trying to find the Mets game on the radio. Bud had told me earlier in the day, as we walked through City Hall, that from a certain angle, it looks like William Penn is in a pronounced state of excitement up on his perch overlooking the city. As we drove away, toward the art museum, I could see what he was talking about, and I said this must have delighted generations of Philadelphians. It made us laugh, too.

Over the next couple of weeks, Bud showed up twice at my apartment with hoagies he'd carried back from south Jersey. The first batch was from the White House, a famous establishment in Atlantic City, and the second was from the Primo's he'd told me about, in Wildwood, where he eats their **Nonna's Veggie** sandwich with eggplant, broccoli rabe, sweet roasted peppers, and sharp provolone. The Italian hoagies just kept getting better.

The **White House** version had a hot pepper hash to perk it up, and Primo's was just primo. This small sample told me it's all about the meat, and also the relative sharpness of the provolone, the sharper provolone bringing the best results.

CONTRIBUTION

Chris Lyons is a restaurant publicist based in Boston. With the customary economy of language of many Bostonians, she provides invaluable help in deciphering some of the unusual terminology and culinary customs in Beantown, starting with the sandwiches.

A BOSTON FOOD GLOSSARY

What They're Called in the U.S.A.	What They're Called in Boston
Subs, hoagies, heroes . . .	Grinders
Hard rolls	Bulkies
Soda	Tonic
Beer	Bee-ah

Just for the record:

◆ Grinders are *hot* submarine sandwiches, anything that gets heated first in a hot oven, like meatballs or sausage.

◆ Lobsta rolls: Always served on a square hot dog bun that has been buttered and grilled. Two versions: with a touch of mayo (cold) and nothing else; or sautéed in butter (hot). These yummy specialties can cost up to twenty-five dollars. Beware of the under-ten-dollar lobster roll.

QUESTION: WHAT IS . . . ?

Brown bread?

Can be made at home using an old tin can and a steamer. Offered at Durgin-Park, our oldest restaurant. Brown bread can be used as a base for a wonderful turkey stuffing.

Indian pudding?

Great sweet dessert made by cooking cornmeal with molasses for hours. Hard to find nowadays.

Clam chowder?

The only type we care about is made with cream, bacon, and potatoes; it's ubiquitous. (See also clam cakes, clam balls, clam stew, clam pie, clam bellies versus clam strips.)

Boston baked bean candy?

Hard and sugary and sold in cute boxes.

Made with cranberries?

Relish, chutney, juice, jam, jellies, preserves, sauce, muffins. Muffins made with a mixture of blueberries and cranberries are called **Sweet 'n' Sours.**

Egg creams, bagels?

Up here, we don't know from them.

The **St. Paul Sandwich** of St. Louis is one of the more unusual around. When I wanted to find out about it, I contacted Thomas Crone for some information. By accident, and much to his own amusement, Thomas has become the local authority on the St. Paul sandwich. He wrote a story about the St. Paul for a Web site a few years ago. Television producer Rick Sebak read the story, and when he came to St. Louis for his *Sandwiches That You Will Like* program for public television, Sebak had Thomas Crone and Crone's friend Kurt Groetsch act as his St. Paul scouts.

Thomas tells me the basics of the sandwich are an egg foo yong patty (a mix of eggs, bean sprouts, and minced onions), served on white bread that has been slathered in mayo and then topped with a pickle, tomato, and lettuce. (There might also be meat, which could be beef, pork, or duck.) You can pick up a St. Paul at any one of dozens of storefront Chinese places, mostly in the south of the city, and they'll set you back from $1.20 up to $2.50 "But never more," Thomas says. (Questions that came to mind, such as "Why this sandwich?" and "Why here?" remained unanswered.)

Kurt Groetsch recalled the film shoot at the Kim Van Chinese Restaurant in the Fox Park neighborhood of the city. Kurt and Thomas ate two

QUICK BITE

Years of French occupation of Vietnam prompted local adaptation of the Gallic baguette into the **Bánh Mì.** It can be found in this country under this name, or as simply a Vietnamese sandwich made with various meats, pork, chicken, or pâté with different vegetable accompaniments. Look for Bánh Mì where there are large concentrations of Vietnamese people: northern California, Orange County, Texas, and so on.

St. Pauls for the program. "And I was spoiling for a third," says Kurt. Kurt likes to take his sandwich with hot chile pepper and sweet-and-sour sauce. The white bread is a key component. The Kim Van restaurant used hamburger buns for a time, but for Kurt, it just wasn't the same. "You need to come away from the table with pieces of bread stuck to your front teeth," he says. He favors Wonder Bread or something similarly "squishy."

Soon after William Ford took over as executive chef of the Mayfair Bar and Grill at the Roberts Mayfair Hotel in St. Louis, he decided to reintroduce some of the hotel's old-time dishes, like the Mayfair Steak Diane. This favorite of the late fifties and early sixties he began to serve table-side in the restaurant.

QUICK BITE

Thomas Crone mentioned other local sandwiches: the **fried-brain sandwich** at Ferguson's Pub and the **tripe, snout, and pig's ear** sandwich at C&K Barbecue. I tried snoot from Smoki O's in St. Louis when they cooked on tour in New York City, and this crispy crackling treat is also available in a sandwich.

Built in 1925 and home to a speakeasy during Prohibition, the hotel created a dish for hungry drinkers—a filling, upscale, one-plate, knife-and-fork meal they called, tongue in cheek or not, a **Prosperity Sandwich.** For his version, Chef Ford takes a thick piece of sourdough, piles it with ham, turkey, bacon, asparagus, and broccoli, pours a sharp cheddar cheese sauce (the original called for a Mornay sauce) over it, adds some Parmesan cheese, and finishes it up under the broiler. The sandwich is very popular—it's the number two seller at lunch. Chef Ford says he'll keep it on the menu as long as he's at the hotel.

QUICK BITE

Back in England in the seventies and eighties, I used to love a good **cheese-and-onion sandwich** with cheddar cheese and as thick a wedge of raw onion as I could stand. (Because it was England, the sandwich's other elements were probably butter and white bread.) It's similar to a **ploughman's lunch,** a staple of English pub food that includes the renowned British delicacy the pickled onion.

    I'm reminded of this by book editor Cassie Jones, who nominates the **Limburger cheese-and-onion sandwich** on rye bread, served on a sheet of wax paper, with an Andes chocolate mint as a chaser, from Baumgartner's Cheese Store and Tavern in Monroe, Wisconsin. "Not to be missed," Cassie says.

On the menu at Bartolino's restaurant on the Hill, the Italian neighborhood in St. Louis, you'll find a version of the Prosperity Sandwich as part of the lunch menu. When I call the restaurant, the Prosperity Sandwich is described to me as an open-faced turkey sandwich with cream sauce, bacon, and melted cheese ($7.95), which sounds a lot like a Hot Brown (see page 267) and less like the Mayfair Hotel original. At Bartolino's second location, Bartolino's South, there's a **Veal Prosperity,** where a veal cutlet and ham replace the turkey. Just across the river, in Waterloo, Illinois, Gallagher's serves a Prosperity with ham and turkey, but does so on an English muffin. If there's a family tree of these sandwiches, the Mayfair Hotel would be at the root. William Ford is from Binghamton, New York, where the sandwich of choice is the spiedie (see page 268). "I could live off those," Chef Ford says.

—————

On three separate occasions I was given unsolicited testimonials about the quality and singularity of the sandwiches created by Primanti Brothers in Pittsburgh. What is notable about a Primanti Brothers sandwich is that it comes with French fries. So what? The French fries are *inside* the sandwich, between the pieces of Italian bread, along with coleslaw, tomatoes, and various other fillings. Of all the variations offered, I was pointed toward the **Capicola Primanti's sandwich.**

I talked to Rick Sebak, a producer at WQED in Pittsburgh and an expert on Primanti Brothers and other local fare. He has reported on a sandwich called **The Devonshire,** which is another variant of the open-faced turkey sandwich, this with bacon and tomato topped with grilled cheese, created near Devonshire Street in Pittsburgh and sold at the Union Grill. At the Union Grill, you can also try a **Pittsburgh Salad,** made with steak if you choose. The feature of the Pittsburgh Salad is the presence of . . . French fries, which in Pittsburgh not only go in sandwiches but on salads, too. If you like, have your steak cooked **"Pittsburgh rare,"** which means charred on the outside and rare within, like black and blue. Pittsburgh Rare is also the name of the fancy-looking steakhouse at the Sheraton Station Hotel in Pittsburgh.

Then there is **The Slammer,** a sandwich made with **chipped ham.** The Slammer originated at the Isaly's in Westview, in Pittsburgh. (Isaly's used to be a large dairy chain in the Midwest.) The Slammer was made with chipped ham grilled with onions on a homemade roll and named for the sad patrons of the magistrate's office, across the street from the restaurant.

From the kitchen of the Brown Hotel in Louisville, Kentucky, comes the **Hot Brown,** a richly decorated open-faced turkey sandwich that has a very similar sensibility to the Prosperity. The Brown Hotel helpfully publishes a recipe on its Web site, and you should really try it out. At Thanksgiving, I handed the recipe to my brother-in-law Buzz, who is a professional chef. I saw the sandwich as a good way to get rid of some of the turkey leftovers, but it was so much more than that. The hotel recipe calls for roux with an egg, Parmesan cheese, and whipped cream added. This is poured over the turkey resting on toast and then placed under the broiler. Slices of bacon are added as adornment. "It's just a Mornay sauce," said Buzz, who made a round of these delicious, rich sandwiches in about three minutes. The Hot Brown is definitely a knife-and-fork sandwich. You can find it beyond Louisville—Bobby Flay's Bar Americain, in Midtown Manhattan, has the Hot Brown on its lunch menu.

Also originating in Louisville, with potential to be spotted around the time of the Kentucky Derby (the first Saturday in May), is the local item called **Benedictine,** which is made with cucumber and cream cheese and which can be used as a dip. ("Ghastly green but good," says Georgia Orcutt of Benedictine.) Everything tastes better with bacon, and Lilly's restaurant in the city offers a **bacon-and-benedictine sandwich,** available with a cup of soup for ten dollars.

To continue this diversion around the course of the Kentucky Derby there is something called Derby-Pie, which the maker says originated at the Melrose Inn in Prospect, Kentucky, more than fifty years ago. Nonproprietary recipes, such as a **Kentucky chocolate pecan pie,** describe a rich pecan-pie-like dessert with chocolate chips.

And, finally, the Pendennis Club in Louisville is said to be the place where the cocktail the old-fashioned was first poured. (The cocktail you might more readily associate with the city is Derby Day thirst-quencher the mint julep.) Also first mixed at the Pendennis Club, in 1881, is **Henry Bain sauce,** put together by a waiter named Henry Bain, who pretty much emptied the club kitchen cupboard in so doing. Recipes call for chutney as a base, with ketchup, Worcestershire, Tabasco, and hot sauces, with A-1 steak sauce thrown in. The sauce needs a strong meat to hold its own in the face of all this: steak or venison might work.

SPIEDIES

David Joachim, author of *A Man, a Can, a Plan* and *The Tailgater's Cookbook,* went to graduate school in Binghamton, New York. Binghamton, Endicott, and Johnson City make up the "Triple Cities," where the **spiedie** sandwich is the local favorite. Each year, it's celebrated during the first week of August, with a Spiedie Fest and Balloon Rally. One year, a hot-air balloon landed in the Joachims' back garden. I don't know if David was grilling at the time, but he's added the spiedie to his repertoire and kindly given us the recipe from *The Tailgater's Cookbook* (published by Broadway, 2005).

The feature of the spiedie is the marinating of the meat you grill for the sandwich.

You can use different marinades and different meats. The sandwich may have begun life in Endicott, when an Italian immigrant named Augustine Iacovelli made a grilled-lamb sandwich with meat he marinated in a vinegar-based sauce. According to this story, the name derives from the Italian word *spiedo,* which is the name of the spit or skewer the meat is grilled on.

You can buy special spiedie marinade, but David Joachim points out that it's basically Italian vinaigrette, so he makes his own. Feel free to experiment with your own recipes, using different vinegars and different meats. (You can, for example, replicate the original sandwich by using cubed lamb shoulder meat and adding some fresh or dried mint to the marinade.) David's recipe for **chicken spiedies** uses a white wine vinegar.

2½ to 3 pounds boneless skinless chicken breast

1 cup extra-virgin olive oil

Juice of 2 lemons

3 tablespoons white wine vinegar

6 bay leaves, finely crumbled or chopped

6 large garlic cloves, minced

1 tablespoon salt

1 tablespoon dried oregano

2 teaspoons dried basil

2 teaspoons dried thyme

1 teaspoon ground black pepper

6 to 8 steak sandwich rolls

David suggests cubing the chicken and mixing up the marinade a couple of days ahead of time, and storing the chicken in most of the marinade in a Ziploc bag in the fridge. Set aside a small amount of marinade, which you'll use for drizzling over the meat during the grilling. The chicken will be whitish from the marinating process. Grill it on a medium-hot grill until it's cooked through but still moist (to about 160°F). Spiedie purists say you should cook the meat on a skewer, but David skips this stage. Put the rolls on the grill for a second, brush with marinade, and then unite with the chicken for your spiedie. You can throw some onions, peppers, and mushrooms onto the grill to put on your sandwich, which can also be adorned, should you so choose, with mayo or cheese.

CORNISH PASTIES

Michigan's Upper Peninsula has been a site of ore and mineral mining for thousands of years. In the 1840s, Europeans settled here to dig for valuable commodities like copper. One of the most productive areas, the Keweenaw

QUICK BITE

Also from New York State is the **beef on weck sandwich,** found around Buffalo and of German ancestry. The "weck" refers to the *Kimmelweck*, which is a round roll, like a Kaiser, with salt and caraway seeds on top. The sliced roast beef can be served au jus and slathered with horseradish for a super-hot finish. Beef on weck is served at locations like the famous Schwabl's, in West Seneca, New York.

Peninsula, which juts into Lake Superior, became known as Copper Country. Mining specialists from Europe flooded into the area, among them Cornishmen, veterans of the tin and copper mines in the far southwest of England. Included with the remembrances of home they brought with them were Cornish pasties—not accessories for Victorian strippers, you understand, but the local meat pies. Cornish pasties are baked with as much legend and lore as any prepared foodstuff around.

From its regional roots, the Cornish pasty (with a short *a* as in "ass-ty," not "ace-ty") has become popular all over Britain. The basic pasty is a rounded short-crust pastry pie, crimped along one rounded edge, usually the top side, and filled with beef and potatoes that have been cut into small cubes, sometimes with other root vegetables like carrots and turnips added. But practically anything, be it savory or sweet, can go in a pasty. This occasioned one of the pasty myths that held that the Devil wouldn't cross over the river Tamar that divided the county of Devon from Cornwall because he was afraid the Cornish would bake him in a pasty.

I was turned on to the fact that Cornish pasties took hold in the Upper Peninsula by Eric Villegas, the chef/owner of Restaurant Villegas in Okemos, Michigan. We talked a bit of pasty. I said I remembered being told the pie was designed so it could withstand being dropped down a mineshaft. The womenfolk would heave a hot pie down to hungry miners, the crust would break the fall, and the filling would survive. This tall-sounding tale Eric hadn't heard. He did know that the correct way to eat the pie was to hold it along the ropelike crimping. Miners wouldn't get the pasty's body dirty that way. Also, the miners would carve their initials on one end of the pie and eat the other half. When they came back for a snack, they knew which pie was theirs. Eric also said the pies would be filled with

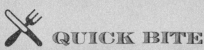

QUICK BITE

You'll find Cornish pasties among the selection of pies at Myers of Keswick, in downtown Manhattan. (Myers is where we've bought our Christmas bangers and Cumberland sausage. See page 85.) Meat pies are at the very heart of English popular cuisine, and Myers has 'em all: **chicken and mushroom, steak and kidney, curried lamb, pork pies, shepherd's pies**, and **sausage rolls** and Scotch eggs. The last two aren't pies as such—a sausage roll is a jumbo pig-in-a-blanket, and the Scotch egg is a hardboiled egg rolled in sausage meat and breadcrumbs and fried, essentially an inedible curiosity, even worse in reality than it sounds.

a savory end and a sweet end packed with dried fruit, to provide a two-course meal in one package. (Neither of us mentioned that it was bad luck for some reason to take a pasty with you out to sea, which I read about subsequently.)

Eric Villegas likens the Cornish pasty to the **Salteña,** which is from Bolivia, the country of his parents' birth. A Salteña uses a different kind of dough and is made with a brothy gelatin. The pie is fully cooked ahead of time and, in cooling, the broth firms up and suspends whatever filling is used. Come time to reheat the Salteña, the gravy melts deliciously.

Eric referred to the pasty by its colloquial name, Cousin Jack's Mouth Organ. Cousin Jack was a name used for Cornish miners, and the mouth organ came about because you eat a pasty much as you play a harmonica, from end to end. Where there was a folkloric Cousin Jack, there was invariably a Cousin Jenny, the wife whose job it was to bake the pies, hence the name of Cousin Jenny's Gourmet Pasties, a flourishing specialty store that operates in Traverse City, Michigan. Cousin Jenny's proprietor, Jerilyn DeBoer, knows well the origins of the pasty. In the 1840s, Michigan's Upper Peninsula was a frontier region with multiple deposits of not just copper but other minerals, such as iron ore, creating boomtowns like Hancock, Houghton, and Marquette. Along with the Cornish came other European settlers, including what became the largest concentration of Finns outside the homeland (of which, more overleaf.)

Jerilyn had even more pasty lore. From the first, pasties were primarily filled with leftovers, so the name comes from a contraction of "passed day's meal." The miners packed the pasty in their pocket as they left home and heated them up on the backs of their shovels. "Love letters from home," they were called.

Jerilyn's family had owned a pasty shop a while back, and she ate a pasty a couple of times a week. She was once a dental technician but left that line of work and started up her own shop with her husband, Nicholas, in 1979. Jerilyn works from three in the morning to two in the afternoon in her store, a block from Lake Michigan. She bakes eight types of pasty, each using a flaky pastry crust made from flour, margarine, and water surrounding a filling cut into the small cubes I'm familiar with from home. You can start the day with a **breakfast pasty** (with hash browns, sausage, bacon, ham, and cheese) or try a **vegetable pasty** (seven veggies with cream cheese and cheddar, available in a whole wheat crust), or the **steak and cheddar,** the **French** (with scalloped potatoes, cheese, green onions, and sour cream), the **chicken** (basically an enclosed chicken pot pie), or the **German** (Swiss, ham, and sauerkraut). These pasties are all a far cry from those I recall from my youth. As with most things, this is no doubt a positive.

RUNZA

You're most likely to find a **runza** at the restaurant chain of the same name, centered in Nebraska. I found one in New York City in my son's backpack whence I unloaded it after a day of school. Wrapped in aluminum foil and frozen, the runza had been driven straight down Route 80 from its point of origin in Wahoo, Nebraska, and through the Lincoln Tunnel by my son's Cornhusker music teacher, Robert Kennedy. (Robert and his wife, Donna, did have other business in the state than just trafficking in runzas.) Robert said that Husker football fans getting together outside Nebraska to watch games might have runzas shipped in, together with some of the state's favorite, **Valentino's Pizza** (forty-one locations in Nebraska and neighboring states).

The runza had a life before it was a Runza—it has a similar lineage to the bierock and the pierogi, being an Eastern European/Russian filled roll. "A Runza sandwich is a delicious blend of fresh ground beef, cabbage, onions, and special spices all baked inside homemade bread," says the blurb from the Runza restaurant people.

Per Robert's instructions, I kept my runza frozen after it was delivered, and microwaved it when I was ready to eat. The filling is completely enclosed, so you have no hint of what is within till you take a chunk out of it. I liked it. There's some bite provided by the cabbage, and the seasoning takes the meat over the bland line. As the sandwich had sat in a cooler for a day's driving, then been frozen and reheated, it had stood up remarkably well. There are seventy Runza restaurants, almost all of them in Nebraska. The nearest one to where I live would be the first one you hit on Route 80 out of New York City, in Council Bluffs, Iowa.

SANDWICHES AND PIES SUMMARY

RUN, DON'T WALK, FOR . . .

- Anything from Philadelphia: The **pork and greens** sandwich with broccoli rabe from Tony Luke's in Philadelphia. Peppery, sharp, fantastic.

- **Jim's cheese-steak** with Provolone and onions: A great sandwich, and this saves you from having to choose between Pat's and Geno's.

- A **hoagie** from Primo's with all the fixin's.

- A Kentucky Hot Brown sandwich: Not tough to make, very tough to resist.

IF YOU'VE NEVER TRIED . . .

- A Cornish pasty: Good whether from England or from Michigan.

17

DELI FOOD, SALADS, AND CHEESE

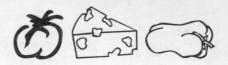

"Harry was always good company," said May Southern,
who would soon marry Bess [Truman]'s brother George. Harry,
she said a lifetime later, never complained about anything unless there
were onions in the potato salad. "Harry didn't like onions."
—David McCullough, *Truman* (1992)

There are a number of landmark Jewish delicatessens in New York City. One of the most famous is Katz's Delicatessen, on East Houston Street in Manhattan. (If you don't know it for the food, this was where Meg Ryan showed Billy Crystal how to fake an orgasm in *When Harry Met Sally*.) This is a place that isn't afraid to toot its own horn. "New York's Oldest and Best Delicatessen" is what they tell you here. Katz's is certainly the oldest, founded in 1888 a few years into the era of massive immigration into the United States. In the forty years after 1880, approximately twenty-three million people immigrated to the United States, many of them through New York City. Three million or so of these immigrants were European Jews, and hundreds of thousands of them settled on New York's Lower East Side.

Significant institutions of Jewish immigrant life were gradually established. Yiddish theater arrived with a performance by young Boris Thomashefsky on East Fourth Street in 1882. The great Eldridge Street Synagogue opened in 1887, and the *Jewish Daily Forward*, under its pioneering editor Abraham Cahan, started publication in 1897. By this time, Katz's Deli had been operating for ten years. There were many other delis round here then, but only Katz's remains, soaked in history. Here, they say, originated the slogan "Send a salami to your boy in the army," which was coined during World War II, when three sons of the owners were serving.

Visiting Katz's is not something for the terminally meek. Be brave when approaching the counter. My feisty Scottish friend Sean managed to get into an argument with a fellow patron here. You can take a seat in the functional dining room or you can engage with one of the countermen. If you don't know what to have, it's probably safest to order one of the gigantic hot sandwiches on your choice of bread (or split one with a friend; they really are huge). Katz's cures its own **corned beef,** which is hand sliced. There are sandwiches with **pastrami, brisket,** and **knoblewurst** (garlic-infused beef sausage), and the **Reuben sandwich** with corned beef, Swiss cheese, and sauerkraut. With a pickle on the side, any of these would be a good choice.

Katz's ships, and not just a salami to your boy (or girl) in the army, but knish, cheesecake, bagels, **bialys,** and their extraordinary meat: sliced brisket and beef, turkey, corned beef, and pastrami: 1-800-4HOTDOG (446-8364) / www.katzdeli.com.

This part of New York has changed dramatically in the past few years. For one thing, some people would have you refer to it as LES, not the Lower East Side. Near Katz's on East Houston Street, the Sunshine movie theater moved into an old Jewish vaudeville theater whose company had vacated fifty years before. South of Katz's are the recent young hipster destinations on Rivington Street, including Schiller's Liquor Bar, which does a terrific **fish-and-chips** and other fine fare amid the cacophonous tocsin of the young and splendid at play.

Just to the west of Katz's Deli is the Yonah Schimmel Knish Bakery, which has been here since 1910. Next door nowadays is a Howard Johnson. The knish is a kind of potato dumpling wrapped in pastry and baked or fried. They can also be filled with various vegetables or meat or cheese. At Yonah Schimmel you can examine the knishes and strudels and other baked goods on display in an ancient glass case. I've had knishes that were so dry you felt you might choke to death getting them down. At Yonah Schimmel, however, I liked the **red cabbage knish,** which was very moist and sharp-flavored and not bland at all. I liked the **spinach** also. The other fillings available at Yonah Schimmel are kasha, vegetable, mushroom, cabbage, and broccoli.

Ship Yonah Schimmel knishes by the dozen: download the form from www.knishery.com and fax to 1-212-477-2858.

QUICK BITE

David Kamen is an associate professor at the Culinary Institute of America, in Hyde Park, New York, one of America's oldest and most prestigious culinary schools. David says, "If you are coming to New York, especially Queens, you can't miss Ben's Best Deli on Queens Boulevard and Sixty-third Drive, where you will find the best **corned beef** and **pastrami on rye** and potato knishes that ever existed."

Ben's Best sells kosher heroes, cocktail party nibbles, and giant containers of spreads serving up to thirty people: 1-718-897-1700 / www.bensbest.com.

Artie's menu includes traditional deli favorites like **flanken** (beef on the bone in mushroom and barley soup), **liver and onions,** various chicken soups, and **stuffed cabbage.** There is the Reuben sandwich, which Artie's offers with corned beef or pastrami, and with corned beef *and* pastrami, along with the sauerkraut, grilled Swiss, and Russian dressing, and also in a turkey, chicken, brisket, and vegetable version. The restaurant thoughtfully extends this largesse to other dishes. A **Two Pastrami Dog Deluxe** is a frank with pastrami. The **Knishpuppy Deluxe** promises a frank inside a knish. Most decadent of all is a **Pastrami Burger Deluxe,** a half-pound burger with grilled pastrami laid over the patty.

Artie's does catering, like the "My Son's Becoming a Doctor" special, and will ship the "Displaced New Yorker Care Package" for you, which includes the essentials—homemade pastrami, salami, rye bread, sour pickles, mustard, and **rugelach** (a Jewish pastry): \1-212-579-5959 / www.arties.com.

Barney Greengrass ships sliced meats, fish (including whitefish and **sable** and oestra caviar, if you fancy): www.barney greengrass.com.

I spoke with Lévana Kirschenbaum, co-owner of kosher restaurant Levana and author of *Levana's Table: Kosher Cooking for Everyone*, and asked her for a deli recommendation. She talked fondly about the world-famous Second Avenue Deli, which closed in 2006 over a rent increase. (There were soon reports that the deli would be replaced by yet another branch of a major bank. In twenty years' time, every single retail property in Manhattan will be either a bank or a drugstore.) Lévana told me about Mr. Broadway, on Broadway between Thirty-seventh and Thirty-eighth streets. Lévana says the **pastrami sandwich** is "fabulous." As for the coleslaw, "I don't know what the heck they put in it. It's out of this world."

As for delis in other parts of the city, many people on the Upper West Side swear by Barney Greengrass, which has been around since 1924. The **whitefish** is famous. My family likes the upstart Artie's Delicatessen, which has only been around since 1999, so shoot me. They bring you a big bowl of coleslaw and a selection of pickles and peppers right off the bat, which might stop you from overordering. The **potato pancakes** are crispy and fluffy alike. Bet you can't eat just two. Artie's will cut you **extralean pastrami,** for a small premium. This may not interest purists, but if it is a choice between extra-lean pastrami and no pastrami at all, which would you rather have?

If you're going to Yankee Stadium, a good place to know about is the Court Deli in the Bronx, between the Bronx Courthouse and the stadium, which my baseball buddy Gary likes to hit before the game. Yankee fans line up here for the pastrami sandwiches and hot dogs and carry them through security in transparent plastic bags. The food is good; much better than the stuff inside the stadium, where the dogs can be wan and beer may well have passed ten dollars a pop by the time you read this.

PREPARED SALADS

In her book *Perfection Salad*, Laura Shapiro details the rise of the prepared salad that came about during a period of revolutionary change in American kitchens, the turn of the twentieth century. Fresh salad was an unmistakable sign of an upper-class household. The middle classes, keen to show off the increasing number of gadgets and processed and prepared foods available, began organizing messy raw ingredients into futuristic salads.

Frozen cream cheese and hard-boiled egg yolks mixed with mayo and rolled in cottage cheese was a **golf salad.** A pear half stuck with almonds was a **porcupine salad.** The mania for neat salad reached a height with the use of gelatin. When the Knox Company put granulated gelatin on the market in 1893, it became a much easier product to use, and soon everything was being suspended in it.

In the first decade of the twentieth century, the **Perfection Salad** was put together, a mixture of cabbage, celery, and red peppers bound in plain and then tomato aspic. *James Beard's American Cookery* says that a Perfection Salad won third prize in a competition sponsored by the Charles Knox gelatin company in 1905. Mrs. John E. Cooke of New Castle, Pennsylvania, won a hundred-dollar sewing machine. The recipe includes sugar, vinegar, and lemon juice in the gelatin, with shredded cabbage, celery, and pimiento

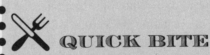

QUICK BITE

It was in the late-nineteenth-century era of prepared salads, in 1893, to be precise, that the **Waldorf salad** made its first appearance. A mix of apples, nuts, celery, pineapple, and mayonnaise, it demonstrates two other trends: the appearance of dessert foods in savory dishes, and the ubiquity of mayo.

to be suspended. It says the Perfection Salad should be served on a bed of greens, aka actual salad.

Salads like this are not merely historical curiosities. They live on to this day. On her weblog *Making Light,* Teresa Nielsen Hayden wrote a fascinating piece on some of the food of Mormon Utah (http://nielsenhayden .com/makinglight/). Teresa was brought up in central Arizona as a member of the Church of Jesus Christ of Latter-day Saints. Mormon people currently make up over 60 percent of the population of neighboring Utah (a number that is trending down). Nielsen Hayden has outstanding LDS credentials because her great-great-grandfather was once imprisoned with Mormon founder Joseph Smith. Nielsen Hayden now lives in New York, where she edits science fiction books and runs her blog with her husband.

The *Making Light* piece featured a number of extraordinary salads from the author's youth, made with pudding mix or Jell-O, all of which sound almost unbearably sweet. **Orange Sherbet Salad,** for example, features orange gelatin, whipped cream, orange sherbet, and canned mandarin oranges and pineapple. Then there's **Candle Salad.** Picture this: "We dipped our bananas in Dream Whip and rolled them in crushed cornflakes before placing them upright in their pineapple rings and sticking half of a red maraschino cherry onto the tip." If you can't imagine what this looks like, check out the linked picture. As the author notes, "It takes a very, very

QUICK BITE

Chef William Ford of the Mayfair Hotel in St. Louis is custodian to more than one of the city's traditional dishes. In addition to the Prosperity Sandwich (see page 265), Chef Ford is also serving the **Caesar salad with Mayfair Caesar dressing,** which would go nicely on the side of the sandwich for lunch. The recipe for the 1937 dressing is a well-guarded secret. Ford knows it, as do his two predecessors in the kitchen, and that's it. When he leaves the hotel, Ford will tell the next chef. Local restaurants make Mayfair Caesars, but they don't know the real dressing recipe, Ford says. He's been offered money to spill the beans, but he won't tell. (Caesar salad, by the way, is not an American dish, hailing instead from Mexico. Legend is that it was created by an Italian-born restaurateur named Caesar Cardini in Tijuana in the 1920s.)

clean mind to think that up." I think this might be a spoof, but these are, Teresa assures me, genuine recipes from a family cookbook. (Teresa says a friend looked at the book and asked her mother, "What is it about *marsh-mallows?*")

QUICK BITE

As for commercially available gelatin salads, in Virginia, the Ukrop's store-brand **Strawberry Creme Salad** is a sweet treat—sweet but not too sweet, with some acidity, and generous chunks of fruit. The salad is a layer of strawberry/pineapple-studded gelatin, then a thin lode of cream cheese, finished with another layer of gelatin. As far as these sweet salads are concerned, I have no problem with the dishes themselves, I just don't know what you're supposed to eat them with. I probably should stop thinking of gelatin salads as a *salad* as such, but rather as a condiment, like cranberry sauce—then, no problem. I'll take my strawberry creme salad on the side, thank you. Nice big helping. I was surprised I liked it, and you might be, too.

Theresa and I speculate about Utah's stereotypical, yet real, fondness for Jell-O (the official state snack), which shows up in a lot of these salads. She rattled off a number of ideas: gelatin is always the same, it's always good, and you don't have to heat up the kitchen to make it, which is a plus in a place like Mesa, Arizona, where she grew up and where she has seen a temperature of 123°F. It's also cheap, which helps in the often large Mormon family. I added the point I'd heard Francine Segan make about Perfection Salad in a lecture on dessert: it's possible to divide gelatin salads exactly evenly, which might also be a plus with a large band of kids to feed. For the Mormons who went west, it was hard-going for a long time, and perhaps the frugality of the fifties-style use of gelatin has resonated.

On *Making Light* you can read the story of Teresa Nielsen Hayden's excommunication (the official word) from the LDS, seemingly for asking too many questions about women's rights back in ERA days. Now she attends church suppers at St. Augustine, in Brooklyn, a multiethnic church with services in English, Spanish, and Haitian Creole. To represent her traditional cuisine, Teresa often brings a **salad of Jell-O with strawberries, bananas, and pineapple,** and every time, someone transfers the dish to the dessert table. But it's not a dessert, she says. Whether or not the Jell-O dish is a dessert depends on whether it has Cool Whip on it—Cool Whip, it's a dessert; no Cool Whip, not a dessert.

━━━━━━

According to James Beard, Fannie Farmer was one of the judges at the contest where Perfection Salad came in third, and her *Boston Cooking-School Cook Book* includes a recipe for the still popular **coleslaw:**

> *Select a small, heavy cabbage, take off outside leaves, and cut in quarters; with a sharp knife slice very thinly. Soak in cold water until crisp, drain, dry between towels, and mix with Cream Salad Dressing.*

Also in her book you will find **Hot Slaw,** which I for one had never heard of. (The "cole" in *coleslaw* refers to the cabbage: *koolsla* is a Dutch cabbage salad, and the name came from there. It's not a variant of *cold*.)

> *Slice cabbage as for Cole Slaw, using one-half cabbage. Heat in a dressing made of yolks of two eggs slightly beaten, one-fourth cup cold water, one tablespoon butter, one-fourth cup hot vinegar, and one-half teaspoon salt, stirred over hot water until thickened.*

My favorite coleslaw is simply the "**slaw**" that's served with pulled pork in North Carolina: cabbage, onion, vinegar, sugar, black pepper, and salt.

━━━━━━

I turned to Valerie Phillips of the Salt Lake City *Deseret News* to see if she could shed any light on Utah's thing for Jell-O. It turns out that Valerie played a role in the whole business. She writes, "It happens that I'm the food writer who first 'broke' the story that Utah was the lime Jell-O capital of the world—back in April 1994, after talking to a Jell-O sales rep who noted that lime Jell-O sells so well in Utah." Valerie's story in the *Standard-Examiner* received a lot of attention. So did the news, in 1999, that Salt

Lake City had fallen behind Des Moines in national Jell-O consumption. A campaign was mounted involving different constituencies, including the two groups guaranteed to devote time and energy to a cause like this: college students and, naturally enough, the Jell-O manufacturers. The idea was to buy enough lime pudding to return the Jell-O crown to Salt Lake. T-shirts and Jell-O pins were made. Kraft spokesperson Bill Cosby came to town and lobbied state lawmakers to officially enshrine the wobbly foodstuff as the state snack. And in 2001, for better or worse, this is what came to pass.

MANGO SALAD

In the summer I love to make a simple **salad** of **mango,** avocado, red onion, cherry or grape tomatoes, and cilantro with lime juice and olive oil. For four adults I'll use one mango (or two if they're extra good), two avos, half a medium red onion, a punnet of tomatoes, and half a bunch of plucked, thoroughly rinsed cilantro.

Prepare the mango(es). Slice the fruit round its widest point with a sharp knife angled so you're clearing the pit inside. Set aside the half without the pit and cut the pit out carefully. Cut each half of the mango crosswise so you have three-quarter-inch squares cut in the fruit. Then take each end of the half and open it out so the squares are splayed out and ready to be cut off at the base.

After halving, cut up the avocado(es), using the same method but cutting into smaller squares. Then halve or quarter the tomatoes and slice the onion finely. (You'll be putting all the ingredients in a bowl as you go along.) Chop up the cleaned cilantro leaves and squeeze the juice of a lime over the salad and add a little olive oil. I find that this salad goes beautifully with chicken or fish done on the grill.

POTATO SALAD

There's no such thing as really bad potato salad. So long as the potatoes are not undercooked, it all tastes pretty good to me. Some potato salads are sublime, some are miraculous and some are merely ordinary, but I have yet to taste any that was awful.

—*Laurie Colwin,* Home Cooking *(1988)*

With a couple of variations, **potato salad,** you might think, is potato salad. Eggs or no eggs; mayo or oil and vinegar. And no onions, President Tru-

QUICK BITE

Also go to Teresa's *Making Light* site for two recipes for **Funeral Potatoes**, a baked dish that in one version combines potatoes (or, canonically, Tater Tots) with minced onion, a can of mushroom soup, sour cream, grated cheese, butter, and cornflakes. "It tastes really good," Teresa says. It's "fast, easy, and consoling," which fits the bill for something whose name derives from its function as a dish to bring to wakes.

man. Teresa Nielsen Hayden tells a story that illustrates how distinctive this simple dish can be. She was traveling west with a friend, and they planned to make a stop at Teresa's family's home in Mesa. The friend asked what they'd be having to eat. A barbecue, he was told. Immediate family only, so about thirty-five people. They'd be having Teresa's mom's potato salad, which, Teresa said, is the best potato salad in the world. C'mon, says the friend. Everyone's mom makes the best potato salad in the world.

At the barbecue, the friend takes a bite of the potato salad and gets a strange look on his face. "Pretty good, huh?" Teresa says, and the guy replies, "This is *exactly* my aunt's potato salad." Later, the man asked some questions around his normally reticent family and discovered that his own family was Mormon a generation or two back, which he never knew, a fact uncovered by a potato salad recipe. What was it about the potato salad? It has more eggs than a German potato salad, Teresa says, with pimentos and chopped pickle and a very different balance. What potato salad carries your fingerprints?

HOPPING JOHN

Potato salad is one of the great holiday staples: we make it to go with cold cuts on days after the major holidays. Another holiday dish is **Hopping John**—black-eyed peas cooked in a hambone-based stock and vegetables served over rice.

In many Southern homes, Hopping John is served each New Year's Day with the toast that the more black-eyed peas one eats the more prosperous will be the coming year. I like to perpetuate this custom wherever in the world I find myself, and invite friends for Hopping John, **hot cornbread,** *and* **pecan pie**—*welcome* *and simple after rich indulgences from the holidays. But I don't stop there—it's one of my favorite dishes anytime.*

—*Ronald Johnson,* The American Table *(1984)*

TOASTED RAVIOLI

Joe Bonwich of the *St. Louis Post-Dispatch* talked about local specialty **toasted ravioli.** It seems that Italian restaurants in St. Louis all serve toasted ravioli, "toasted" here being a euphemism for deep-fried. The legend is that an order of ravioli fell into a deep fryer some years back in an un-named restaurant and the result turned out to be delicious. Let's be honest. What food-stuff isn't delicious deep-fried? I suspect this was no accident, Your Honor.

By chance, just hours before I spoke with Joe Bonwich, I had set out a box of **Raffetto's Cheese and Spinach Ravioli** for our family's dinner. That night, after the ravioli were cooked, I took a couple of the plump pillows—this ravioli is superb—and sautéed them

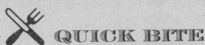

QUICK BITE

I'm reminded of the legend/story of the invention of potato chips, about which event there are more details. George Crum, a man of Mohawk and African American ancestry, was chef at the Moon Lake Lodge in Saratoga Springs in 1853. A particularly fussy customer sent his fried potatoes back because they were too thick. Crum went at the potatoes with his peeler, shaved them thinly, fried them, and sent them back as if to say take that. But the man liked them, and what were first called "Saratoga chips" came to be.

lightly in olive oil, which isn't going whole hog by any means. Golden and slightly crisp on the outside and hot and steaming within, they were quite excellent. So you can pick up ravioli at your local deli and easily make a version of this dish yourself. (I bought my Raffetto's ravioli at Fairway, but you can go to the Raffetto's store on Houston Street and pick it up there.)

A few days after trying my own toasted ravioli, I got to talking on the subway in New York City with a very nice lady who was on her way with a group of friends to Carmine's Restaurant, on the Upper West Side. (Carmine's serves giant family-style platters of delicious Italian American food, notably a wicked **chicken Parmigiana,** so I was glad to see she was taking eleven friends with her.) Clearly not from New York (she had spoken politely to a stranger—me—on the subway), she told me that her group was visiting from St. Louis. I promised to mention Zia's restaurant, where the daughter of one of the other ladies works, so there goes. Zia's does a **toasted seafood ravioli** stuffed with shrimp and crabmeat that sounds pretty good. Toasted ravioli is highly adaptable: another St. Louis restaurant featured a chocolate ravioli with a raspberry coulis. As for the original, Joe equated toasted ravioli with a Philly cheese-steak: it's good if you grew up on it.

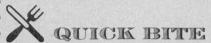

QUICK BITE

Toasted ravioli is one of St. Louis's culinary ambassadors. At Blue Smoke, the New York City barbecue restaurant of St. Louis native Danny Meyer, toasted ravioli is on the menu as a starter. Filled with a little smoked pork, coated in breadcrumbs, and fried, the ravioli is good dunked in some of the marinara sauce that comes on the side.

QUICK BITE

Chef Ford of the Mayfair Hotel in St. Louis tells me he recently came across another St. Louis pasta specialty—mostaccioli, a baked dish he hadn't encountered anywhere else. It's also the name of a type of pasta, which according to Barilla is like penne only longer and with a smooth surface. I asked Barilla if the pasta had a special profile in the state of Missouri, or anywhere else for that matter. They said no, and went on: "Mostaccioli originated in southern Italy, some say Naples, and most likely originated from small, square hand-rolled pieces of pasta dough, joined together at two of its diagonal corners—like another shape called garganelli. *Mostaccioli* is Italian for the whimsical 'little mustaches.'" For the record, Bartolino's South restaurant in St. Louis does have **baked mostaccioli** on its lunch menu.

CHEESE

America produces a lot of cheese. The state of Wisconsin led the nation in cheese production in 2005, making 2.4 billion pounds of cheese, with California a close second, at 2.14 billion pounds. So it's clear Americans eat a lot of cheese, too. Unfortunately a lot of it is American cheese. How did processed cheese come to hijack an adjective that covers all the cheese made in this country? It casts an unfortunate linguistic shadow over the whole industry because there's a lot more to American cheese than American cheese.

Steven Jenkins has been buying cheese for Fairway Market in New York since 1980. I attended a lecture on cheese and wine given by Jenkins at the first Hamptons Wine and Food Festival. Jenkins gives a fantastic lecture. Go hear him (or read his food blog, at www .fairwaymarket.com). To say he was passionate and infectiously enthusiastic does him a disservice. What he said about the food of Sicily made me want to move there permanently and spend my life eating, and I've never even visited the place.

Jenkins talked about great peasant cheeses: **Parmigiana**

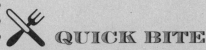

QUICK BITE

According to the *New York Times*, California is fast catching up on America's Dairyland, Wisconsin, in cheese production, having already passed it in milk totals. Wisconsin turned to the dairy industry in the mid-nineteenth century when soil conditions and pests compromised the wheat crop. German and Swiss immigrants led the cheese charge, and by 1910, the state had passed New York for the national lead. New York State now sits fourth, behind Idaho and the big two of cheese.

Reggiano, the greatest of cheeses; the **Burrata,** from Puglia, which is, he said, "like a gland, like eating an angel's pancreas"; and Comté, Le Chevrot, Torta de Cesar, and so on, none of them, alas, American. As an aside, Jenkins pronounced **Jamon Ibérico** as the "World's Single Greatest Edible Substance."

Turning to Jenkins's book, *The Cheese Primer*, which is the only book on cheese you'll ever need, I looked for some American greats: "With the exception of Jack cheese, which originated in California, and Brick and Colby, which originated in Wisconsin, American cheeses are imitations or adaptations of the European originals."

Even jack cheese, Jenkins tells us, was created by David Jacks, who was a Scotsman, near Monterey in the 1890s. Brick cheese came from Wisconsin and was invented by one John Jossi, who took a Limburger curd and squeezed it between two bricks to make a cheese that was like Limburger in flavor but firmer. It is, Jenkins says, "usually a pungent, tangy, semi-soft rindless cheese dotted with numerous small holes." For its part, Colby cheese is like a mild cheddar.

Within the range of American cheeses that are adaptations of European originals lie thousands of fabulous cheeses. There is a well-appointed market with upscale stores located inside Grand Central Terminal. On our way to the crosstown shuttle, Kara and I checked out the Murray's Cheese Shop stand, an outpost of the store's main location, on Bleecker Street in Greenwich Village. Murray's was running a promotion on American cheeses, and we asked for three for the weekend: one smelly, one cheddar, and one blue. The first, I chose. The World Cup was on, and I couldn't resist a cheese called **Hooligan**. I blanched a bit when the half wheel I ordered cost more than $21.00 (per pound, it was $25.99). I hoped this hooligan wasn't beating me up in the wallet for nothing.

Murray's prints an informative little blurb on the cheese's label. Hooligan was described as "a delightfully stinky washed rind cheese from Colchester, Connecticut," that's made by a mother-and-son team on the Cato Corner Farm. Next we picked up a **Cheddar Grafton Four-Star** for $12.99 a pound, a raw Vermont Jersey cow's milk cheese aged a minimum of four years. "Nutty and extremely sharp," promised the label. Third was an **Oregon blue** from the Rogue River Creamery, who have more than seventy years' experience making cheese. Aged a minimum of ninety days, the cow's milk wheel "tastes of smoked meat with a light underlying vegetal tone and a sweet burnt sugar finish on the palate." For $21.99 a pound.

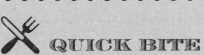

QUICK BITE

Marialisa Calta likes the "extraordinary" **Fernwood** cheese from the Willow Hill Farm, located on Hardscrabble Road in Milton, Vermont. Check out Sheep-cheese.com for outlets selling Willow Hill Farm's award-winning sheep's and cow's milk cheeses. Can we get some **Blue Moon**? It's a "creamy mild sheep milk blue that begins with a bit of tang and finishes with buttery blue earthiness," but they make it only once in a blue moon. Fernwood is a cow's milk cheese described as a "washed rind, unctuous soft cheese made from Brown Swiss/Dutch Belts' milk."

Murray's Cheese has a selection of more than 150 cheeses available, and its own Cheese of the Month Club: www.murrayscheese .com / 1-888-MY-CHEEZ (69-24339).

 Cato Corner Farm: 1-860-537-3884 / www.catocornerfarm.com.

 Rogue River Creamery: 1-866-396-4704 / www.roguegoldcheese .com.

With our guests, we started on the cheeses before dinner, accompanying them with crackers and the recommended fruity red wine. I enjoyed the cheddar and the blue—the first was as sharp as advertised, and the blue had a lot of bite. But I kept coming back for more of the Hooligan. It was impressively smelly. Kept overnight inside its wrapper in the fridge, it managed to perfume the whole kitchen via the subtle wafts of air occasioned by the opening of the fridge door. The aroma was concentrated in the rind, which was thick and salty. Inside, the cheese was beautifully smooth and creamy. If you can find it, you gotta try it. This truly was a sweet and tender hooligan, and it killed me all weekend with its kindness.

QUICK BITE

According to the American Cheese Society, "'washed rind' is used to describe those cheeses that are surface-ripened by washing the cheese throughout the ripening/aging process with brine, beer, wine, brandy, or a mixture of ingredients, which encourages the growth of bacteria." The Hooligan is washed twice a week with a buttermilk/bacteria mix and with brine.

WATCH OUT FOR . . .

As a general rule, it's sensible to cut down on the amount of fat we eat. It's also important to remember that not all fat is created equal. The fat to avoid as much as possible is **trans fat.** Trans fatty acids, or trans fat, is found in hydrogenated fats, liquid oils to which hydrogen has been added so that the fat remains solid at room temperature. (Margarine has a lot of trans fat.) Trans fats are used in many processed foods, where they help extend a product's shelf life—foods like prepared baked goods, snacks, muffins, cakes, cookies, microwave popcorn, chips, and so on.

Trans fat is particularly bad because it raises the LDL levels of cholesterol in the blood (that's the *bad* cholesterol) and also lowers levels of HDL (the *good* cholesterol). HDL is helpful against heart disease, and the double whammy of high LDL plus low HDL can point to risk of coronary heart disease. Our bodies have no use for trans fats at all. They build up in the body over time, and there's no safe level. Avoiding trans fat has become much easier because, since 2006, food packaging has been required by law to include trans fat information. Also watch out on labels for the key words *hydrogenated* or *partially hydrogenated,* indicators of trans fats.

Cholesterol is a naturally-occuring substance manufactured in our bodies. We need it for the integrity of our cell structure, among other things, but too much of it is bad for us. Waxy cholesterol can accumulate in our arteries where thick plaque can form, blocking blood flow to the heart (causing a heart attack) or brain (a stroke). Measurably high cholesterol levels show an increased risk of heart disease. Our bodies create as much cholesterol as we need, but we ingest cholesterol, too—it's part of saturated-fat animal products ranging from meat to cream. For more information, go to the American Heart Association Web site (www.americanheart.org), where the AHA maintains a heart-healthy grocery list.

We also hear a lot about saturated fat, which can also raise LDL levels. So watch out for the amount of meat you eat, especially red meat, also dairy products and some oils, so-called

(*continued on next page*)

tropical oils: coconut oil, palm oil, palm kernel oil, and cocoa butter, all of which have saturated fat. We're encouraged to replace saturated fat in our diet with more healthful, unsaturated fat. These are monounsaturated fats like olive and rapeseed oils; nuts and seeds like hazelnuts, almonds, and cashews; and avocados. Polyunsaturated fats are found in other seeds and oils: sesame and sunflower seeds, corn and soybeans, and so on.

Among the polyunsaturated fats we need are omega-3 acids. In *Newsweek,* Dr. Dean Ornish said omega-3 fatty acids "may reduce your risk of sudden death by up to 80 percent and may significantly lower your triglycerides and reduce inflammation." He suggests you take three grams of fish oil a day. There are different types of omega-3 acids and two key ones: EPA and DHA are found in oils from fish like salmon, mackerel, halibut, sardines, and herring.

It's important that everyone finds out his or her cholesterol levels and talks to a doctor about the results. I address my high cholesterol with medication and get in some exercise a few times a week. (I completed the New York City Marathon in 1999 but stick to lower-impact, and a lot shorter, exercises these days.) If you've read this far in the book, you'll know I'm not a vegetarian, but I try to strike a balance in my diet. Something I hope we've emphasized in this book is fresh food with a lot of fruit and vegetables, but with variety, too. As for me, I'm not going to say, "I'm never eating a donut again," but if I have only three in a year, that's okay.

DELI FOOD, SALADS, AND CHEESE SUMMARY

RUN, DON'T WALK, FOR . . .

- A sandwich from an old-style Jewish deli in New York City.
- Your mom's **potato salad.**

- A **cheese,** like Hooligan, from a small supplier sold to you by someone who knows his stuff.

IF YOU'VE NEVER TRIED . . .

- A knish, from **Yonah Schimmel** in New York: much more interesting than it looks.
- A gelatin salad: much less unappetizing than it sounds.

18

EATING OUT

Breakfast

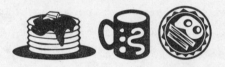

*Bosch sat at the counter at the Original Pantry drinking coffee, picking at
a plate of eggs and bacon, and waiting for a second wind to come.*
—Michael Connelly, *The Black Ice* (2003)

If you sit at the counter, breakfast at the Original Pantry in Downtown Los Angeles might be the best eating deal in all of America. It's not just the food, which is good; it's not just the portions, which are generous; it's not just the price, so low it scarcely seems feasible; it's not just the service, which is attentive; it's not just watching the hash-slingers, which is mesmerizing; it's not just the feeling of history, because you feel like you're eating with the many thousands who have gone before; and it's not just beating the long line outside waiting for a table. It's all of it.

I knew about the Original Pantry from reading Michael Connelly's peerless Harry Bosch novels. According to Connelly, Bosch once ate in the place entirely alone, thereby single-handedly maintaining the restaurant's record of never being without a patron. Harry Bosch is about as stand-up a guy as you're ever going to come across. If he recommends a place, it should be good enough for any of us.

At nine thirty one Sunday morning, my friend Rick and I showed up at the corner of Ninth and South Figueroa for breakfast. Dispiritingly, when we parked the car, I could see a throng stretched across the whole storefront and round the side of the restaurant. I abhor lines. I see a line, and my instinct is to abandon ship immediately, whether I'm food shopping, buying popcorn at the movies, or flying out of town on the holidays. On closer inspection, it turned out that there were two separate lines, both of them long: one for the diner and one for the bakery attached, where the food's the same as in the restaurant next door. I asked a woman on security detail if either was a fast line, and she suggested I go inside and wait for a seat at the counter. That queue had only three people on it. Bingo. So what may have been a thirty-minute wait went away just like that.

Once seated, Rick and I had no need of a menu. (There are no conventional menus here anyway; your choices are displayed on plastic panels and chalkboards attached to the walls.) To Rick's left, in the last seat at the counter, a man was eating an impressive assembly. I asked for what I saw he was having—**scrambled eggs, bacon, wheat toast, potatoes, a dish of salsa** on the side, and coffee. Rick asked for a **ham omelet,** potatoes, and **sourdough toast.**

Once we ordered, we sat back and watched the show. The counter is clamorously busy. Eggs and potatoes are cooked on burners either side of a wide grill. The potatoes start off in a mountainous pile in one huge pan, and then get moved to another pan on the other side of the grill to brown. On the griddle, pancakes—white and buckwheat, plate-size and silver-dollar—jostle with ham slabs, pork chops, bacon, and steaks. Thick slices of sourdough are ladled with bacon grease and pressed onto the hot surface. The two cooks work quickly and precisely and keep a clean grill. Fabulous cooking smells rise up and perfume the air.

We're served quickly, and each of my four plates demands immediate attention. First a chunk of the bacon, double-thick, crunchy, and super-savory, then a bite of toast, then a piece of the brown mantle of the crisp potatoes, and, finally, a dash of the hot salsa, whose hot bite tops and tails what has come just before. My coffee cup is refilled regularly. The server negotiates with a man who's trying to parcel out seats at the counter for his family of five when only ones and twos are ever free. "*Yo la tengo,*" the waiter says to the cook. "Don't worry 'bout it." I watch the cooking and the to-and-fro of people, and I am extremely content to be exactly where I am, doing exactly what I am doing.

Meanwhile, Rick is talking to his neighbor, who says he eats here often. The regular fills Rick in on some Pantry etiquette (adjust your tip if you're sitting awhile) and menu advice (come at night for an **open-faced turkey sandwich**) and repeats some of the Well-Known Facts about the place. After the Original Pantry opened in 1924, it has never closed. For this reason, there's no key for the front door. Maybe that's true, maybe not. It is true that the restaurant is owned by the former mayor of Los Angeles, Richard Riordan.

Our breakfast neighbor tells a good story about eating breakfast here once seated between a couple who talked over and around him his whole meal. Reasonably enough, he suggested that they sit next to each other so he wouldn't be piggy in the middle, but they refused; this was how they liked to sit. To my right, a man orders three eggs over easy, white potatoes, and a New York steak that he asks to be taken off the grill quickly. An all-underdone meal.

Our check came in at a laughably light $14.40, payable at a caged-off till by the door, and we left $6.00 on top of that, for we had lingered a little. From the counter, you only want to watch the cooking, so on our way out, I looked around at the décor, or nondécor: tables, chairs, some paneling, the menu items spelled out on the walls. Stepping outside, Rick and I frankly marveled at the food to each other. Rick said it was the best ham omelet he'd had since camp at the age of nine. A lawyer by training, Rick is someone who speaks with precision. It was a good omelet, then. Rick corrected himself—what he ate at camp wasn't an omelet; it was scrambled eggs and ham. With that, today's omelet ascended a minor pinnacle.

A Pantry breakfast will set you up beautifully for the day. Rick and I had a plan to go to the Grand Central Market, some blocks north and east of the restaurant. We had the car available across the street. But having just eaten what we had just eaten, Rick and I did what a couple of New Yorkers would do. We decided to walk.

━━━━━━━

After my first visit, I couldn't wait to go back to the Original Pantry. I went with the whole family the second time, around midday on a Monday, when there were no lines. The lunch menus were up on the wall—sirloin tips with noodles, ham hocks with beans, country-fried steak, and so on—but I stuck to what I'd had for breakfast with Rick. Sam had **roast chicken with peas and mashed potatoes,** and Lindsay, **spaghetti and meatballs.** Both ate imperially well. Kara had an American cheese omelet, and liked it fine.

I picked up a little pamphlet on the way out, together with a couple of coffee cups so I could take a piece of the Pantry home with us. There's more Pantry lore in the booklet: how Dewey Logan, "a dishwasher from Denver, started [the Pantry] with five employees and a hot plate" in 1924. The restaurant has seating for only eighty-four patrons but claims it can serve twenty-five hundred to three thousand people daily.

The Original Pantry is a perpetual-motion machine. We sat at a table for our breakfast/lunch, but I got glimpses of the work going on at the counter. On the way to the bathroom, I peeked in at the kitchen and the steaming vats of whatever it was bubbling away on the stovetop. Customers pinged in and out of the place, eating in just a few minutes, which helps explain the high totals for daily customers. We were hardly malingering (there was some chocolate cake involved in our meal), but it felt a little like it. There's an entry in the Pantry booklet I liked that characterizes the place for me. When the restaurant moved to its present location, in 1950, it served lunch at the old location and dinner at the new one. I can't wait to go back again. Who knows? Perhaps I'll see someone who looks a bit like Harry Bosch.

There's a special pleasure in finding a great breakfast place, somewhere like the Original Pantry or the Ajo Café in Tucson. The Ajo Café is a small freestanding building by the side of the road close to Tucson Electric Park, spring training home of the Chicago White Sox and the Arizona Diamondbacks. My family visited on a weekday morning, and after a drive past downtown from our hotel, we were a hungry bunch. The menu showed the usual breakfast items, with some southwestern touches. Our friendly server recommended the French toast to Sam, and that is always an easy sell. He'll eat two or three slices of the version we make at home with challah bread; here, he ate two full grown-up servings of the homemade toast that came sprinkled liberally with powdered sugar, before it was covered in syrup.

Kara essayed a cup of **biscuits and sausage gravy** that was thick and rich, as well as a plate of eggs and bacon. I had a **green chile omelet** with some bacon and salsa on the side. I often like Tabasco with my eggs, and

QUICK BITE

Upstairs at Eli's Vinegar Factory, on Manhattan's Upper East Side, the Sunday brunchtime **French toast** is a raft of bounty. Crispy at the crust; inside you wonder where the bread went, because it's almost a soufflé, not quite a flan and well past the quotidian French toast.

Eli's will ship you its **Brioche Braid** loaf to make your own French toast, and other fresh baked breads, overnight, plus coffee cakes, croissants and other breakfast foods and more: 1-866-254-3547 / www.elizabar.com.

salsa performed the same spicy function here. Green chile is a terrific accompaniment for omelets or scrambled eggs. It gives breakfast dishes like this an extra dimension when you're eating out west.

Our Ajo Café breakfast was terrific and a lot of fun. All the staff were sociable and welcoming, and the coffee was good and plentiful. These are essential elements for a successful diner. Fortune has truly smiled on you if you have found a place like the Ajo Café within walking distance of where you live.

New Mexico–styled chile is not a condiment, not meant to enhance, as with a dab of salsa. New Mexico chile is a sauce meant to enrobe enchiladas, burritos, soft tacos, and huevos rancheros lavishly.
—*Katherine Kagel,* Cafe Pasqual's Cookbook (1993)

At seven forty-five on a beautiful crisp Santa Fe morning, I was sitting at Cafe Pasqual's enjoying a strong cup of coffee. Cafe Pasqual's is one of the best-known places in town, with a reputation that's spread far beyond Santa Fe, and a cookbook to go with it. The smallish room is very bright and cheery, with colorful paper *picatas* strung from the ceiling. You can buy the cookbook at the cash register, together with knickknacks like calendars and tote bags bearing the image of Emiliano Zapata. The stuff is all good quality, and you're not overburdened by the commercialism. And the food's great, so why should I care?

My breakfast took the substantial form of the **Chorizo Burrito,** made of homemade chorizo with scrambled egg and home fries in a whole wheat tortilla with green chile and melted jack cheese ($13.75). I separated out some morsels of the sausage to try on their own, and they had a lovely spicy bite. The real joy was in making forkfuls of the burrito slathered in the fabulous smoky chile and piquant cheese. This was, I thought, the burrito gone up-market, with fresh and top-notch ingredients and expert preparation. I had a full day's eating planned. But any thoughts about pacing myself for the day's rigors went out the window (as they would at other points during the day), and I ate the whole glorious zeppelin.

———

Vacationing one time in Las Vegas, I asked the concierge of the Hard Rock Hotel if there was anywhere in "Old Vegas" where our party might have breakfast. In this particular setting, which is a temple to cosmetic rejiggering, the question was asked semi-ironically. I'd wanted to go to the Sands Hotel (1952–1996), but it was shut, awaiting its imminent implosion. We went to the breakfast buffet spread at the Desert Inn (1950–2001) instead. It was quiet, relaxed, and very pleasant, unlike the Hard Rock Hotel, which we found loud and exciting but not quiet, relaxed, or particularly pleasant. Alas the relative sanctuary of the Desert Inn is no longer available either. As is customary, the place was imploded to make way for something grander before it could reach a dignified late middle age.

———

"Business isn't so good anymore," Lefty said. "If you want to open a bar try Greektown. Or Birmingham."

My father waved these objections aside. "Bar business isn't so good maybe," he said. "That's because there's too many bars around here. Too much competition. What this neighborhood needs is a decent diner."

—*Jeffrey Eugenides, Middlesex (2002)*

As we mentioned before, countless diners around the country have been set up by Greek Americans. In the 1920s, Sam Armatas opened five "Coney Islands" in and around Denver, the third of them on Curtis Street in the city. This particular restaurant closed long ago, and eventually the only remaining Sam's was No. 3, in the east Denver suburb of Aurora. But

Armatas's son and two grandsons reacquired and reopened the Sam's on Curtis, so now there are two Sam's No. 3s, and nothing else 1 through 5.

When my brother-in-law Craig married his now-wife Heather in Denver a couple of years ago, my family took in some of the local attractions on the wedding weekend. We went to a Rockies game, a typical Coors Field encounter that finished 10–11 despite neither starter seeming to pitch particularly badly. Although it was empty and quiet, the Red Rocks amphitheater was magnificent to behold. For a couple of mornings, the extended family ate in the hotel where we were all staying, but for the last breakfast, we moved the party down the street to the local diner, Sam's No. 3.

This was breakfast, so I wasn't having any of the advertised Coney Island specials: hot dogs, burgers, or chili. But twenty-one different breakfast burritos were on offer, some including gyro meat and feta cheese, another, the "poppa's as big as a house burrito," promising six eggs with everything up to Mount Olympus thrown in. My **Denver Burrito** was modest in comparison, stuffed with three eggs (scrambled) and home fries, with diced ham, onions, and peppers, and smothered with green chile. To me, this was a revelation. I may have had breakfast burritos with better green chile subsequently, but this great big breakfast just made me happy. I wondered what had kept us, and wished I'd eaten at Sam's the other mornings we spent in Denver. When you're out of town, checking out the neighborhood places beyond your hotel can pay unexpected dividends.

I've never had, in three or four trips to Denver, the meal I nearly always have when I eat breakfast at a diner in New York, namely, a **Western** or **Denver omelet** (these days made with egg whites). When it's cooked up nice and crisp with thin-cut ham, onions, and green peppers, an egg-white Western omelet with a few bites of home fries and a piece of wheat toast is a fine morning repast. There is, on the other hand, little that's more inedible than a watery, undercooked egg-white Denver omelet, which I've had the misfortune to experience once or twice. But never, either good or bad, in Denver.

I had been anticipating my first plate of **scrapple** for a considerable time. Even before I'd started writing about eating, scrapple had been a topic of discussion over the years around the family dinner table. My father-in-law, a native Philadelphian, conceded that, yes, he had eaten scrapple when he was a kid. Kara remembers him eating it when she was a kid herself, when her mom would buy it as a treat. "It stunk up the house,"

QUICK BITE

There's a British breakfast specialty that I've seen on a couple of hotel breakfast menus in the United States: **kedgeree.** It's a decadent mix of cooked rice and fish, often smoked haddock, with hard-boiled eggs. It's thought to have been cooked up by Scottish soldiers (hence the smoked haddock) in India (thus the curry powder It's often cooked with) in the nineteenth century. There's a simple recipe for "kegeree" in Mrs. Beeton's *Book of Household Management* (1859–1861), the most famous early Victorian cookbook from Great Britain:

Ingredients—Any cold fish, 1 teacupful of boiled rice, 1 oz. of butter, 1 teaspoonful of mustard, 2 soft-boiled eggs, salt and cayenne to taste.

Mode—Pick the fish carefully from the bones, mix with the other ingredients, and serve very hot. The quantities may be varied according to the amount of fish used.

Time—¼ hour after the rice is boiled.

Average cost, 5d. [pence], exclusive of the fish.

Smoked haddock is also called **finnan haddie** and is one of the Scots' gifts to the world of food. It's served for breakfast at the oldest restaurant in Utah, the Lamb's Grill, in Salt Lake City, which has been going since 1919 (firstly, in Logan, Utah, and from 1939, in the capital). The restaurant is proud of its longevity, and not much has changed here since 1939. The chairs in the main dining room were imported from Vienna in the twenties. The Lamb's Grill serves other venerable restaurant relics like beef Stroganoff and tournedos of tenderloin.

Kara recalls warmly. The pickiest of the picky eaters in the family would grimace and groan when talk turned to scrapple, and I'd make a mental note: I have to get myself some of that.

And now here it was, on location in the Down Home Diner in the Reading Terminal Market in Philadelphia, a browned, rectangular comestible sitting defenseless on a plate before me, with some scrambled eggs, home fries, and wheat toast for company. I hovered, knife and fork at the ready.

The Down Home Diner has been open since 1987. It certainly looked the part: a counter flanked by lightly colored wooden booths with red seats and a real jukebox at the entrance. I was here with my friend Bud, and he noticed the machine was actually playing records because the Patsy Cline forty-five was skipping. At each table was a giant bottle of Tabasco, another good sign, as was the cranky command printed on the menu: MINIMUM TWO PERSONS IN BOOTHS/39-MINUTE LIMIT.

Bud and I had set off for Philadelphia from New York at eight in the morning. We were held up by some thick traffic on the New Jersey Turnpike before we'd even reached Newark. Bud's itinerary called for us to start at the Reading Terminal. Now and then, as we were moving around the city, Bud would point out some old haunts, the book and record stores, and the site of the old Gimbel's department store where Father Christmas would climb in through a window in the façade every year to cap off the parade. In his youth, Bud would come into the city through the station by the market from his home to the north.

There has been a market in this location since 1893. Spruced up in recent years and subsequently thriving, the market looks great. It was after ten thirty when we sat down for breakfast. With just a cup of coffee each for sustenance, we

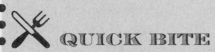

QUICK BITE

Location, location. The ferry to Bainbridge Island near Seattle offers lovely sound and sea views and the promise of a great breakfast at the Streamliner Diner, right near the ferry stop.

were hungry. I asked for scrapple, eggs, and toast; Bud, partly for my benefit, or so he claimed, ordered the **Creamed Chipped Beef on a Raft.**

Expectantly, I cut into my chunk of scrapple. The piece was about three-quarters of an inch thick. The crispy, fried outside layer resisted the knife, which sliced the softer center through to meet the other side. In the mouth, the scrapple had a sharp initial crunch. The taste was savory but not overwhelmingly meaty—there was a lot of sage in the seasoning, and the binding meal was pleasantly leavening. So scrapple turned out to be a subtle, almost understated dish and not harsh at all, as I was half expecting. Bud told me you can eat your scrapple either with ketchup and salt and pepper or with syrup, so it has that breakfast-sausage adaptability.

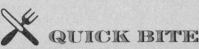

QUICK BITE

In Baltimore, my friend Will recommends Lexington Market for breakfast. He picked up crab cakes from one stall and eggs from another, and had himself a good meal of **crab cakes and eggs.** Faidley's in Lexington Market is famous for its crab cakes and also for selling raccoon and muskrat when they're in season.

Mine came with a little pot of strawberry jam, which went well with the superior heavily grained toast.

Of what scrapple actually consists has been a longtime mystery to me, and it's probably better it stays that way. I suppose you can say it's a delicious pork breakfast loaf, in the same way that a frankfurter is a noble and popular sausage that tastes great in a bun. By the time I ate some scrapple, I figured I knew well enough. At the Down Home Diner there's a T-shirt for sale that reads EAT MORE SCRAPPLE. A scrapple recipe lists ingredients: cornmeal, buckwheat flour, seasoning, meat broth. "Meat broth" is surely a coy euphemism. I decided to peek, and a quick Internet survey finds various versions of the meat: pork shoulder, side, liver, "head meats, skins, tongue, trimmings," intestines, and other offal. There may be truth in all of these, there's everything in here but the squeak. It tastes good, so "don't ask, don't tell" worked better for me.

Bud noted that his creamed chipped beef, or creamed dried beef, wasn't white, as it usually is (being beef in a béchamel sauce), but was more like beef and sausage gravy. Either way, it was very good. The gravy soaked into the white-bread raft for a warm, peppery, delicious mix that was gummable but still carried a very grown-up taste. Before tax, Bud and I

QUICK BITE

From *How We Cook in Tennessee* (1906) comes a recipe for **souse.** It tells you to soak a pig's head and feet. Chop the meat and add salt, pepper, red pepper, and sage. "Press with weights in a bowl. Fry up in hot fat for breakfast." Souse makes scrapple sound genteel.

paid $13.55 for breakfast, and we also had our parking ticket validated, which would save us a few bucks later on. Thus was an already great value meal made greater value still.

QUICK BITE

In Cincinnati you can find **goetta,** a scrapple-like breakfast loaf. Some Cincinnatians make it at home, out of pork and beef, pinhead oatmeal (unrolled oats), and onions. Some like it smoked; others cook it in a loaf pan, then cut it into slices and fry it up. Neighborhood butchers also make goetta, and the commercial manufacturer of it in Cincinnati is Glier's. For the last few years, Glier's has sponsored a Goettafest that celebrates (and promotes) all things goetta—goetta pizza or fudge, anyone?—across the river from Cincinnati, in Newport, Kentucky.

CONTRIBUTION

Marjorie Druker is the chef and owner of New England Soup Factory. ("We serve outrageously interesting flavors that you can feel all over, inside and out.")

I was doing some foliage touring in Mason, New Hampshire, recently and came across a place called Parker's Maple Barn. It's an out-of-the-way place popular with families and motorcycle enthusiasts. They produce their own maple syrup and serve pancakes that are just enormous, bigger than your face. What I really love are their **maple babyback ribs** *that they serve for breakfast. They are tiny and tender, with just the right sweetness. Their breakfast platters are like an old-fashioned country breakfast. The toast they serve is thick and fat, and they bake the bread themselves.*

Another breakfast place that I adore is called Arthur and Pat's. It is located in Marshfield, Massachusetts. Marshfield is not a very fancy place, and neither is the restaurant, but the food always blows me away. It's a brother-and-sister team, and if you go, get the **Ohmygod Platter.** *It's poached eggs on a bed of thin and crispy potato pancakes topped with smoked salmon, capers, and crème fraîche; hence the name. It also has at the corner of the plate a small* **mesclun** *salad that is perfectly refreshing with this meal. I love a place that serves a salad with breakfast. Who ever heard of it?*

 All the hours it is open, Parker's Maple Barn will sell you their breakfast. Online, they'll sell you maple syrup, maple coffee, and attractive-looking cedar furniture: 1-800-832-2308 / www.parkersmaplebarn.com.

———

The Los Angeles Farmers Market at Third and Fairfax is airy and spacious and is a great place for meandering, which you might do inadvertently because it's easy to get lost. And that's okay, because there's nothing here that isn't worth a little of your time. It's also a great place to get a good breakfast.

In the market, Rick and I window-shopped at Magee's House of Nuts and Littlejohn's English Toffee House. After wandering past the Pampas Grill, a Brazilian churrascaria—a self-service buffet—that was still warming up, then Bryan's Pit Barbecue (where you can get an interesting-looking Texas Salad for $7.75), a French crêperie, the Gumbo Pot, and Moishe's Middle Eastern, Rick and I decided to take our breakfast at the Kokomo Cafe. We also eschewed **funnel cakes** at the Country Bakery and a smoked salmon–laden bagel from Phil's Deli in the process. Tomorrow's always another day.

QUICK BITE

In Asheville, chef Laurey Masterton says, her favorite morning spot is Early Girl Eatery.

"John and Julie [Stehling] make good Southern food in a modern-ish way. They use local products from the many farms here. My favorite thing to eat there is the **Southern Breakfast.** Two over medium, bacon (thick and baked with brown sugar, I think), grits (stone-ground white grits), biscuits (which they serve with locally produced jams), and coffee. Very good."

"Al fresco is the fun way to dine," they say at Kokomo, and it is indeed extremely pleasant to sit out under the awning, sipping from our pints of fresh orange juice and listening to the California sound track (Beach Boys, the Monkees, the Righteous Brothers, et al.), anticipating a hearty feed. My **Red Turkey Hash** was terrific—turkey with potatoes, onions, and beets, which colored and flavored the whole dish. It went perfectly with scrambled eggs. Rick's **Breakfast Burrito** with scrambled eggs, double smoked bacon, tomatillo sauce, and cheddar was also very good. With one cup of coffee, we spent twenty-four dollars.

I've also had the **Chicken and Waffle** at Kokomo's, a vanilla waffle with marinated southern fried chicken. The thick waffle was great, with voluminous little crenellations for the syrup and cinnamon butter, and the chicken was just the right side of greasy. If Kokomo was at the end of my block, and it brought the Southern California weather along with it, I could happily eat there every day.

DIM SUM

[Guangzhou (Canton)] is the home of dim sum (literal meaning "heart's delight," or, "to touch the heart"), famous beyond China's borders because they were carried by Cantonese immigrants around the world.

—Ken Hom, Taste of China

We pulled into the parking lot of the East Manor Restaurant in Flushing, Queens, at 10:15 on a Saturday morning. We tucked into our first dim sum around 10:21. One of the numerous joys of dim sum is that there's no wasted time with menus or long waits for your order to arrive. Food is brought to you on a steady succession of wheeled steam trays that you either accept or decline as they are offered. You can also go and pick up dishes yourself, at the serving stations where they are cooked. The dim sum are small dishes like dumplings, fish balls, tiny tarts, little plates of ribs and chicken feet and fried pork skin, puddings, and rice gruel. At the East Manor there were so many different dishes to try. We were a large party with different likes and dislikes, eating at different rates. Kids tend to get to dessert more quickly than grown-ups. That's all okay, because you can eat what you want in any order you like. This was certainly the first time I had **beef tripe with jalapeño** immediately preceded by a dish of **mango pudding**.

We and our friends Paula and Bob brought our families together at the

East Manor. Paula is Chinese American and ably guided us through the food, about which Bob is also very knowledgeable. First Paula ordered our tea, a vital component of the meal, choosing **chrysanthemum tea,** with tiny pieces of flower floating in it and rock sugar on the bottom of the pot slowly releasing sweetness. It was lovely. The small teacups drain quickly, and everyone refills his neighbor's cup when he sees it's empty. It's customary to tap your fingers a couple of times to say thank you in return. If you want more tea, turn the pot lid over to show a waiter you're in need of a refill. There were so many staff flitting around the large dining room that none of our wants went unfulfilled for long.

Paula took us to the long table at the front of the room where hot dishes were being auditioned. I asked her what the big character up on the wall behind the table meant, and she said it was the symbol for luck, repeated back-to-back, so it says "double luck."

It's good to start off with some leafy vegetable. We selected **pea greens** that were poached for us and served with a bowl of **oyster sauce.** Then there were bowls of duck feet (a lot of work, said Paula), **curried fish balls,** beef tripe, fried pork skin, **glutinous rice with filling,** and **congee with thousand-year-old egg, scallions, and pork.**

Together we picked out some dishes and sat down. We asked for a lazy Susan for the table: it's a key accessory. It's also fun for the kids to pass the food round the table that way. In steady succession, more food was offered to us: **shrimp dumplings, garlic-chive dumplings with fish, steamed barbecue pork bun,** pork-filled pastries, bright green **sesame paste buns** . . . I grappled with the glutinous rice filled with dried scallop, peanuts, mung bean, and salted egg yolk, which has a grainy consistency and an intense flavor. Many of these dishes are Cantonese, southern Chinese, where rice predominates, said Bob, who talked about dim sum variations he had tasted in Vancouver and Hong Kong. Never mind that, I was having trouble keeping up with what was right in front of me.

At some point, we had **steamed pork ribs** with black beans and jalapeño, **shu mai**—steamed open-faced dumplings made from wonton skin with pork and shrimp decorated with shrimp eggs. I ate some *juk,* the congee or rice gruel, with preserved egg. Paula said this is an acquired taste, but I liked it—thick and savory and flecked with the egg. To make preserved eggs, they are boiled and buried in lime, not perhaps for a thousand years but long enough for the white to turn an obsidian color and the yolk a dark green and for the egg to develop an aura of ammonia, like a stinky cheese rind. The curried fish balls were good. Made of a bound liquid, they're of a surprising consistency, bouncy in the mouth. Some green peppers stuffed with fish I liked a lot. Tofu skin wrapped round bamboo shoots, pork, and shrimp I missed; fried tofu with shrimp I tried.

Paula waved away the desserts for a while. After watching one particular corner over her shoulder for some time, she jumped up and took us over. A batch of **dan tat** were just coming out of the oven. Dan tat are little egg custard tarts that are fantastic eaten hot. They're everyone's favorite, which is why there's a small melee at the oven door when they're ready. All the pastry was rich and superbly flaky. There's no dairy in Chinese cooking (most Chinese adults do not have the lactase enzyme that allows the body to digest milk products), so the pastry is made with lard. Which is why it tastes so good. But dan tat is extra special, a beautiful deep yolky yellow, hot and sweet and melt-in-your-mouth.

Paula said we were early, and not every dish was out yet. We'd seen even more food on another lap round the edge of the room, the vat of steaming squares of poached duck's blood, fried crullers, live buffalo carp, and crabs in their tanks.

By now we were eating dessert dishes, too: squares of wobbly coconut jelly you have to impale on two chopsticks to eat, the sweet mango pudding with coconut, and wonderful **steamed rice crêpes** with sweetened soy sauce. The last can come with shrimp or beef, but these were unadorned. Slippery folds of soft silk, they're hard to manipulate, too, but they slid right in. Delicious.

Suddenly Paula called out, "Here comes the pig!" **Roast suckling pig.** We called some over. The rich fatty pork has unbelievably crisp skin. It's set on a bed of pickled daikon to cut the fat. Just divine. A couple of picks at what was left, and I was done. I was determined to split the check, but Paula grabbed it. Throughout the meal, the card we'd been given was marked with a little stamp every time we ordered a dish. We had accumulated a lot of stamps. When I protested, Paula and Bob told me we were their guests. Because I was going to write about the meal, she told me I could look at the check. Including service, the bill was $109.18, which I couldn't believe. A lot of the dishes were two bucks; my gallon of tea cost fifty cents. What a great meal. Looking at the debris on the table, I saw there was one last *dan tat*. I offered it to everyone and then, with their permission, finished it off.

EATING OUT: BREAKFAST SUMMARY

RUN, DON'T WALK, FOR . . .

▦ Breakfast at the counter at the Original Pantry in Los Angeles. A little breakfast theater, and less of a line.

▦ A **breakfast burrito** at Cafe Pasqual's in Santa Fe is a civilized way to start any day.

▦ **Red turkey hash** at Kokomo Cafe in Los Angeles, where you can plan the rest of your eating day in the most amiable surroundings.

▦ **Dim Sum** at the East Manor in Flushing, New York. With the Original Pantry, the best *Eat This!* meal bargain I had. Dim sum's designed for lots of people—get some friends together and try it. Kids can try stuff they've never had; friends can hang out and eat. Good times.

IF YOU'VE NEVER TRIED . . .

▦ Scrapple. There's nothing to be afraid of.

19

EATING OUT

Lunch and Dinner

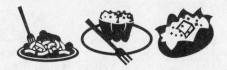

*The lunch was delicious. Trina and her mother made a clam chowder that
melted in one's mouth. The lunch baskets were emptied. The party were
fully two hours eating. There were huge loaves of rye bread full of grains
of chickweed. There were wiener-wurst and frankfurter sausages. There
was unsalted butter. There were pretzels. There was cold underdone
chicken, which one ate in slices, plastered with a wonderful kind of
mustard that did not sting. There were dried apples, that gave Mr.
Sieppe the hiccoughs. There were a dozen bottles of beer, and, last of all,
a crowning achievement, a marvellous Gotha truffle. After lunch came
tobacco. Stuffed to the eyes, McTeague drowsed over his pipe, prone on his
back in the sun, while Trina, Mrs. Sieppe, and Selina washed the dishes.*
—Frank Norris, *McTeague* (1899)

*Bad dinners go hand in hand with total depravity,
while a properly fed man is already saved.*
—Estelle Wood Wilcox, *Buckeye Cookery* (1880)

Many factors come together to help us decide what we're going to have for lunch or dinner. When we're entertaining, many of us will stick with what's familiar, which often means preparing the food we grew up with. Take the late-nineteenth-century picnic that the fictional Swiss German Sieppe family puts on in Schuetzen Park across the bay from San Francisco for McTeague, a young dentist of Polk Street. Novelist Frank Norris mocks the unassimilated German family whose daughter is being courted by the apparently respectable but doomed dentist McTeague. (*McTeague,* by the way, is a great book with a wild ending.) From the tastes of home the Sieppes have strayed not an inch. I have to say, this meal sounds pretty good to me, though we'll skip the postprandial smoke, and I'd hope the men would help out doing the dishes.

I love talking to chefs to hear about the interplay of influences they recognize in their cooking. The chef might play off features of the culinary heritage he was born into. She'll inevitably be swayed by the traditions of the locality where she's set up shop. And a vital consideration will be the fresh ingredients that are readily available to the chef, at markets in town, from farms in the adjoining countryside, and often in the garden that the restaurant maintains for its own vegetables and herbs. My appreciation of the food I eat increases when I know a little about its various contexts.

What follows is a tiny sampling of meals from various parts of the country: from Miami through Atlanta to San Francisco and Tucson, via Okemos, Michigan. There are a few detours, including one to Hawaii for a plate lunch. This food demonstrates how easy it is to travel round the world gastronomically without ever leaving the country. Would that I had

QUICK BITE

My friend Ivan is a big fan of the Mountain Brauhaus in Gardiner, New York. On a fall weekend, he and his family drive upstate to go apple and pumpkin picking and to have lunch at the Brauhaus outside New Paltz, with its views of the climbers shinning up the Shawangunk Mountains. Ivan always picks the **Jaeger Schnitzel,** the sautéed breaded veal cutlet with onions, mushrooms, and sour cream, and an order of red cabbage on the side. If he takes some of whatever is on tap that day, his wife, Patty, will be the designated driver home so Ivan can take a nap.

more time to eat more of this—I couldn't even get to all the food I wrote about here. I relish the feeling that there's so much more food to try. Question is, where to start?

JANOS WILDER'S TUCSON

At his restaurant, Janos, chef Janos Wilder has been feeding the happy residents of Tucson and its visitors since 1983. In 1998, Janos moved to its attractive location at the Westin La Poloma Resort and Spa, and in 1999, Chef Janos opened J Bar, a more casual version of the original restaurant, in the same building. My family had a couple of terrific dinners at J Bar, where the dishes feature the food of southern Arizona, Mexico, and the Caribbean, expertly put together by Chef Janos. We already mentioned the Oaxacan Avocado, Date, and Tangerine Salad (page 34). See if you can pick out the influences here:

- **The Original Jerked Pork with Cranberry Habañero Chutney,** cilantro, chili slaw, chorizo, black beans, smoked poblano, crema [sour cream], and flour tortillas ($14).

- **Yucatan-style Plantain Crusted Chicken** with Green Coconut Milk Curry, roasted corn vinaigrette, pineapple rice, and cilantro chili slaw ($14.50).

Janos took the scenic route to Tucson. As a teenager growing up in California, he worked in a pizza parlor, and kept cooking even as he earned a political science degree from Berkeley. After school, he was a chef at a restaurant in the mountains in Colorado and one in Santa Fe, and then studied French cooking in Bordeaux at one- and two-star Michelin establishments. French food remains Janos's first culinary love.

Janos and his wife, who is from Nogales, settled in Tucson. Janos said he wanted to keep eating French food, but a stronger imperative for him was being faithful to the tradition he'd learned there. "The

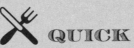

QUICK BITE
As part of his hunt for ingredients, Janos went on a search for native seeds. Check out NativeSeeds.org, which seeks to conserve the ancient indigenous and early agricultural seeds of the southwestern United States and northwestern Mexico. The company currently grows 350 varieties at its farm in Patagonia, Arizona.

heart and soul of French cooking is the relationship between the chef and the gardener," says Janos. "The best are the things that are closest to you." Janos started to explore what grew in southern Arizona. When he was planning his own restaurant, he advertised for gardeners before he advertised for restaurant staff.

So, using refined French techniques, it is local and regional ingredients like mesquite flour and blue cornmeal that feature in Janos's cooking. Janos has also delved deep into his wife's native Mexico, specifically into the Oaxaca region, arguably the culinary heart of the country, he says. Janos leads fund-raising tours to Oaxaca for native seed searches and takes big bags to bring produce back with him. He says that Oaxaca has its own microclimate and, as a result, grows specific and unique produce, like its squash, greens, and chiles. He can't get the same ingredients in Tucson, so he adapts what he has for the specifically Oaxaca-inspired dishes.

Take the **Smoked Tomato and Pasilla de Oaxaca Soup** with tortilla shards, Manchego, and toasted corn puree, as described by Janos himself. The pasilla, a small, smoky, black chile, works with the corn vinaigrette against the richness of the creams and Manchego cheese in the soup. Corn and tomatoes are natural complements to each other, and the tortillas provide a textural context. Janos adapted a recipe from Susana Trilling, a longtime exponent of Oaxacan food, to make his **Oaxacan Bread Pudding** and ancho (chile) caramel ice cream with Almendra (almond) sauce. I love this pudding.

────────

Monica Flin opened El Charro Café in Tucson in 1922. Today El Charro has branches round the region selling quality Mexican standards. El Charro's signature dish is **Carne Seca,** seasoned air-dried beef that's desiccated in a container on the roof of the restaurant. The popular Mexican restaurant dish the chimichanga is said to have been invented in Tucson, and El Charro features a Carne Seca Chimichanga. I decided to order one to get a taste of both specialties. El Charro has received its share of media attention, and it chose to celebrate this in its menu, thus the *USA Today Chimichanga Platter* ($17.95), which has History Channel and Food Channel logos flanking the description of it. The dish is described as an oversize chimichanga with guacamole, picco de Charro, sour cream, chile Colorado, and tomatillo verde.

The massive red cylinder that arrived could comfortably have fed our table of six and perhaps the whole restaurant. The Carne Seca is dry, salty, and good and tasty, but this quantity of it was too much for me. I liked the **Bahia Tacos** better and the **Beef Tamale** best of all, washed down by an **Elegante Margarita**.

For J Bar, his newer endeavor, Janos says he threw out the French and looked at grilled meat, fish, and poultry. The beef of the ranches of the Sonora is indicated in dishes like *carne machaha,* carne asada, and stews like *ropa vieja*. Janos traveled a little farther, to the Caribbean, for the jerked pork dish he created for the opening of J Bar. The spicy pork is livened up even further with his deliciously hot cranberry sauce. Working in harmonious concert with the smoked poblanos, the sauce cuts the richness of the meat.

I have unfinished business at J Bar, where at happy hour Janos serves a **J Dog,** inspired by Sonoran hot dogs like the ones served at El Guero Canelo (see page 233). Janos uses expensive Big City Reds for his franks, and serves them with chorizo, black beans, diced onions, mustard, and

QUICK BITE

While looking at Utah food, I heard there was a lot of fishing in the state, which surprised me for some reason. Acting on a tip-off, I called Barb Hill to talk to her about a trout dish she serves at her Snake Creek Grill in Heber City: **Blue Cornmeal Crusted Red Trout,** which is served with chipotle sauce, poblano chiles, and pureed avocado. On the side are choro and calypso beans. Sounds good, yes? Barb and her husband, Michael, have run the restaurant since 1998. They have an organic garden that produces in the summer bounty like zucchini (for a risotto) and heirloom tomatoes and cucumber. I'm very happy to talk with Barb, but I'm mistaken about the provenance of her trout: she buys her fish from Idaho.

Now, Idaho is famous for its freshwater fishing. Ashton, Idaho, farmer Clen Atchley (see chapter 2) enjoys fishing for trout in Idaho's Snake River and in the lakes it feeds into. He looks mostly for **rainbow trout** and **German browns.** Some he eats, he tells me; some he throws back.

crema. He picks up his rolls from two bakers in South Tucson: El Triumpho and Alejandro's.

I also have to visit Janos's newest venture, for which he is consulting chef, the five-star Kai, at the Sheraton Wild Horse Pass Resort, outside Phoenix. The hotel is operated by the Gila River Community, and Janos has worked with the Mericopa and Pima Indians to celebrate the heritage of the Gila River. Before the river dried out through overuse, the Gila River region was the breadbasket of central Arizona. As in Tucson, Janos is taking local ingredients, in this case salmon and buffalo, and expressing them through modern cooking and meal preparation.

MICHIGAN'S MAGICAL MITT

Chef Eric Villegas of Restaurant Villegas in Okemos, Michigan, has been my guide to a few Michigan specialties (Cornish pasties, for example). His fund of local and international food knowledge is vast, limitless even. Eric was given a solid grounding in good food by his parents. He was born and raised in Saginaw; his parents were immigrants from Bolivia and they provided him with a solid South American eating background. His father, a physician, would take the family to eat where *he* wanted to go, and as a result Eric was exposed to adult food on adult menus from an early age. (Parents take note.) Culinary school and restaurant work, including training in France, came, followed by Restaurant Villegas and Eric's own public television program, *A Fork in the Road*.

Restaurant Villegas features a broad array of Michigan produce in its dishes. Eric talks about the "magical mitt" that is his mental image of the state of Michigan. (If you hold up your right hand, palm facing you, and picture a bulky catcher's glove, you'll see what Eric means. You can also make an Upper Peninsula using the back of your other hand held back and to one side.) Eric refers to the produce that comes from the corresponding area on the mitt: the fruit from the left side up to the pinky, cranberry bogs in the south of the state, sugar beet from around the thumb, and industrial manufacturing from Detroit. He mentions products like Vernor's soda and Superior and Better Made potato chips. (I look up Better Made and see that they use Michigan potatoes eight months of the year. I'm very curious about their **Curry and Garlic** variety—that's one variety, not two.)

Eric says there isn't a cuisine of Michigan in the same way there is a California or East Coast style of cooking. It's more about the wealth of local agriculture, wild game, and fish. (Here Villegas makes an interesting point about Waverly Root's books—Root wrote *The Food of France*, *The Food of Italy*, and *Eating in America*. Does that mean that in this country, there is a focus on the consumption more than the creation?)

As he works on his TV show, spending a couple of days with asparagus farmers, for example, he'll be developing recipes. Talking to Eric about food, which is hugely pleasurable, I see that he loves to be inventive. He'll take Hawaiian tuna that was in the ocean twenty-four hours before and make a **teriyaki** using Michigan maple syrup. Eric buys hard cider from Almar Orchards in Flushing, Michigan, and makes a **cheese fondue** in traditional French style using the cider. Says Eric, "The cider is sweet, which American palates like, and it complements the astringent American cheese."

Amid all this creativity, there are enduring Michigan classics, like the various lake fish: whitefish, perch, walleye. All round the Great Lakes, they're caught and cooked very simply—planked, perhaps, or in fish fries.

There's a recipe for **planked shad** in Fannie Farmer's cookbook that involves oven-baking the fish set on a "buttered oak plank one inch thick." "The Planked Whitefish of the Great Lakes has gained much favor," Ms. Farmer notes. **Walleye pike** and lake perch are featured on the menu at Myron and Phil's, in Chicago, where novelist Adam Langer favors the **relish tray.** And all round the lakes, there are Friday Fish Fries in the summer, such as that at Quivey's Grove in Madison, Wisconsin, where you can pick up **lake perch lightly breaded, fries, and coleslaw** for a good end-of-the-week dinner.

As you've probably noticed, the definition of what is local is changing all the time. Two miles from Eric's restaurant is an indoor saltwater shrimp farm, operated out of a barn surrounded by expensive homes. This facility enables Eric to put up a sign advertising fresh shrimp as if he's a roadside tomato stand, and to serve a dish like **Ceviche of Russ Allen's Michigan White Shrimp with Pears.** There's an initiative to bring pawpaws to Michigan, Eric says, and another, by nearby Michigan State University, to reintroduce chestnuts, which died out under a blight in the 1920s and 1930s. Eric points out that a lot of farming used to be centered on the chestnut: pigs ate them, colonists ate them, and they're featured in a lot of old recipes. "Now we don't know what they are," he says.

Eric is also able to get Great Lakes buffalo. Buffalo is a lean meat whose taste profile Eric likens to venison. "I use the 'hanger steak' simply grilled, served with our dried tart cherry Worcestershire sauce as a nice thin steak sauce, with pommes frites for a Michigan-inspired **Buffalo Steak–Frites,"** Eric says. "I 'ice smoke' the buffalo tenderloin and grill to order for a fancy entrée. I use the round, which I also ice smoke, to make a very elaborate entrée chili using the buffalo suet as the fat."

Then there's the local ostrich. The ostrich is a versatile bird (see page 75). Eric will prepare an **Ostrich Tenderloin** (pan-searing it like a steak). Or you may find **Ostrich Jerky, Ostrich Fajitas,** Ostrich Steak Frites. Eric stays away from the shoulder and legs because he finds you have to add so much fat that the meat loses its personality. An ostrich sausage would have to include up to 20 percent pork fat, and the flavor will overshadow the original. "Then," Eric says, "it might as well be a muskrat sausage." Is that something I need to look into?

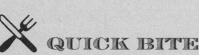

QUICK BITE

Eric Villegas likes to pair expensive and exotic ingredients with more workaday accompaniments. It makes the food affordable and provides an exciting twist to something familiar. Hence his **French Fries with Black and White Truffle Aïoli.** The Kellogg's headquarters is in Battle Creek, Michigan. When Kellogg's people came to Eric's restaurant for dinner he served them **Foie Gras pan-seared with a Kellogg's Corn Flake Crust.** I don't think you'll find the recipe for that on the side of a cereal box.

TACO NIGHT

In the Grand Central Market in Los Angeles, I relished my fish taco (see page 336). Farther south, in San Diego, a place more readily associated with the dish perhaps, Maria Hunt told me, "There are good **fish tacos** all over town. Some of the best fried ones are at a San Diego–based seafood restaurant chain called the Brigantine. They put club soda or something in the batter that makes it really crisp. For grilled fish tacos, I like El Pescador, the seafood market and tiny eatery (with four tables, it's not big enough to

QUICK BITE

My Scottish correspondent Robin McMillan likes La Superica Taco in Santa Barbara. "It's on Milpas, which is my favorite street name in America," he says. "And it's turquoise. And it's hit-and-miss, but it's cooler than the other side of the pillow, and the **Poblano Peppers Stuffed with Cheese** were great."

be called a restaurant) on Pearl, in La Jolla. They will make grilled tacos out of any fish that they have fresh that day. The grilled fish tacos at the Fishery in Pacific Beach are also good. FYI: fish tacos usually come on a flour or corn tortilla, with a slurry of white mayonnaise-based sauce, shredded white cabbage, and fresh chunky tomato salsa. Some places add cheese, but that's not traditional."

Maria Hunt says that **papas locas** can be found at nearly any of the taco stands called Roberto's, Alberto's, or Rigoberto's around San Diego. "Basically they are nachos that are made with French fries instead of corn tortilla chips," says Maria. "Also commonly found at little Mexican restaurants is the **torta,** a big, puffy, but substantial roll with a tan, floury exterior that is used for sandwiches. There's something comforting about the way the fillings—often grilled chicken or carne asada, shredded lettuce, tomatoes or salsa, beans, and avocado—seem to settle into the roll. They use the torta rolls for all the sandwiches at El Pescador, mentioned earlier.

Finally, "**rolled tacos** are also everywhere, and one of the cheapest meals around at $1.79 for a trio. Rolled tacos are corn tortillas filled with ground or shredded beef, a mixture of ground beef and rice, or sometimes chicken or fish (rarely, though), and fried until crisp. The trio is topped with shredded iceberg, creamy guacamole, salsa, and a sprinkle of shredded yellow cheese. I like the ones from the Los Panchos chain, especially washed down with a **Jamaica** (the sweet-tart hibiscus drink from Mexico)."

Patty Pinner is the author of *Sweets: A Collection of Soul Food Desserts and Memories*. "Here in Saginaw," Patty says, "we African Americans have our own specific twist on the Mexican taco. I think of it as . . . *when salsa meets soul*. There is a Mexican bakery that we all frequent for fresh-baked *taco bread*. (That's what we call it.)

"The basic meats used for the filling are the standards: ground beef and ground turkey. The secret's in the way the meat is seasoned. People season differently. The variations enter in when it comes to the salad (lettuce, tomatoes, etc.) that's also a part of the filling. Also, some people stuff their tortilla (taco bread) with the meat filling, pin the tortilla ends together with a toothpick, then deep-fry it. After which, they add the salad. They swear that's the only way to do it.

"I made chicken tacos for supper last night. I used six or seven skinless, boneless chicken breasts. I 'soaked' the meat overnight in a marinade of garlic powder, onion powder, seasoned salt, coarse black pepper, poultry seasoning, chili powder, cumin seeds, smoke sauce, and a packet of taco seasoning. The next morning I boiled the chicken, let it cook to the touch, then shredded it. I stuffed my taco shells with the chicken and my salad. I always add a pat of butter to the oil that I use to deep-fry my shells.

"In my opinion you haven't had a taco until you've had a **Soul Taco** from Saginaw, Michigan."

FRIED CHICKEN AND PEACH COBBLER

I had only a few hours to spend in Atlanta, so I had to pick with care where I was going to go. I decided I could drive out to Weaver D's in Athens for an early lunch and rumble back into the city for an extremely early dinner at Mary Mac's Tea Room. If I could squeeze myself into one of the Varsity Drive-Ins and the Majestic Diner, too, then all well and good.

I called John Kessler, food writer at the *Atlanta Journal-Constitution*, before I left. John expertly traversed a huge swath of food history and geography in a very few minutes. I should think of Atlanta like Los Angeles writ small, he said, with its great interpreters of other people's cuisines, such as Alabaman Scott Peacock at the Watershed Restaurant (see page 240) and the city's growing contingent of good ethnic restaurants: Brazilian, Korean, Mexican, southern Indian, northern Indian. John raved about fresh-baked Brazilian breads, which didn't quite fit my bill, and also talked about the Georgia version of Brunswick stew, with bits of the whole hog thrown in with ketchup and canned corn, which did. I felt as if I'd made decent choices for my trip.

——————

Among John Kessler's numerous nuggets were: the **West Indies salad,** made with crabmeat, chopped onions, oil, and vinegar, found on the Alabama Gulf Coast, and the **fried dill pickles** (sliced, drenched in cornmeal, and fried) that Georgians like to eat with their barbecued pork.

John quickly took me around the area—the Low-Country cooking of South Carolina with a lot of rice dishes, which is best found in Charleston; the mountains of northern Georgia, where the country is close to Tennessee and North Carolina and the peanut-loving areas I mentioned earlier (see page 29). Don't forget the Big Pig Jig barbecue contest in Vienna, John said. Finally he came home to Atlanta, to the famous **Carrot Soufflé** from the teashop at Rich's Department Store.

——————

Dexter Weaver of Weaver D's is famous for the line "Automatic for the People," which adorns the sign outside his restaurant in Athens, and which was used as the title for an album by Athens natives REM in 1992. "Automatic" informs a whole philosophy, one that Mr. Weaver outlines in his book, *Automatic Y'all*, in which he generously includes some of the recipes he uses for his fabulous food. With food this lovingly crafted, there's nothing automatic about the cooking in the regular sense of the word.

For a while I was concerned about making it to Weaver D's at all. The Georgia Bulldogs were playing football in Athens the day I was visiting. I called ahead and asked how many of the ninety thousand fans would be heading for the restaurant. Weaver told me to "Come on down. We'll give you a number." With this in mind, I made sure I arrived hours before the game kicked off. Already the twisting streets of the town were thick with traffic. Bulldogs fans were tailgating wherever there was open ground. Weaver D's is in a modestly appointed white building down near the Oconee River, where textile mills used to process locally produced cotton. Fortunately, I didn't have to take a number, and from the sanctuary of my table I could watch football fans come in and eat, or take out trays of chicken for their tailgate parties.

Weaver told me he cooked what the spirit told him each day. The special was two pork chops for eight dollars. His spirit took me there and beyond, to a plate heaped with a **fried pork chop, fried chicken, potato salad,** and **squash casserole.** I had to turn down his mac and cheese because if I'd started in on a second plate I'd have been in serious trouble. Of the four parts of lunch, the squash soufflé was the surprising highlight. While looking at the recipe in Weaver's book later on, the listing of the goodly helping of cheese, butter, and eggs speaks volumes. The pork chop was thin cut and crisp; the chicken was perfectly cooked and not heavy, as fried chicken can be. In Weaver's book, by the way, he says he seasons his chops and chicken with the same mix. It must be in the touch. I washed the food down with sweet tea. "Sweet" doesn't quite do it, either, for the tea or for the **lemon meringue pie** (Mama Alice's Old-Fashioned Lemon Pie). They both hit high C perfectly.

Alongside tourist types like me making the trip and the football fans, there were longtime regulars taking early lunch. How can you tell someone's a regular? When they go back into the owner's office to retrieve the bottle of **hot pepper and basil vinegar** they keep at the restaurant. Dexter Weaver is terrific company to spend a little time around as he presides over the store, answering the phone and fussing over the food. He was opening Sunday, he was telling people, which he didn't always do. The food's definitely worth the drive out into the Piedmont from Atlanta.

I realized after I left Weaver D's that I had only one more meal in me that day. I drove back to Atlanta and noodled around the Jimmy Carter Presidential Library and Museum.

QUICK BITE

At the Blue Ribbon Brasserie on Sullivan Street in New York City, I followed the recommendation of one of my dinner companions and had the **fried chicken.** He hadn't had it here before and neither had I, and we were both blown away. The whole combo was great: crisp, spicy chicken (lots of paprika, not greasy), buttery mash, thick gravy, and some bright, sharp collard greens to keep you honest. The Blue Ribbon is a favorite SoHo spot for late-night eating: you can get a great meal here every day from four in the afternoon till four in the morning.

The museum is terrific, with rack after rack of memorabilia and thoughtful displays and a full-size replica of the Oval Office. Very nicely done. The grounds are lovely—a real oasis in the center of the city. As I walked back to my car, I saw a couple of guys fishing in the ornamental lake, which is probably not what it is intended for.

Unusually for me, I killed time quite successfully. I parked by the Plaza Theater, near the Majestic Diner on Ponce de Leon, and walked around the treasures in Beaver's Book Sale. At the characterfully weathered Art Deco Majestic Diner, I asked for a take-out menu to use as reference but they didn't have any. So I made my way to Mary Mac's and my 4:00 p.m. dinner.

I wasn't the only person eating at that most in-between of times, but the place was by no means half-full. I sat in the largest of the rooms, a pleasantly open and inviting space. The take-out menu says that Mary MacKenzie opened Mary Mac's in 1945, and the succeeding proprietors have continued her ways. The staff treats patrons like they're guests for dinner at their house, the blurb says, and judging by my personal sample of one visit, it's actually true. I'd have been very happy if my very amiable server had sat down and joined me for dinner.

John Kessler had told me that if I was going to Mary Mac's, then I'd get acquainted with pot likker, which is the water the collard greens have been cooked in, served with a piece of corn bread. Beyond that, I struggled with the menu. I had to complement what I had at Weaver D's—no more squash soufflé. But what to have? At Mary Mac's, you write your own order on a chit. Perhaps it's a cunning ruse to get you to order more than you need. It certainly worked in my case. I put down a whole mess of stuff. To start, **fried green tomatoes,** then **fried select oysters** with **turnip greens** and **cheese grits** on the side and **Georgia peach cobbler** to finish me off. Hurricane Katrina had knocked the oysters off the menu, so I substituted **fried gulf shrimp.** And **fried okra** stood in for the greens. To drink, naturally I had what the menu describes as "Table Wine of the South (Sweet Tea)."

I was brought my bowl of **pot likker with corn bread.** About the last thing I needed was a bowl of soup with a big piece of corn bread, but I ate it down easily enough. By no means a throw-in, pot likker has a strong and interesting flavor. But pairing the shrimp with the okra/grit combo didn't work as a meal choice, with the double crunch of the shrimp and the okra together with the softer grits. I seem to have some kind of ordering mishap whenever I try grits. The shrimp were plump and most succulent. I decided I should add fried green tomatoes to the list of Things I Like.

Looking at Mary Mac's menu now, I reckon I should have had a country-fried steak and gravy and something sweet on the side—**Bartlett Pear Salad,** perhaps. Before I left Mary Mac's I did get my fruit fix with

QUICK BITE

In Maine, cookbook editor Michael Flamini favors venison at Arrows, in Ogunquit; the **wood-oven roasted mussels** at Fore Street, in Portland; and the **fried clams** at Fisherman's Catch, in Wells.

My friend Seana loves Arrows. She says the tasting menu is "just perfect." A highlight was husband Roger's mojito, which was flavored with different types of fresh mint from the restaurant's own bounteous garden.

the peach cobbler, whose pastry was delicious and whose syrupy peaches were sublime.

I could have sat in the tea room for hours, but I headed for the Varsity Drive-In on North Avenue, the world's largest, it is said, where they sell more Coca-Cola than any other eatery in the world. The place seemed huge indeed, and I'm sure it's good, but I'm sorry to say, I drove in the Drive-In and drove through and out the other side. I was just as full as I wanted to be.

If you want good old-fashioned Pennsylvania Dutch home cooking, then go to the Country Table restaurant in Mount Joy, Pennsylvania. The entrées are simple: roast beef, roast turkey, baked chicken, salmon cake, crab cake, liver and onions, and the like. I chose **Oven Baked Hamloaf with Gravy** ($8.25), and Kara went with **Smoked Shankless Ham with Pineapple Filling Topped with Pineapple Glaze** ($9.25). As is often the case, I quickly became covetous of my wife's dinner. My hamloaf, made with minced meat, was ever-so-slightly too sweet for my liking, and a little one-paced texturally. Kara's ham, double-dipped in pineapple (pineapple filling is stuffing with pineapple), and also sweet, was a nice piece of fresh meat.

QUICK BITE

Another dish that might be described as old-fashioned (Marialisa Calta calls it "old-timey") is the **Salt Pork and Milk Gravy** at the Wayside Diner in Montpelier, Vermont.

The side dishes were more interesting, and each was very good. My **Real Mashed Potatoes with Gravy** was thick and rich. My first experience of the local chow chow was very pleasurable. The variety offered by the mixed pickled veg in chow chow makes it a perfect side dish (see page 110). Because I didn't know what they were, I ordered an extra side of **Red Beet Eggs.** What they are is a hard-boiled egg pickled in beet juice, and extremely tasty they are, too. Kara had, and liked, the home-made baked beans and coleslaw, and we both helped Lindsay out with her **Baked Macaroni and Cheese.** Kara doesn't usually take mac and cheese with breadcrumbs, but this was terrific. Other homemade sides: pepper cabbage, pickled beets, and stewed tomatoes.

This is a friendly place, and very hospitable to kids. At the end of the meal, ours each got a wooden nickel they could exchange for a **snickerdoodle**—a cinnamon sugar cookie—in the Bake Shoppe and Deli next door. As a ploy to get us to visit the bakery, it was successful, but we resisted the multiple temptations. Back in the restaurant, I satisfied my stimulated sweet tooth with a fine **Black Raspberry Crumb Pie.**

Here are two accounts of a Hawaiian lunch. Bethany Fong brings us the **plate lunch:** "The simplest way to describe a plate lunch would be Hawaii's version of a box lunch. There is probably a restaurant (usually take-out) that sells plate lunches on every block of Hawaii. If not every block, you can usually find one wherever you are. The components of a plate lunch are simple: rice, entrée, and salad. Entrées can be a variety of things, but classic choices include hamburger steak, **chicken katsu** [Japa-nese fried chicken], barbecued chicken—but don't think chicken with Western barbecue sauce; it is a shoyu-based marinade similar to teriyaki sauce but *hot*—beef stew, chop steak, kalbi [Korean ribs], tonkatsu [Japanese fried pork], etc. The classic accompaniment to a plate lunch is macaroni salad, basically a concoction of macaroni, lots of mayo, and salt and pepper. If you want to get fancy you can add carrots, hard-boiled egg, peas. Plate lunches are a way of life here. They can be eaten at any time of the day and are usually sold in two sizes: regular and mini."

And Susan Volland says, "Put away the poi and shun the hotel luau and go have lunch on a paper plate with two scoops of rice from a plate lunch truck; grab some Spam musubi to go; long for **Zippy's chili;** and always snub a Krispy Kreme in favor of a warm **Malasada.** Talk story." (A Malasada is a kind of Portuguese donut first sold at Leonard's Bakery in Hawaii in the 1950s. You can get Malasadas from the source: Leonard's is still going strong.)

One of the handful of most memorable meals I've ever eaten was the wedding banquet of my friend Deborah Kwan and her husband of a couple of hours, Erik Cosselmon, in San Francisco. It was an extremely festive and social occasion. The banquet at the Four Seas Restaurant, in Chinatown, followed Chinese tradition, with dishes made of expensive ingredients to demonstrate the generosity and standing of the bride's parents. Other food has special meaning for the new bride and groom: "peanuts" in Cantonese sounds like "fast birth," for example. And there are eight savory dishes in total because "eight" in Cantonese sounds like "success." The significance of the shark's fin, sea cucumber, and abalone is mostly in the fact that they cost a lot.

QUICK BITE

I wanted to pass on a piece of dining etiquette from *Eighteen Colonial Recipes*. Along with a recipe for "Calcutta Curry" is this piece of advice: "Curry should always be eaten with a spoon. Only globe-trotters use forks." So now you know.

Wave after wave of platters were presented, each groaning with some opulent and exciting dish. Deborah missed most of it while changing into a succession of ever-more-stunning wedding gowns. I tried a good serving of everything. The magnificence of the whole fish is something I recall well. Beautiful presentation; wonderful flavor. Try dishes like these and open a whole new world of Chinese food. These were the dishes:

- **Oyster Tumble with Lettuce Shell**
- Sea Cucumber and Abalone over Greens
- **Sautéed Squab with Mushrooms and Vegetables**
- **Shark's Fin Soup with Dried Scallops**
- **Golden Fried Crispy Skin Chicken**
- **Prawns with Honeyed Walnuts**
- **Braised Stuffed Whole Duck**

- Steamed Whole Gray Sole
- "Posterity and Prosperity" Sweet Consommé
- Wedding cake

———

Antonia Allegra, speaker, culinary coach, and the author of *Napa Valley: The Ultimate Winery Guide,* recommends the Depot Hotel in Napa, which has been around since the twenties, for its **Malfatti.** "Imagine the inside of a raviolo poached and served with a tomato sauce," says Antonia. "You have a malfatti (meaning 'poorly made' in Italian). People go to the restaurant (which is located in a used-car lot) with plastic containers to take home malfatti for dinner later in the week.

"Taylor's Refresher, a hamburger joint that was started in 1949 (I believe), is now a hot spot serving **ahi tuna burgers, duck confit tacos,** Chinese chicken salad, blue cheese burgers, and more. They also serve beer and wines in 375-milliliter bottles, including top-name wines from Napa Valley wineries." (Taylor's Refresher has restaurants in St. Helena, in Napa Valley, and in San Francisco.)

From the Bouchon Bakery, try a **pain au raisin,** a delicious raisin "Danish" baked in the true French way. Bouchon Bakery, the next-door Bouchon Bistro (great **oysters and French fries**), and French Laundry are all owned by Thomas Keller, the famed chef.

———

ROPA VIEJA

When it comes to eating, South Florida may be best known for three things: Cuban food, the riches of the sea, and Key lime pie. The family was in Miami and we had a little time for exploratory eating. If you have the kids along and just two meals to play with, you sometimes have to do the obvious—have lunch at Versailles, in Little Havana, and buy dinner from Joe's Stone Crab, in Miami Beach (see page 216).

There are approximately 2.4 million people in Miami-Dade County, an area that includes the city of Miami and the metropolitan area north to Fort Lauderdale, and about 30 percent of the population is of Cuban ancestry. The fact that Miami's best-known Cuban restaurant bears the same name as the palace of French royalty is an oddity. Just think of it as "Versai-yes," not "Versai."

We drove down and found a parking space in the small lot of the Versailles Bakery and made our way to the restaurant. Here and there on the sidewalk were groups of men, talking and drinking coffee, just as we'd been told there would be. This is the most noticeable thing about Versailles: how social it is. Inside a small café selling pastries (*pasteles*) and cigars were more men talking and drinking *cafecitos* (Cuban coffee in tiny cups). In the restaurant itself were tables of businessmen, older gentlemen, and a few families, including obvious tourists like us. Next to us were a couple of men who were joined by a third after they started to eat, and much later by a fourth. Versailles is clearly a place where residents of Little Havana can show up and find someone they know.

The Versailles menu—we were given the English version—is very long. I wanted to try as much as possible, within reason, so the "Cuban Samplers" were ideal. I took the **Criollo** (native), with a **Cuban sandwich** on the side. Kara had **Ropa Vieja** and took a Malta to drink. We ordered empanadas, but they didn't come, which, given the amount of food we ate,

was probably a blessing. First came a basket of **Cuban garlic bread:** thinly sliced, toasted, lightly flavored, and definitely more-ish. Quickly the rest of the food followed, which saved us from the garlic bread. Kara's stew was terrific. *Ropa vieja* means "old clothes," so called because the shredded beef that makes up the bulk of the dish is said to resemble torn-up rags. You can get *ropa vieja* in thousands of Hispanic restaurants around the country. The English menu said the beef came in "Tomato Creole Sauce," but in Spanish it read "*con Cebolla, Pimientos Verdes, Tomate y Vino Seco.*" Either way, with rice and beans and fried plantains, it is a rich stew worthy, dare I say, of Louis XIV.

My sampler plate was laden with goodies. Yellow rice (*Arroz Amarillo*) and black beans; my own *ropa vieja* (which tasted just as good as my wife's; I checked); **fried pork chunks** (which definitely taste better in Spanish: *Masas de Puerco*); a ham croquette; yucca; and the wonderful **Plátanos**

QUICK BITE

Check out the Cuban food at Carmine's and the Columbia in the Ybor City neighborhood of Tampa. The Columbia is home to the **1905 Salad**—ham and Swiss, tomatoes, and olives with grated Romano and garlic dressing that is tossed tableside.

Maduros—fried sweet plantains, which are wickedly good. I washed my food down with a domestic beer. Kara's Malta soda tasted like fizzy Ovaltine—which is not surprising, as both are malt drinks—yet it was heavy, more a meal in itself than something to drink with one.

Having seen the dessert menu already, I was eager for some **dulce de leche,** described here as "sweet curd pudding." For years, my friend Ivan and I went to the Cabana Carioca, a Brazilian restaurant on Forty-fifth Street in New York that is now, tragically, no more. We'd have a couple of caipirinhas (Brazil's national cocktail), the garlicky chicken special, and then share a *dulce de leche* (or *doce de leite*) *con queso*. Brazilian *dulce de leche* is caramelized condensed milk; the Cuban version is the milk curds, which are rough and almost gritty, and a different animal entirely. They do share a toothy sweetness. At Versailles, I saved room for at least one serving of **flan**—rich, creamy, and a perfect puddingy consistency. Kara and I topped off lunch with a Cuban coffee, which is to a Starbucks espresso what malt liquor is to 3.2 percent beer. I never have trouble sleeping after caffeine, any time of day, but I'm sure this drink to many people would simply taste of insomnia in a cup.

Thus jolted and revived, we headed out, past the café and bakery, lighter only sixty dollars (kids' meals included). I'd be very happy to go back with someone who knows the town and the culture and the language. We drove down Calle Ocho, the main drag of Little Havana. We were headed for El Rey de las Fritas, which has subsequently been forced to move east by an expansion of Miami's downtown business district into Little Havana. Few places are static. So many Nicaraguans now live in this area, for example, that they style part of it Little Managua.

━━━━━━━━━━

We talked to Edwin Froelich about alligator in chapter 3, but where can you get it for dinner? In the wild, alligators live in the southeast, in Florida and Georgia, and also in Texas and Louisiana. Since 1987, the alligator is no longer an endangered species (the American crocodile is endangered) and it's not difficult to find restaurants that sell gator if you have a yen to try some. Alligator Alley, a restaurant and music venue in Oakland Park, Florida, will sell you Gator Bites, Gator Scallopini, Buffalo Gator (like Buffalo wings), and Gator ribs.

Prejean's restaurant in North Lafayette, Louisiana, serves up

Cajun food and music: catfish, crawfish, fried oysters, and a provocative-sounding **Smoked Duck and Andouille Gumbo.** Prejean's has a webcam trained on the dining room. I've checked in a few times, when I was thinking about the gator, and subsequently. Each time I was happy I could confirm that the restaurant was open and seemed to be doing a brisk trade. Now I feel that I know the place, and I hope a particular table I've singled out will be available when I visit.

The restaurant advertises a fourteen-foot gator called Big Al, who sits, stuffed, in the dining room. Big Al was caught in the Grand Chenier swamp, and Prejean's serves an **Alligator Grand Chenier,** in which the gator is stuffed with crab and shrimp. You can have this covered with crawfish étouffée if you like. Gator is also available grilled or fried, with gator sausage, but I'm in for the Grand Chenier (with a dessert of **Gateau Sirop,** spicy Cajun syrup cake), provided someone else wrestles the alligator for me.

A COUPLE OF QUESTIONS FOR CHEF VICTOR MATTHEWS

Multiple award–winning chef Victor Matthews, who has been a U.S. culinary ambassador, cooks his wonderfully inventive meals at the Black Bear Restaurant in Green Mountain Falls, near Colorado Springs. In 1997, Chef Matthews was declared "The Youngest Four Star Executive Chef in Louisiana History" by the *New Orleans Times-Picayune*.

What dish says the Rockies or Colorado to you?

"It is vital that people know the power coming from this area. The lamb of Colorado is legendary. Right now it is on New York, Paris, and Tokyo menus. It has a bigger eye . . . less of that off 'lamby' flavor. The majority of America's golden and organic potatoes come from the San Luis Valley, and most of the buffalo production for America is local. Colorado has organic mushrooms, escargot, Biodome-raised tilapia, and organic striped bass. We have two of America's championship cheeses, and everyone knows how good the beer is."

I'd love to hear what you think the key dishes are in New Orleans.

"Number one, no matter what, worldwide, is gumbo. Other famous dishes include étouffée (four different official spellings), boiled crawfish, blackened steaks and seafood, and many others. Less famous are **macque choux,** fried gator, **turducken,** and **rémoulade.** Creole and Cajun influences can also creep into anything . . . such as seafood pastas or my new favorite, **spicy Caesar salad.**"

How easy is it to get to your restaurant in the winter?

"Interestingly, it isn't that bad. The road is a highway [Highway 24 West], and it is plowed and sanded quickly if there is snow. Only a couple days a year are difficult. I like it best in winter because of the huge fireplace [Colorado's second biggest]. We have so much fun it is silly."

SOUTHERN EXPOSURE

A few years ago, I made the drive from south Florida to eastern Long Island with my brother-in-law Buzz and his parents' golden retriever. The aim of the exercise was to get the dog and the family car to point B as quickly as possible, which meant traversing much of the length of I-95. These runs north and south follow the same pattern: early start, overnight stop, early start. Good eating along the way is not a concern. Even halfway decent eating along I-95 is no one's priority, and people refuel themselves much like they fill up their cars, from the nearest retailer by the side of the road. The road passes through some of the most interesting food territory in the country, but you have to go out of your way a little to find the food itself.

Driving up from south Florida, Buzz and I stopped in Emporia, Virginia, a truck-stop town off I-95 that has a Hampton Inn that takes dogs. Nearby, there's a Shoney's, an Applebee's, and so on, but we asked the Hampton Inn receptionist if there was an actual restaurant anywhere, and she told us about the Squire House in town. Getting to the Squire House involved a few extra miles of driving, but it was definitely worth the effort. Walk in the door of the restaurant and find yourself in what resembles a Victorian club, old-fashioned fixtures and fittings, very comfortable, luxurious even. What did I eat that night? It was a nice piece of fish (I have no idea what). When I telephoned, most recent, I was told the prime rib is the house specialty.

A couple of years later and I volunteered for the southbound leg, which took place soon after Labor Day. I was on my food quest, but job number one was getting the dog home. If I was planning some eating stops, I was going to have to be selective, with no huge detours away from I-95 and no stopping every eleven miles for a different kind of pulled pork. I thought we might visit three places. I knew we'd be leaving Southampton around 4:30 a.m. Figuring fifty miles an hour net, I estimated where we might get to at what time and looked for restaurants nearby.

I made a rough plan. I wanted to begin with Ed Mitchell's barbecue joint in Wilson, North Carolina, for a late lunch. Then, if we could make it to Savannah by dinnertime, I thought I might sneak off to the Lady and Sons, Paula Deen's famous southern cooking emporium. Next day, for breakfast, we could stop off at Azalea's Café, in St. Augustine, on our way through Florida. At Azalea's I was interested in the **Jalapeño Cheddar Grits** I'd read about. And along the way, we could also stop for some boiled peanuts.

If you look at it one way, my planning was spot-on. My mileage estimates—which put us into Wilson around lunchtime and Savannah at eight o'clock at night and near St. Augustine in good time for an early breakfast—were right on the money. Problem was, all three restaurants were closed. The biggest personal disappointment, and embarrassment, was Ed Mitchell's. I'd eaten Mitchell's sublime pulled pork in New York in the summer, and I very much wanted to try it in situ. I'd pulled directions off the Internet, but we got slightly lost and had to be put right at a gas station. I felt bad—this was adding time to the trip, but I couldn't just drive by. Of course, when we got to the restaurant, it was thoroughly shuttered. I felt like a total rube, even if the people back in the gas station hadn't known either, or hadn't cared to tell me.

———

In Asheville, North Carolina, check out Laurey's Catering downtown, whether you want to eat lunch or organize a party. Laurey Masterton calls what she makes "gourmet comfort food." Apart from the locally baked bread, it's all made on the premises, using local produce.

"To name a couple of our specialties," Laurey says, "I'd point to our **Baked and Fried Chicken,** which I'd suggest eating with

Richard's award-winning **Sweet Potato Salad,** which is probably our most popular salad. Richard was experimenting, trying
to make sweet potato chips. He accidentally overcooked the
potatoes but, when he sampled them, was delighted to find
them quite interesting in a charred sort of way. He added **Sour-
wood Honey** (a local specialty, which is a strong honey like a
buckwheat honey) and some lemon, and there you have it. I'd
recommend fried green tomatoes, too. They are pan-fried with
cornmeal and are tangy and intriguing. Relishes are big around
here. Chow chow is a pickle-and-mustard concoction that is a
regional specialty. We don't make this but sell it in the 'gourmet-
to-go' section of the shop. For dessert I'd suggest one of our
Mingus Bars, which is like a pecan pie with a shortbread crust
and some chocolate chips tossed in. *Really* good!"

You can also check out the Web site (www.laureysyum.com)
and see what's for dinner. (How good do Fig and Chevre Stuffed
Chicken Breast or Stuffed Summer Peppers with Hickory Nut
Gap Beef sound? Hickory Nut Gap Farm raises grass-fed beef in
Fairview, North Carolina.)

Just down the road from Mitchell's, Buzz and I pulled into Parker's
Barbecue restaurant. The simple low building looked like it had been here
forever—since 1946, it turned out—and, thank goodness, it was open.
Parker's is a local institution that doesn't deserve to be just the place you
drive by looking for Mitchell's. Judging by the **pulled-pork sandwiches**
we ate on the trunk of the car, this is a fine establishment and a destination
in its own right. Now I was a double rube for not having found out about
Parker's. The sandwiches were made of hamburger buns with a good helping of pulled pork, with coleslaw on top. The pork was tender and moist;
the slaw, tart and vinegary. It made a great sandwich. I also bought a tub of
Brunswick stew to take back on the road. The sandwiches, the stew, and
two Diet Cokes ran to a grand total of $10.17. (You can take out a gallon of
Brunswick stew for $10.75.)

While we were eating our sandwiches at Parker's, an eighteen-wheeler
pulled into the parking lot. The driver said that, in fact, Mitchell's had
been shut for months, even before I ate the pork in New York in June. The
Internet is great, of course, but if you really want to know, call ahead. You'd
think someone would have told me that.

QUICK BITE

I'm sorry to say, as far as checking ahead is concerned, I haven't learned my lesson. Recently, I have swung by Union Square in New York for the farmers market on a day it was closed. I also made a very long-anticipated trip to the cart on Fifty-fourth Street whose German sausage won a "Vendy" Award and was voted the best in the city. I wanted to try the sausage and I also wanted to be able to write, as everyone who wrote about the award did, that this was the best wurst in New York. Right as I walked up, the cart was being pulled off its station. And these two mishaps took place on the same day.

I did get a menu for the cart, and for the rest of the Hallo Berlin group of restaurants of which it is a part. The menu made me hungry, and it made me laugh, too. The sausages are given an accompanying German auto as part of the description: wienerwurst is a Volkswagen; bauernwurst, an Audi; a brat is a Mercedes. Then the Berliner Currywurst is a Porsche; a Smoked Andouille Brat with Cheese, the absolute top-of-the-line Maybach; while boiled bockwurst is a Trabant, the old East German jalopy. I sated my appetite at the burger joint at the nearby Parker Meridien Hotel, so my misadventure ended happily after all.

I've committed to memory the fact that the Union Square Market is open Monday, Wednesday, Friday, and Saturday. On a visit one fall morning, I saw heads of the extraordinary **romanesco,** a member of the *Brassica* genus that includes all the cabbages, mustards, and collard greens. The beautiful romanesco looks as if it had been grown in a lab from quartz crystals. It is variously called the romanesco cauliflower and the romanesco broccoli (cauliflower and broccoli are other *Brassicas*). At Union Square, I saw both monikers.

The Hallo Berlin Wurst cart is open Monday–Friday, 11:30 a.m.–3:30 p.m. Another day, I picked up a tasty **bauernwurst,** a pork/beef sausage set in a hard roll with sautéed onion, red cabbage, and sauerkraut. The companion car for this wurst, the Audi, is a good analogy.

I had gleaned by this time that the Lady and Sons in Savannah was closed for a post–Labor Day spruce-up. The next morning was a night's sleep and hundreds of miles away when we pulled out of Wilson, but I thought I'd make a call to Azalea's to find out what time it opened. I would have hated to show up too early. No need to worry about that—a recorded message told me that Azalea's was closed, too. By the time we got to Gateway Boulevard, the motel strip outside of Savannah, I was too beat to think of driving into town to eat. If I had, I figured, the town itself would have closed.

Before we looked for a motel that would take the dog, we gassed up at a Shell station, where I read a sign advertising boiled peanuts inside in the shop. Here they were, delivered right to my car door. I went inside to make my buy, but the very kind attendant told me she'd just put the peanuts on to cook. They were still frozen solid.

I did get my boiled peanuts, at 5:15 the next morning. These were presumably the selfsame peanuts from the night before, now defrosted and heated through. Buzz couldn't find his glasses, and it was pitch-dark, so I had to take the first shift driving. Buzz wedged the polystyrene container in front of the gear stick, where I could reach the nuts. I ate the peanuts one-handed without being able to look at them. They'd swelled up considerably, and I was sure I did too, with all the sodium in the brine. Once out of the shell, the meat was quite soft and intensely savory and, surprisingly, quite delicious. They're well worth going out of your way for. As we drove by the exit for St. Augustine and the closed Azalea's Café, my serving of boiled peanuts didn't seem like such a bad consolation prize.

POSTSCRIPT

A couple of months later, I wanted to check in with Azalea's to see if it was open and to ask how the grits were doing. I called, and the chef-owner Sandy Krebs answered, "Great Food, Groovy People." Sandy told me she'd taken her usual vacation but had to keep the restaurant closed to get something seen to. But now she was in great form. I asked about the grits, and Sandy, who is from L.A. but has lived all over the country and in the Virgin Islands, said they were her concession to running a restaurant in the South. I told her what I was writing, and she said that most people think American food is burgers, fried chicken, and barbecue. I momentarily felt chastened, but when she said there's so much more out there, I was relieved—yes, that's exactly what I was finding out. "We're so *diverse*," Sandy said with feeling, promoting the word, and the idea contained within it, just beautifully.

So what should I eat if I were coming in today? There's a **salad of garlic roasted beets, feta cheese, and avocado over organic field greens with basil vinaigrette.** A new American classic, Sandy said, and good enough to eat. Sandy said she was sorry I hadn't been able to come by before but she hoped I would sometime. I sincerely hoped so, too. I told her I was glad everything was groovy again. I bet that's the first time I ever used that word, and I meant it, too.

EATING OUT: LUNCH AND DINNER SUMMARY

RUN, DON'T WALK, FOR . . .

- ▣ Whatever Dexter Weaver is cooking today at Weaver D's in Athens, Georgia.

- ▣ **The Original Jerked Pork with Cranberry Habañero Chutney** and **Oaxacan Bread Pudding** at J Bar, in Tucson. Good food like this is informed by numerous sources and crafted with skill and care.

- ▣ A good **pulled-pork sandwich** like the one at Parker's in Wilson, North Carolina. A good, quick lunch dish, pulled pork and slaw is a world-class combination.

- ▣ **Doing your homework.** Before you run *or* walk someplace, make sure it's open.

IF YOU'VE NEVER TRIED . . .

- ▣ **Pot likker with corn bread** and **fried green tomatoes,** as at Mary Mac's Tea Room in Atlanta. A fine way to start a good meal.

- ▣ **Grits.** Worth persevering with, probably.

20

STATE-BY-STATE

Farmers Markets, Festivals, and Fairs

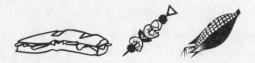

*Prior to the twentieth century, public markets were a major
component of American retailing. As late as 1918, the U.S. Census
Bureau noted that there were 237 municipal markets in 227
cities with populations greater than 30,000 inhabitants.
At that time New Orleans contained 23 neighborhood markets,
Baltimore had 11, New York City had 9, and Pittsburgh 6.*

—Alexander Garvin, *The American City: What Works, What Doesn't* (2002)

The big-city market might seem like an unusual place to visit on vacation, but I love them. Some of the old markets, like Reading Terminal Market, West Side Market in Cleveland, and Grand Central Market in Los Angeles, are housed in what can be quite magnificent buildings. The space within hums with action. Stall by stall, they're full of excellent food adventures and fantastic bargains. If nothing else, there'll be a selection of places for your lunch. You don't have to spend a dime: there's always something to see. Go to Pike Place Market in Seattle and watch the fish vendors sling their wares to, or at, each other. (I know this is something of a Seattle cliché, but it is fun to watch. And Pike Place Market is just wonderful.)

 Pike Place Market's City Fish carries an offer called "Two Socks in a Box," two Copper River sockeye salmon filleted and delivered anywhere in the United States, plus a big selection of fish and shellfish: 1-800-334-2669 / www.cityfish.com/products.htm.

In New York City, I'd far rather spend time poking around Chelsea Market than going anywhere near Midtown, where you and two million of your closest friends can duke it out for space on the sidewalk. At ten years of age, Chelsea Market is relatively new but is housed in its own historic building, where the National Biscuit Company, manufacturer of Oreos, Fig Newtons, and **Mallomars** (don't you love Mallomars?), used to be housed. This is a fun place to hang out. It also has free WiFi access, which is a beautiful thing.

The time my friend Rick and I spent in Los Angeles, including visits to Grand Central Market and the Farmers Market in West Hollywood, demonstrated how enjoyable gastro-tourism can be. Rick and I traveled around town with little other purpose than to try out various eating places. Rick, who has probably been to Los Angeles fifty times on business, said he went to parts of the city he'd never been before, and he now has a fresh appreciation of the place.

In this spirit, if you're following your stomach round Los Angeles, the

QUICK BITE

In San Francisco, pick up pupusas at Las Palmas market in the Mission District (or tacos, or masa for your own tamales). Or Cuban and Puerto Rican food, including **Mofongo,** the amazing mashed plantain and garlic dish, Cuban sandwiches (ham, pork, cheese, and pickle), and frozen fruit drinks at El Nuevo Frutilandia.

And Joanne Weir says, "Don't miss the **crispy grilled steak burrito** at La Taqueria in the Mission . . . A fun place, lively, and truly San Francisco." The district is named for the Mission Dolores, built in 1776, the oldest building in the city.

Farmers Market in West Hollywood and the Grand Central Market downtown are both can't-miss places. In each, you could work your way through the menus at the restaurants and food stands for weeks and have whole cuisines left over to work on. They're great places to eat in and great places to shop for good, cheap produce—for example, when we visited Grand Central Market, you could pick up five pounds of bananas for a dollar at a number of stalls.

The Grand Central Market is housed on the ground floor of the Homer Laughlin Building, an L.A. antique that's ancient by local standards. (It was built in 1897.) Across from one entrance is the site of the Angels Flight funicular railway, which is currently idle. Angels Flight is the scene of a memorably undignified murder in Michael Connelly's novel of the same name. If you take a stroll, as Rick and I did, you can also check out the curves on the stunning Walt Disney Concert Hall, designed by Frank Gehry, and then swing back down to the market.

The Grand Central Market is noisy, busy, and full of life. It's packed tight with food stands like El Gaucho, home to Argentine food and ninety-nine-cent empanadas, and Sarita's Pupuseria, specializing in the stuffed-tortilla dish, the **pupusa,** from El Salvador. There are Chinese and Japanese places, a Hawaiian and a Mongolian barbecue stand, Mexican food at Tacos Tumbras a Tomas, Thai food, pizza, kebabs, and so on.

Roast to Go has been operating in the market since 1952. The front of the stand is packed with steaming trays of meats for your taco or burrito, many of them tubular and smooth, indicating an intestinal origin. Other specialties are listed as gorditas, tortas, *sopes, flautas,* and tostadas. I had to have a taco—it was on my list—but it hadn't been even an hour since my

QUICK BITE

Cleveland's West Side Market is at the corner of West Twenty-fifth and Lorain in the Ohio City neighborhood. The market is open Monday, Wednesday, Friday, and Saturday. You must check with all these markets, because many of them are open less than seven days a week. If you're going for one special item, check with the individual vendor, because some may not be open all the hours the market is running. Online, my eye strayed to Reilly's Irish Specialties at the West Side Market and the thought of 150 varieties of pierogis at the Pierogi Palace.

massive breakfast at the Original Pantry. There was so much to choose from: roasted pork or beef, chicken, brains, beef cheek, lamb, and *buche*, described as "hog maw," which is pig's belly. Meekly, I went for some fried fish.

My Roast to Go **fish taco** plate was heavily laden, with a substantial slab of battered fried fish and piles of lettuce, onions, tomatoes, hot sauce, cilantro, and *queso cotija* (salty cheese) resting on top of two corn tacos. I couldn't eat the whole thing, but it was fresh and good, with sharp flavors, and it cost only two dollars. The market seemed full of good deals, like the cheap bananas and other fruit, and more than one stand for dried goods, all manner of chiles, dried shrimp and dried whitebait, and the like. The shopping and the window shopping are good here, and the eating is great. At the end of your visit, if you feel like you've overdone it with another stop at the taco stand, someone at Jones Grain Mill will check your blood pressure for $1.50.

━━━━━━━━

Olvera Street in downtown Los Angeles houses a pedestrian-ized Mexican market that attracts a lot of tourists. The oldest house in L.A., the Avila Adobe, dating from 1818, is here, and Olvera Street is in the historic center of the city, near the old plaza. There are local people as well as tourists, picking up Mexican soccer shirts and wrestling masks, perhaps, and buy-ing food to eat in one of the tiny restaurants that line the street. We checked out a couple of **chicken taquitos** and a **tamale** from Juanita's and ate the food on a bench in the plaza.

Down the hill from Olvera Street is Los Angeles's magnificent Union Station. Inside, Rick pointed out the huge beams running across the ceiling. We decided that each is made up of the wood of one tree. Well, old-growth trees that size probably don't exist anymore, Rick surmised. He and I wanted to continue our dis-cussion about forestry over a drink at the Traxx Bar, in the sta-tion, but, alas, the bar was shut.

━━━━━━━━

The stately redbrick building housing the Lancaster Central Market is very easy on the eye. There's been a market on this site since the 1730s, and the Romanesque Revival market building itself dates from 1889, making this the country's oldest publicly owned farmers market in continuous operation. The market is open Tuesday, Friday, and Saturday, when it closes at two o'clock. We rushed to get there before closing time one Saturday and had a very successful visit. (That was nothing compared with how well we did at the wonderful Cultural History Museum Store nearby, or rather how well they did when we were there.)

In the market, from Ruth Thomas, I bought sweet corn and peaches (see page 52). Ruth sent me across the aisle to Wendy Jo's Homemade for a **shoo-fly pie,** which was delicious. We looked round Stoltzfus Baked Goods, Kiefer's smoked meats and cheese, the Pennsylvania gristmill, and S. Clyde Weaver smoked meats and cheeses of East Petersburg, where you could buy pigs' stomachs (six dollars each). I picked up some excellent subs from here, which, seeing as we were in Pennsylvania and not so far from Philadelphia, I told myself, were hoagies. We washed them down with the local Turkey Hill iced tea. It is the S. Clyde Weaver **Italian Sub** that single-handedly turned my son, Sam, on to the delights of hot peppers, and for that, I shall be grateful for ever more.

Farmers markets come in many shapes and sizes. The USDA maintains a great resource, a list of farmers markets state by state: www.ams.usda .gov/farmersmarkets/map.htm.

Small markets of just a few stalls seem to be popping up all over New York City. Many are open only one day a week. On these days, it's as if the farm is bringing the farm stand into the city. Check where you live for information. It's worth looking, because there might be a stand closer than you think. Sam and I were taking a bus on the weekend across 110th Street in Manhattan, toward our neighborhood, when I spotted a small collection of stalls by the entrance to Morningside Park. I had no idea there was a Saturday market here. To Sam's evident displeasure, we got off the bus we'd waited some time to catch and did some shopping.

The largest of the three stands was from the Migliorelli Farm, in Tivoli, New York. I made a quick note of what they had on offer, all of it grown on the farm:

Apples (Gala, McIntosh, Ginger Gold, Honeycrisp, and Macoun), peaches, red beets, golden beets, white beets, carrots, radishes, sweet corn, beefsteak tomatoes, plum and yellow tomatoes, arugula, mizuna (Japanese mustard greens), basil, cilantro, bok choi, tat soi (a dark salad green), broccoli rabe, red chard, Swiss chard, kale, collard greens, mustard greens, Kirby cucumbers, zucchini, white potatoes, eggplant, flat beans, green beans, and Bartlett, Bosc, and **Seckel pears** (tiny, sweet pears with a lovely purplish color to them).

This was one of seventeen markets organized in Rockland and West-chester counties and in the boroughs of New York City by Community Markets, an organization that started work in 1991. Whether the market is a couple of stands in the street or a permanent building housing ranks of stores, the principles of local goods brought to you fresh are just the same.

State tourist authorities can be a good source of food informa-tion. Take the initiative put together by the state of Alabama, which designated 2005 as the Year of Alabama Food and se-lected the "100 dishes to eat in Alabama before you die." Down-load the PDF file of the one hundred dishes here: www.tour alabama.org/yof/YOFbrochure.pdf. Big Bob Gibson's B-B-Q is there (see page 237). The state helpfully enumerates the older restaurants, like Pete's Famous Hot Dogs in Birmingham.

These are some dishes that caught the eye: **fried catfish** and coleslaw (and fried dill pickles) at Ezell's Fish Camp in Lavaca, out on the Tombigbee River; at the Sahara Restaurant in Montgomery, I might try the West Indies salad John Kessler told me about (see page 318), and at the Cotton Patch Cafe in Eutaw, the **drop biscuits** received official state approval.

The promotion also extolled the virtues of the local produce: **scuppernong** grapes, for example, and the Alabama tomato (usually the **Globe** variety). The reputation of the local tomato prompted a statewide competition to find the best tomato-based dish. The winner would be served on the menus of sixty restau-rants. The prize went to chefs John Hamme and Bradley Czajka of Ariccia Restaurant at The Hotel at Auburn University. They won five thousand dollars at the Alabama Food Festival held at the Pepper Place Market in Birmingham for their **Alabama Warm Tomato Tart.**

STATE FAIRS

State fairs are huge business. The biggest, the monthlong event in Dallas, draws about 3 million visitors. Minnesota's fair, which has been running since 1859, attracts up to 1.7 million people. That's another feature of many of these fairs, the fact that they've been staged so long, since the 1840s in a few cases. The fairs were agricultural shows in origin, and the local farm economy still plays an important role. As does food.

Checking out the various online literature of state fairs, I see that there are clearly some interesting gustatory experiences awaiting the intrepid visitor. Some of the dishes possess what might be called shock value (certainly more than much nutritional value), as vendors compete to come up with more and more outlandish creations. That isn't to say they won't taste good. And a trip to the state fair is presumably a day out when we can let things go a little.

[See contact information for details of America's state fairs.]

The food directory for the Iowa State Fair, in Des Moines, is an impressive document. The list shows individual foods, who supplies them, and where they are located on the fairground. Brats you can get from nine locations, hot dogs from twenty-one. Then there are the **cheese curds** and **cheese-on-a-stick.** Plus **elephant ears** (fried-dough treats) and **pickle dogs.** The most alarming dish is a drink: Red Bull Smoothies.

Cheese-on-a-stick isn't the half of it. In fact, if you are one of the one million visitors to the fair, you can get all your meals served to you on the end of a stick. According to the organizers, here are the impaled foodstuffs you can expect to find:

Pork chops, dill pickles, corn dogs, cheese, Cajun chicken, caramel apples, chili dogs, beef, cotton candy, veggie corn dogs, turkey drumsticks, nutty bars, chocolate cheesecake, hot bologna, chocolate-covered bananas, taffy, fried pickles, honey, wonder bars, deep-fried Twinkies, meatballs, Ho-Ho's, and fudge puppies (waffles drenched in chocolate sauce).

The Texas State Fair has held a contest for its concessionaires (the Big Tex Choice Awards) and awarded prizes for Best Taste and Most Creative for new state fair products. The latest winners were: Shirley London, first place for Best Taste with Fried Praline Perfection ("Guaranteed to melt in your mouth; plump coconut and pecan pralines are battered and fried to a rich golden crust and served warm with powdered sugar"); and Abel Gonzales, first place for Most Creative with **Fried Coke** ("Smooth spheres of Coca-Cola-flavored batter are deep fried, drizzled with pure Coke fountain syrup, topped with whipped cream, cinnamon sugar, and a cherry. The product is served in souvenir contoured glasses"). Oh my.

The Texas fair folks listed new items for the 2006 fair, revealing impressive ingenuity in the art of calorie delivery. Some standouts:

- Candy Apple Turnover: "A flaky turnover, filled with apples, crushed red candy and brown sugar, is deep fried and topped with powdered sugar." (Granny's Funnel Cakes)

- Deep-Fried Cosmopolitan: "A delicious fried pastry is filled with rich cheesecake and topped with a sweet & tangy cranberry glaze and a lime wedge. Served on a stick." (Desperados)

- Donkey Tails: "Large all-beef franks, slit on one side and generously stuffed with sharp cheddar cheese, are wrapped tightly in a large flour tortilla and fried until golden brown. Served with mustard, chili, or Ruth's salsa." (Ruth's Tamale House; **Donkey Tails** have a life beyond the fair: they're on the menu at Tolbert's in Grapevine, Texas, for example)

- Fernie's Fried Choco-rito: "A flour tortilla—stuffed with marshmallows, coconut, candy bar pieces, caramel morsels and cinnamon—is dipped in pancake batter and deep fried to a crispy, crunchy outside and sweet, gooey inside. Drizzled with honey and topped with whipped cream." (The Dock)

- The Fried Pancake Sundae: "Tasty country sausage bites wrapped in a light pancake batter, deep fried to perfection, topped with whipped cream, lightly glazed with hot fudge sauce and finished with a cherry on top. Pineapple and strawberry glaze options available." (Smokey John's BBQ)

- Wedgee: Frozen chocolate-covered Wisconsin cheesecake-on-a-stick offered in Turtle (caramel) and Key lime flavors. (Weiss Enterprises)

- Melon Monroe: "Honey-dew melon sauce ladled over chocolate chip ice cream, topped with whipped cream then garnished with two fried-dough, shaped 'legs' filled with a special caramel sauce. Served fresh out of the fryer." (Midway)

STATE MEALS

Like other states, Oklahoma has an official bird (the scissor-tailed fly-catcher), a state animal (the buffalo), and a tree (the redbud). Many states have adopted various foodstuffs as official state drinks, snacks, cookies, pies, muffins, and the like, but Oklahoma is alone in adopting an entire state meal. Oklahoma's meal, chosen in 1988, was designed to represent the diversity that had come to be characteristic of the state. In full, the Oklahoma state meal is fried okra, squash, corn bread, barbecue pork, biscuits, sausage and gravy, grits, corn, strawberries, **chicken-fried steak, pecan pie,** and **black-eyed peas.** If this is supposed to be one meal, it's an impressive spread.

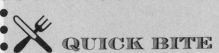

QUICK BITE

A well-known purveyor of chicken-fried steak in Oklahoma City is Ann's Chicken Fry House, which stands along the path of the historic old Route 66. Ann's is also renowned for its **deep-fried peaches.**

Starting with Lynne Olver's terrific Food Timeline Web site, I took a quick detour through the esoteric world of the state-anointed foods. Do you know your state foods, and would you ever eat them? As we mentioned, Rhode Island has a state drink—coffee milk—but not a state food as such, although you could eat the state fruit, the Rhode Island Greening apple; the state fish, the striped bass; and, at a stretch, the state bird—the Rhode Island Red (a hen). (Rhode Island in general and Providence in particular have a lot of interesting food histories. Cindy Salvato runs culinary tours of the Italian Federal Hill neighborhood of Providence. Contact her at 1-401-934-2149 / www.rimarkettours.com.)

Big-government-happy Massachusetts leads the nation in state sweets with an official muffin, dessert, donut, and cookie (the corn muffin, the **Boston cream pie,** the **Boston cream donut,** and the chocolate chip cookie, which is also given official recognition in Pennsylvania). Minnesota favors the **blueberry muffin;** New York, the apple muffin. New Mexico's state cookie is the **bizcochito** (a Spanish, anise-flavored import). South Dakota's state dessert, the kuchen, can be made according to the official state recipe, and there is also a state bread: fry bread.

In 2002, Georgia made grits its "official prepared food." Popcorn is the official snack food of Illinois, the result of a third-grade civics project. **Natchitoches meat pie** is the official state meat pie of Louisiana, which also has a state donut (the beignet) and two official state jellies, **Louisiana sugar cane jelly** and **Mayhaw jelly.** (The mayhaw is a tree that grows in swampy areas and produces a berry that you wouldn't eat raw but which makes good jelly.) Louisiana also favors a state crustacean, the crawfish, and gumbo as official state cuisine. In Texas, **pan de campo** is the state bread, and chili, the state dish. Other states have left this to Texas. Ohio, which has its chili, of course, counters meekly with a state beverage: tomato juice.

Perhaps the cheekiest of these state endorsements comes from Vermont, which in 1999 designated apple pie its state pie. Surely the apple pie belongs to the Union, not to any one particular state? Not only did they try to co-opt a national symbol, but the legislature also tried to tell people how to eat their pie. "When serving apple pie in Vermont, a 'good faith' effort shall be made to meet one or more of the following conditions: (a) with a glass of cold milk, (b) with a slice of cheddar cheese weighing a minimum of ½ ounce, (c) with a large scoop of vanilla ice cream." This, then, is the Vermont state meal, and much less of a plateful than you might get at the state house in Oklahoma City.

FOOD AND OTHER FESTIVALS

While there might be potentially distracting elements at state fairs, like fairground rides and concerts, you can be reasonably sure the focus at a food festival is on the food. Still, there'll be more to do at these events than just eat (Liza Minnelli sang at a recent Norsk Høstfest, North America's largest Scandinavian festival, for example). A town can proclaim its singularity and claim to fame for all to see. Take Wilmington, Ohio, where the **banana split** was invented and where there's been a Banana Split Festival the last few years. Among the main attractions, the build-your-own-banana-split stands. I imagine this event wouldn't be a hard sell for the kids.

The banana split was first made at Ernest Hazard's restaurant in 1907, when the proprietor threw together the split (banana, ice cream, chocolate syrup, strawberry jam, pineapple, nuts, whipped cream, and cherries) one rainy day. No food first is ever unchallenged: Latrobe, Pennsylvania, claims the split comes from there.

FESTIVALS MENTIONED IN THIS BOOK

- Hamptons Wine and Food Festival at the Hayground School, Bridgehampton, New York

- National Cherry Festival, in Traverse City, Michigan
- Chestnut Roast, in New Franklin, Missouri
- Riverside County Fair and Date Festival, Indio, California
- Rhubarb Festival at Kitchen Kettle Village, in Intercourse, Pennsylvania
- Ramp Cook-off and Festival, in Elkins, West Virginia
- International Dutch Oven Society World Championship, Logan, Utah
- Testicle Festival, at the Rock Creek Lodge, Clinton, Montana
- Sheboygan Brat Festival, in Wisconsin
- Madison Brat Festival, in Wisconsin
- OysterFest, in Shelton, Washington
- Mussels Festival in Whidbey Island, Washington
- National Mustard Day, at the Mount Horeb Mustard Museum, Mount Horeb, Wisconsin
- Napa Valley Mustard Festival, in Yountville, California
- International Pickle Day, on Orchard Street in New York City
- Apple Butter Festival, in Berkeley Springs, West Virginia
- Highland Maple Festival, in Highland County, Virginia
- Czech festivals in Omaha, Lincoln, Wilber, and Prague, Nebraska
- Czech Festival, in Yukon, Oklahoma
- Kolache Festival, in Caldwell, Texas
- Chile Festival in Hatch, New Mexico
- CASI International Chili Championship, in Terlingua, Texas
- ICS Chili World Championship, in Omaha, Nebraska
- Original Terlingua International Championship Chili Cookoff in Terlingua, Texas
- LSVN Vegetarian Chili Cook-off, in Austin, Texas
- Annual Brunswick Stew Cook-off, in Lawrenceville, Virginia
- International BBQ Fest, Owensboro, Kentucky
- Burgoo Festival, in Arenzville, Illinois
- Burgoo International Cook-off, in Webster Springs, West Virginia

- Big Apple Barbecue Block Party, in New York City
- Memphis in May International Barbecue Festival, Tennessee
- Spiedie Fest and Balloon Rally, in Binghamton, New York
- Big Pig Jig barbecue contest, in Vienna, Georgia
- Glier's Goettafest, in Cincinnati, Ohio
- Banana Split Festival, in Wilmington, Ohio
- Norsk Høstfest, in Minot, North Dakota
- Danish Days Festival, in Solvang, California
- Danish Days, in Viborg, South Dakota
- Scandinavian Festival, in Junction City, Oregon

There are sweet corn festivals celebrating the harvest all over the country, many of them in August. They'll often offer musical entertainment and kids' activities, as well as steaming vats of sweet corn.

◆ Zellwood, Florida, holds its festival early, in late May, befitting the harvest schedule in the state.

◆ Seventy tons of sweet corn are consumed over the August weekend of the Sweet Corn Festival in Sun Prairie, Wisconsin, which can attract a hundred thousand visitors over its four days of entertainment and activities. Tickets are one dollar.

◆ Millersport, Ohio, has held a festival every year since 1947. It features a parade and a tractor tug pull. (Held over Labor Day weekend.)

◆ The DeKalb Corn Fest, DeKalb, Illinois, in August, gives out free corn on Saturday. It's also one of the last free music festivals in the state.

◆ The annual Cokato Corn Carnival, in Cokato, Minnesota, began in August 1950. It is run every second Tuesday and Wednesday of August.

◆ The West Point, Iowa, Sweet Corn Festival features a Shuck Fest. Family fun since 1952!

◆ The town of Olathe, in western Colorado, hosts its Sweet Corn Festival in August.

◆ For a twist, the Popcorn Festival of Clay County has been held since 2003, at the end of September until early October at Forest Park, in Brazil, Indiana. The festival has its own Ocktoberfest and also celebrates the life of local popcorn entrepreneur Orville Redenbacher (1907–1995) with what is billed as the world's only Orville Redenbacher look-alike contest.

Check the Festivals and Shows section of www.foodrefer ence.com for hundreds of listings.

━━━━━━━━━

If I spent enough time looking at the various festivals, fairs, and markets around the country, there was always a danger that I might learn something. I was reading about the Norsk Høstfest, a giant Scandinavian knees-up at the North Dakota State Fairgrounds in Minot. I came across this sentence in the description: "Indulge in such culinary favorites as Danish Aebelskivers, lutefisk, lefse, Oof-Da Tacos, rice pudding, Swedish meatballs and viking [*sic*]-on-a-stick." Apart from rice pudding and Swedish meatballs, I didn't really know what these things were. Lutefisk, I had a vague notion; Viking-on-a-stick? I wouldn't like to hazard a guess.

With the help of the Internet, I found out what a lot of this stuff was very quickly. With the help of my friend Diane, who is of Scandinavian origin, I found out about even more dishes I'd never heard of and also some leads to the above. Aebelskivers, or *Aebleskiver,* are a kind of spherical pancake from Denmark made in a special pan, and served with jam and powdered sugar. Solvang, in California's Santa Ynez Valley, is the "Danish Capital of America," and the Solvang Restaurant (on Copenhagen Drive) serves **Aebleskiver** and will sell you the pan, mix, and everything you need to make these guys at home. From the restaurant menu I also learned about the Danish Days festival in Solvang in September. There's also a Danish Days Festival in July, in Viborg, South Dakota. All Scandinavia is celebrated at Junction City, Oregon's Scandinavian Festival each August.

🛒 For Aebelskiver kits and more at the Solvang Restaurant: www .solvangrestaurant.com.

Back to the list: *Lefse* are a kind of potato pancake/crêpe/flatbread. Lutefisk is whitefish that has been soaked in lye and is then eaten, curiously, as a special dish all over Scandinavia. Viking-on-a-stick is a state fair kind of snack, I think—a fried meatball fritter. Diane told me that "oof-da" or "uff-da" is what someone of Scandinavian extraction might say if she stubbed her toe and didn't want to swear. Oof-da Tacos is an operation in the upper Midwest that travels to fairs like the Red River Valley Fair in Fargo and the Craft Show in Little Falls, Minnesota, and sells its fry-bread-based tacos.

Diane told me, "My Norwegian grandmother was seventy and a widow when I was born, so she didn't cook a lot. I do remember every Christmas it was a huge treat for her to eat herring and *ekte gjetost* (**brown goat cheese**). Also *krumkaker* [like pizzelle, a cone-shaped cookie made in a special Krumkake iron]. Plus family favorites that I now realize were actually Norwegian specialties. *Agurksalat* [cucumber salad in water and vinegar], *Rabarbrakompott* [**stewed rhubarb**], and lutefisk. As for lutefisk, thankfully no one in my family liked it."

I enjoy food like this very much—I love herring, for example, which is an obvious entry point to Scandinavian cuisine. I've been to Aquavit restaurant in New York City a few times and had a great time eating Chef Marcus Samuelsson's exciting food. Thus did I go off on a pleasing *Eat This!* detour from a thought about a food festival in North Dakota, racking up more entries in my have-to-eat log.

From Deerfield Beach in Florida, Norwill Scandinavian Food will sell you Nordic delicacies. I counted fourteen types of herring, shrimp, meats, **cloudberry** and lingonberry jams, and the wonderful brown cheese that I remember tastes like toffee: 1-866-598-4506 / www.norwill.com.

21

WHY THERE ISN'T A KIDS' FOOD CHAPTER

*It is not wicked sensuality . . . for a little boy to prefer buttered toast
with spinach for supper and a cinnamon bun with milk for lunch. It is the
beginning of a sensitive and thoughtful system of deliberate choice, which as
he grows will grow too, so that increasingly he will be able to choose
for himself and to weigh values, not only sensual but spiritual.*

—M. F. K. Fisher, *How to Cook a Wolf*

remember only a few of the dishes from my elementary school years in
England. One was a meat crumble—a savory crumb with cheese baked
over a layer of minced beef. And semolina, of a very fine grade, served
warm with a dollop of raspberry jam plopped in the center. At a young age
I took a liking to institutional food like this, food that's parenthetical to
the place's purpose. The courses are all wedged onto one tray, and the por-

tions are small, so eat what you like. You also have license to eat fast, like a race for your taste buds.

Into this category I'll place airline food up to circa 2000. Does Kuwait Air still serve a great curry like the one I had on a London–New York flight fifteen or twenty years ago? I know People Express doesn't hand out tasty little sweet rolls anymore because there is no People Express. Even I balk at what you get now on airplanes, at the back of the plane at least, when you get anything at all. The food used to be like a decent school lunch; now it's not really food at all.

Back to school lunch—or school dinners, as we called them, even though we ate them at what I thought was lunchtime. In 2002, the Calhoun School on Manhattan's Upper West Side decided to take on the Herculean (or Sisyphean) task of trying to teach its students how to eat well. The school hired Robert Surles, universally known as Chef Bobo, as executive chef to cook in its Upper School building, which houses Calhoun's grades two through twelve. When he was interviewed for the job, the school's request was simple. As Chef Bobo recalls, "They said they wanted their kids to know how to eat real food. That's all I needed to know."

Chef Bobo says he came to realize that kids could stand his brand of diverse food program simply by watching them eat. The key to what he does at Calhoun lies in rejecting the kids'-menu mentality. Restaurants provide a kiddie menu (chicken nuggets, mac and cheese, burgers, fries) rather than smaller, more affordable, more nutritious versions of the adult menu. So the kids' section in this book is really a misnomer—the kids get to eat the same food as the rest of us, but it just comes on a smaller plate. That's why there isn't a kid's food chapter. We'll listen to Chef Bobo instead.

To Chef Bobo, the staple of kids' menus, the chicken nugget, is a particular abomination. "Any meat that's been processed no longer has any nutritional value," he says. "That's what chicken nuggets are: processed chicken. So there's no nutritional value. They're just bland and chewy." Chef Bobo continues: "We've got to start training kids' palates. That's what I do here. A kid is ready to start doing this as early as three years old. If we can develop that palate, by the time he's in middle school, he's not going to be wanting to eat all that fast food. He's going to be wanting something that's a little more satisfying to the palate. That's what it's all about."

Chef Bobo practices what he preaches. "When I consult with a restaurant on a menu and they ask if they should do a children's menu, I say, 'If you even threaten to do it, I'm walking out right now.' " It's a moment of triumph for Chef Bobo when parents of Calhoun students tell him they no longer need the kids' menu when they go out to eat as a family.

Eating out with the kids is a great way to introduce them to new food. You have to choose the restaurant carefully of course. If the menu has a dish that comes with a lavender foam on it, you're probably not going to find anything they'll eat and the restaurant won't want your kids there either. If the restaurant doesn't have a kids' menu, you'll pay for more than they can eat for a few years, but it's money well spent, I reckon. And many enlightened places won't charge you to split a plate with your children.

At Kate Mantilini's in Los Angeles, there are numerous easy options for children on the lengthy menu. One night Sam and Lindsay went for meat loaf and spaghetti and meatballs. On another night, they switched orders, and both times healthily ate their fill. I love this restaurant, for kids or otherwise. Sit in a wooden booth and read the music in the boxer's gloves in the giant mural on the wall, which features Kate Mantilini dressed as a ballerina in the ring. (Kate Mantilini was a boxing promoter in Los Angeles before the Second World War.)

My **Wild Rocket and Red Chili Pepper Linguini** with garlic, anchovy, lemon, and Parmesan was a big plate of fun. And the signature **chicken pot pie** packed with wholesome peas went down fine. The highlight of one dinnertime came when I asked Sam if he wanted to try some of my appetizer. He said he did, took a bite, said he loved it, and ate three more forkfuls. To my delight, he was eating pickled herring, admittedly herring smothered in sour cream, but herring nonetheless (part of the extra-delicious **Creamed Herring Appetizer** with onions, apples, beets, and sour cream).

This is not to say there haven't been some problems over lunch at Calhoun. What to do about ketchup, for example? Going in, Bobo's great fear was that in order to make his food palatable, kids were going to want to smother it in ketchup. If that happened, he felt he'd have failed. So that was rule number one: no ketchup in the school cafeteria. He recalls the initial hysteria that resulted.

" 'We've got to have ketchup, Chef Bobo,' they said. I said, 'Sorry. Ketchup has more sugar than ice cream, and personally, I'd rather have ice cream.' So they all thought I was going to let them have ice cream. So it was double disappointment."

Two months into the program, the kids had a pretty good sampling of what they were going to get, and were accepting it for the most part. "I was beginning to have parents come and threaten me and say, 'You've gotta give me that recipe. The kid's never eaten that in her life.' That's the kind of threat I like." Then, on Halloween, one of the students came to lunch dressed as a bottle of Heinz ketchup. It was, says Chef Bobo, "an incredible costume."

"She had a sign round her neck reading CHEF BOBO, PLEASE PUT ME ON YOUR MENU. That broke me. I thought she was so clever and so adorable, so I said, 'Okay.' Such times as we have hamburgers—and we do it twice a year, with oven-roasted French fries, which taste better—we put out ketchup. With five hundred kids, we serve less than a gallon of ketchup. So I've broken the ketchup habit. I like ketchup on those things, too, but I don't have to have it on broccoli or Brussels sprouts. I have kids coming back wanting third helpings of Brussels sprouts."

Having conceded about an inch in the war on ketchup, Chef Bobo went on the offensive in other areas. He took more risks and branched out from good wholesome American fare into Italian food, Greek food, Mediterranean, Middle Eastern, Asian, and Latin American food, assisted by chefs of Greek, Lebanese, and Cuban heritage.

Chef Bobo will try out some of his New Orleans favorites (see page 211) on his young charges. One is **jambalaya,** which he describes as a poor man's paella, the great Spanish rice dish. Because of dietary restrictions, he can't put shellfish in his jambalaya—in New Orleans it would include shrimp and oysters—so he uses sausage and chicken and the New Orleans holy trinity (onions, celery, and green pepper) and seasonings like black, white, and red pepper, bay leaf, basil, and thyme.

The day we spoke, the kids (and the staff) were having roast chicken with a tomato and honey glaze with orzo and steamed broccoli. The soup was a vegetarian carrot fennel soup, and the sandwich was Greek salad with feta cheese and roasted tofu.

The day before had been a summer miso soup, a Thai chicken salad wrap, and a Korean-flavored turkey meat loaf with spicy roasted cauli-flower and curried orzo. All I can say is, that's a lot better than my standard Tuesday lunch.

Spicy roasted cauliflower? Dave Lieberman of the Food Network was filming at Calhoun for his show. Chef Bobo says Lieberman tasted the cauliflower and said it was kind of hot and peppery. "I said, 'No it's not,' and he said, 'I can feel it in my mouth.' I said, 'It's not hot and peppery. It's what we call happy mouth. That's what southwestern and Cajun food does. I love spicy southwestern food. It gives you the total experience—the feeling in your mouth, the feeling in your belly. You perspire a little bit, too."

Chef Bobo takes his message round the country. "I think I've got the best job in the world," he says. "If you could have been here yesterday. Dave Lieberman was sitting at a table eating with a bunch of third-graders and they started chanting, 'We Love Chef Bobo,' and it got louder and louder. I thought, Where is that going to happen anywhere else in the world? No-where. I wouldn't trade that in for anything."

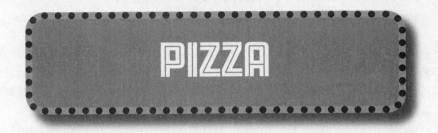

22

PIZZA

*If you have a clam phobia . . . order eight to ten white
clam pizzas at Frank Pepe's in New Haven, Connecticut,
perhaps the single best pizza in the United States and certainly
the best thing of any kind in New Haven, Connecticut.*
—Jeffrey Steingarten, *The Man Who Ate Everything* (1997)

My son, Sam, is a lifelong pizza aficionado, at least since he started on solid food. As he traversed his eighth and ninth years, he got more adventurous about what he wanted to eat. I thought it would be fun to bring him along on some eating trips to expand his pizza world a little. Also, many of the old-style pizza places in New York eschew the slice, so unless you want to tackle a whole pie, come with a friend. Bringing Sam, I wouldn't have to force myself not to eat eight slices of pizza for lunch. I found that four was usually sufficient.

The rain was coming down in unrelenting sheets the Saturday Sam and I decided to visit Grimaldi's Pizzeria on Old Fulton Street, in Brooklyn. It was a hard, heavy, soaking rain. It had already rained through the night and into the early morning and was forecast to keep going all this Saturday, too. When a low cloud comes in close enough to sit on the taller buildings in Manhattan on the weekend, it's usually a day to stay indoors, or, at most, to scurry to the movies. To me, it looked like eating-out weather. So my pizza pal, Sam, and I took the subway down to Clark Street, in Brooklyn, and pushed along Smith Street against the wind, passing Pineapple, Orange, and Cranberry streets, walked across the bridge approaches and down toward the river to Grimaldi's, one of the city's handful of must-visit pizzerias.

I hadn't allowed for the customary weekend subway slowdown, and we arrived later than I wanted. Grimaldi's opens at noon on Saturday, but this day, I felt we'd be in good shape, even at twelve thirty. The weather was terrible, and for some blocks we hadn't seen another soul out on the street. We were going to be fine. But as we walked up to the restaurant, I could see a small crush at the door. I struck the umbrella and walked into the restaurant, which was noisy and busy. I was grateful that Sam and I got the second-to-last table for two. I knew the food would be great because the place was full. Full of kindred spirits, I thought—eaters who went out in spite of the weather, or even because of it.

Grimaldi's helpfully details its house rules on the place mat: "* NO SLICES * <u>NO CREDIT CARDS</u> * NO DELIVERY * NO RESERVATIONS * OPEN SEVEN DAYS A WEEK." A history is also provided. In 1933, when he was ten, Patsy Grimaldi started working in his uncle Pasquale Lancieri's pizzeria, the famous Patsy's in East Harlem. Almost fifty years later, Grimaldi opened his own Patsy's on Old Fulton Street in Brooklyn. In 1991, Lancieri's widow sold the original Patsy's to a realty company that began licensing the name "Patsy's" to other restaurants. In 1996, under pressure from the Realtors, the Grimaldis renamed their Patsy's "Patsy Grimaldi's," or Grimaldi's, which is what it says on the awning outside. On the place mat, you can also read that in 2004 Grimaldi's was voted by Zagat's New York's best pizzeria for the sixth year in a row. (In 2005 and 2006, while finishing second to Di Fara, Grimaldi's scored a heady 26 out of 30 for its food. In 2007, Grimaldi's and Di Fara tied for first.)

Any of this, of course, Sam couldn't care less about. Just bring the food fast and make sure it's good. He was happy to be out on another eating trip with Dad, even if we had to swim to our destination. I noticed Grimaldi's had a television in the way back, and I was happy to see it was showing a soccer match. One–nil Grimaldi's. Otherwise, the walls are lined with the requisite reviews and pictures of celebrities, well known and otherwise. The largest picture is, inevitably, of Frank Sinatra. There is also a rendering of Vito Corleone saying, I'M GONNA MAKE YOU A PIZZA YOU CAN'T REFUSE.

Our eighteen-inch (large) **pie with anchovies and pepperoni** on one half came quickly, steaming hot out of the oven. Because it was cooked in a coal oven, the edges of the crust were blackened in places and there were spots of charring on the underside. Compared with other exceptional pizza, there's more tomato than there can be, and some was spread over rather than under the cheese. A pie was delivered to the table to our right and it looked to be redder even than ours. The diners confirmed they'd asked for extra sauce. In fact, the menu says "Extra Crushed Tomato," and it's tomato rather than tomato sauce that you get on these pizzas. The anchovies and pepperoni were sparsely scattered but made up for their scarcity with a strong flavor. The pepperoni was thick and rounded into tiny crispy bowls. After the magma had cooled on the crust, Sam dug in and downed two slices fast. As he tackled the third, I asked him how he liked the pizza. "Man," he said quickly, "this is delicious!"

I easily finished my half of the pie and helped out with the fourth slice from Sam's side. Sam was right—man, it *was* delicious. With my Brooklyn lager and his soda, the bill was twenty-four dollars before tax. In truth we could easily have shared with Sam's sister and mother, who'd remained dry at home. There were a lot of kids in the place, including a baby in a sling, positioned so he was looking up at Dad maneuvering pizza methodically into his own mouth. The kid was getting some good training, so in another five or six years he could be pinching his own slices with the big kids like Sam.

The rain was still coming down in sheets when we left the restaurant. Down at the end of the street, which ends at the river, is the entrance to the heralded River Café, which is rated highly in Zagat's too. Even in the squall, the entryway was inviting. When you're standing down here on the water, the Brooklyn Bridge looms overhead. The beauty of the bridge is a given in New York City, and from this spot right beneath, you're afforded a fine perspective. The quickest way home was across the river, so Sam and I took a river taxi back to Lower Manhattan. At one thirty, the taxi service was calling it a day at the South Street Seaport stop. Even for ten dollars, it was fun to get out on the water when we hadn't expected to. I made a vow to come back to Grimaldi's and to go both ways by boat.

A couple of subway stations that had been open on our way downtown were now closed for some reason, so Sam and I trudged across the Financial District toward a station that was operational. A commercial was being filmed on Wall Street, which was quiet for the weekend. A pen had been set up, and in it was a small herd of cows. The cows stood about in the rain, uninterested. A few of the humans in attendance were speaking into walkie-talkies but most of the people were just getting wet, like the cows. This was, I thought, a pretty odd and amusing scene: a dairy herd on Wall Street. My seven-year-old son, who is, unlike me, a New Yorker born and bred, was completely unfazed.

From Naples, pizza has made its way to every corner of the globe, usually traveling with migrant Italians. It's been adopted by the locals and then adapted to the new environment. Pizza is a world food, like the hamburger (to beef-eating peoples) and Chinese food; even more so perhaps because it is versatile within every cuisine and culture. In the UK, the "Hawaiian" pizza, topped with specks of ham and chunks of canned pineapple, is very popular, allowing sweet-toothed Brits eating their entrée to get a head start on dessert. In Japan you might find an "Idaho" pizza topped with potato, or even potato salad. In Brazil, green peas may feature; in Costa Rica, coconut. With pizza, anything, or everything, goes. That can be the case here, too. The special at the Happy Joe's chain in the Midwest, for example, is Canadian bacon and sauerkraut.

How do we illustrate the global reach of the pizza pie? The Scandinavian chain Peppes operates a restaurant in Hammerfest, in Norway, the world's most northerly town. (The company also opened a restaurant recently in Shanghai.) The world's most southerly town, Ushuaia, on Tierra del Fuego, in Argentina, has at least three pizza parlors, according to the municipal online directory. There are pizza restaurants in Kathmandu. I googled "Timbuktu" and "Pizza," only to turn up restaurants called Timbuktu in Hanover, Maryland, and Palatine, Illinois. I did read that you can get pizza in Bamako, the capital of Mali, the West African nation that includes Timbuktu. Go online and you find a place in Tehran that'll deliver pizza. And so on.

The pizza in these far-flung places has a chance to be at least as good as the majority of the stuff served in this country. It's familiar, so we're contemptuous toward pizza and our expectations of it are extremely low. Most often it's prepared carelessly, with a heavy hand. The crust is thick and bready. Grease collects in pools across the rubbery surface of the cheese. If there's too much sauce, the cheese and your toppings can slide right off when you try to pick up the engorged, soggy slice. If this is a possibility, if you're not confident that you can hold the slice without spillage, then you have to use a knife and fork, which is just wrong. This is what pizza is like most of the time.

Then you go to somewhere like Grimaldi's, or the original Patsy's in

East Harlem, or Totonno's in Coney Island, or Di Fara in Midwood, Brooklyn, or Lombardi's in the Village. You make the pizza pilgrimage up to New Haven, Connecticut, and pay homage at Sally's and Pepe's. (Visitor to New York, you do all this, and you haven't spent a single minute fighting the crowds in the street malls of Midtown Manhattan.) You seek out the thin crusts where you live, if you can find them, and shun the pretenders: the delivered; the stuffed crusts; the "extra mozzarella"; the manifest sins of the thick, bready pie.

 QUICK BITE

Yes, there's a lot of bad pizza around, but there's plenty of the good stuff, too. How do you find it? Zagat's guides are great resources, and voters often elevate pizza parlors high in the standings. Check out Zachary's Chicago Pizza in Oakland, highly rated for pizza and highly rated overall.

We're obsessed with lists. In its *Life* section, *USA Today* prints "Ten Great Places" for various food (collected at www.10greats.usatoday.com). The 2006 pizza list was compiled by Penny Pollack and Jeff Ruby, authors of *Everybody Loves Pizza*, itself a great resource. It included strip-mall-located Punch Neapolitan Pizza in St. Paul, where you can find "the perfect **Margherita**" featuring San Marzano tomatoes and *mozzarella di bufala* flown in from Naples. Also mentioned, the Cheese Board Pizza Collective, a thirty-strong cooperative in Berkeley that's a bakery and pizza joint making one specialty pie a day. If you dare, go online and see what it is today, and see if your mouth doesn't water wildly. How about **mozzarella, yellow onions, roasted red bell peppers, olive tapenade, and feta?**

The common denominator of the aforementioned Grimaldi's pizza and those that follow is that this is the thin-crust variety cooked in a (usually) coal-fired brick oven. These ovens generate extremely high temperatures that quickly cook the pizza to within an inch of being burned. In a terrific passage in *It Must Have Been Something I Ate,* Jeffrey Steingarten attempts to re-create the optimal pizza cooking temperature in a domestic oven. Coal-fired ovens are *hot,* reaching temperatures just shy of that enjoyed on the surface of Venus. The furnace, up to 850°F, superheats the topping and crisps the crust. If you look underneath your thin-crust slice, some areas of the crust will have the characteristic sooty black burn marks.

(Don't try to look under the crust on a regular slice; the topping is liable to slide right off.) Portions of the edge of the crust may well be charred, too. Lower temperatures invite droop, the mortal enemy of thin-crust pizza.

If your pizza restaurant in Manhattan doesn't have a coal-fired oven now, it never will, because an environmental ordinance forbids the construction of new ones. If they want to open a classic coal-fired brick-oven pizza place, restaurateurs can find a location that has one already (like the Patsy's on West Seventy-fourth Street that opened in 1996), or they are obliged to look outside the borough of Manhattan, which is why Grimaldi's opened up in Brooklyn and in Hoboken, New Jersey.

———

In St. Louis, Joe Bonwich has written about Provel cheese more than once. Provel comes with a trademark, so you know it was conjured up under laboratory conditions. The aim, Joe says, was to create a pizza cheese that would bite away cleanly when it was hot, unlike mozzarella, which can trail hot strings behind it when you draw the slice away from your mouth. Perhaps the name derived from a diminutive of provolone and mozzarella. This was more than fifty years ago, and the companies responsible have passed through various hands and into the wide arms of Kraft.

Provel is used by the local Imo's chain of pizzerias, where the pie is cut into squares rather than regular slices. According to the company, Ed Imo, who opened the first Imo's in 1964, laid tile by day and cooked by night. When it came to cutting pizza, force of habit caused him to cut squares, not slices. There are numerous Imo's in and around St. Louis, in Illinois, and a couple in Kansas City, where we can debate the merits of the three characteristics of **St. Louis pizza**: Provel, cracker crust, and square slices.

———

Sam and I headed across town at a fine early-summer lunchtime for Patsy's, where Patsy Grimaldi had learned his trade. One feature of New York pizza is the small number of mentors whose pupils went on to greatness. The original proprietors of John's, in Manhattan, and Totonno's learned their trade at Lombardi's, the city's oldest pizza joint, of which more later.

Patsy's runs much of the block between 117th and 118th streets along First Avenue. At the top end of the block you can get a plain slice to take out (for $1.50), but Sam and I took a seat in the restaurant. The place dates from 1932. The copy of a photograph, browned with age, accompanies a big portrait of late-period Sinatra on the exposed brick wall. In the photograph is a man I was told was Patsy. He's wearing a suit and a no-nonsense look that he gives straight into the camera.

Sam and I ordered a **pie, half with pepperoni.** "Paper thin crust, tomato sauce, grated mozzarella," said the menu. And that's just what you get. Patsy's old coal-fired oven had given the crust its characteristic look: risen slightly here and there and irregularly charred brown and black. And it was thin. There was more sauce than I expected, but still, when Sam and I picked up a slice and pinched it at the edge to eat, the slice sat straight out just as it should, like a divisional pennant at Yankee Stadium on a breezy day.

My meal at Patsy's was probably the first occasion I'd traveled more than fifty yards for a slice. If you're having it for the first time, proper pizza is a true revelation. *This* is pizza. Call the regular stuff something else. It's anti-pizza: soggy, not crisp; heavy, not light; thick, not thin—the antonym of pizza.

At Patsy's, you're left with a pizza wheel to cleave and serve the pie. I cut, and the two of us worked through our pizza steadily. Happy in his work, Sam gave the pizza the thumbs-up. He ate his full share, four slices—half the pie, minus a couple of shards of crust. He also ate the croutons from my Caesar salad and still wanted ice cream, his coda to many meals we eat away from home. Fortunately, Patsy's had no ice cream. This meant I was obliged to order the homemade **Italian cheesecake.** Ricotta cheesecake can be dry, but this was perfect—the eggs prominent, like a flan, yet with a little sharpness and robust cheesiness. Sam went at it hard, and I reluctantly forced down a couple of forkfuls.

Later, Sam and I recounted our lunch to his mom and sister. I talked at length about the pizza and about the restaurant. We'd all have to go, I said. If we were out on Long Island, we could phone in an order from the Triborough Bridge and pick it up on the way home. The crust! The sauce! The cheese! "So," I said to Sam, doing what you're supposed to do with a kid and trying to ask a leading question, "what was your favorite thing about the pizza place today?" "Oh," he said. "I *loved* the cheesecake."

QUICK BITE

Pizza of the deep dish variety is intimately associated, of course, with Chicago. When as a teenager I'd go into London from my English suburban home, I thought the deep dish at the Chicago Pizza Pie Factory in Hanover Square was about the top meal going. Now, *quel horreur,* there is a CPPF in Paris and also one in Madrid. Chicago's Pizzeria Uno has gone farthest in spreading deep dish from the Second City—it has branches in South Korea and the United Arab Emirates. Adam Langer spoke up for Lou Malnati's Pizzeria in Lincolnwood, Illinois, or Pizzeria Due in downtown Chicago. Malnati's has twenty-four locations around Chicago, in case you can't make it to Madrid.

And if you can't make it to Chicago, **Lou Malnati's** will send you their **pizza.** Their Tastes of Chicago service includes Eli's cheesecake, Vienna Beef's hot dogs, and much more, all available in great Windy City combos: 1-800-LOU-TO-GO (568-86-46) / www.tastesof chicago.com.

Once you've decided you want it, how far are you prepared to go for great pizza? If you live in Brooklyn, or, better yet, around Coney Island, the original Totonno's, on Neptune Avenue, isn't an arduous trip. Dedicated pie hounds could jet into Kennedy Airport and head straight down there. But from Manhattan, specially from Morningside Heights, it's a trek. When I told Sam we were going to Coney Island to get some pizza, he was excited about the subway ride down there. But even for this young train lover, the novelty had worn off after eighty minutes.

We'd left home early and arrived around eleven. Online, I read that the restaurant opened at eleven. I also read that opening hours were not set in stone. Sam was hungry, so we headed straight over to Totonno's. The block up Stillwell Avenue to Neptune was unpromising. Past the auto repair shops and an unofficial graveyard for old fairground rides, we found the restaurant. Here it was, small and square, but it was resolutely locked. The guy cleaning the oven came to the door to tell us he was opening at noon. Obviously, when it comes to opening time, it's best to check with the restaurant itself. And note: Totonno's is closed Monday and Tuesday. I'd been planning to come on a Monday, and a long and sorry trip that would have been.

After a visit to Nathan's Famous, Sam and I sat for a while on the quiet Coney Island strand. We watched as a family, each member fully clothed, messed about in the chilly ocean. A man lay on a towel, reading a novel in Russian and eating peaches one after another out of a black plastic bag. The sun came out, and it became too hot to sit, so Sam and I walked over to the Coney Island Aquarium. We didn't know it then, but this was the last time we'd see the white beluga whales before they were moved to the Georgia Aquarium in Atlanta. At two o'clock it was respectably long enough since we'd had our hot dogs to go eat some pizza.

As we had at Patsy's, we ordered a **pie, half with pepperoni.** I took Sam up to the front of the restaurant, where the *pizzaioli* were making the pies. They worked on a wooden surface supported by a sawhorse. Pre-cut mozzarella, small pans of sauce, a can of olive oil, and a large bowl of finely grated cheese were to hand. Onto the dough, a few slices of cheese were arranged; sauce was sparingly ladled on, followed by a fistful of Pecorino Romano cheese and a drizzled dash of oil. We watched our pie being put together and saw it on its way into the oven. When our pizza emerged, it was scorching hot. The Pecorino had baked down hard and the sauce was little more than a memory. The flavor, once the pie had cooled just a little and we could get it, was intense and strong. You can't adequately judge a place on one visit, of course, but this was a different pie from Patsy's and Grimaldi's even if it was recognizably of the same genus.

 QUICK BITE

My friend Bob told me about a decidedly non-thin crust dish he used to enjoy in his native New Jersey: **panzarotti,** fried-dough concoctions with various fillings from pizza sauce and mozzarella onward and not all pizza-related. Something like a fried calzone, said Bob. (The *Larousse Gastronomique* says panzarotti are Corsican rice fritters made for religious festivals. Two different things, obviously.) Bob ate his panzarotti at Franco's in Westmont, New Jersey, but they seem to have originated at Tarantini Panzarotti in nearby Camden. Italian immigrant Pauline Tarantini, who subsequently trademarked the idea, opened the store in 1963. She had learned to make this kind of panzarotti from her mother, back home in Brindisi.

When we left, a young pizzaiola was taking a break in a lawn chair on the sidewalk. She had looked so accomplished making the pies that I was shocked to learn she'd been working there for only four months. There was still years of experience on hand: Cookie, who served us, is the grand-daughter of the founder.

For comparison purposes, I visited one of the Totonno's branches, on the east side of Manhattan. The restaurant on Second Avenue in the Upper East Side is larger and more spruced up than the Brooklyn original. It has a much fuller menu and is generally grander all around. Except that the pizza, though good, and immeasurably better than most Manhattan pizza, just didn't have the excitement or élan I had found in the Coney Island version.

QUICK BITE

What's the best pizza in your city? In Phoenix, chef and writer Gwen Ashley Walters is a booster of the pies at Pizzeria Bianco. "We have James Beard Award winner Chris Bianco, and his pizza would stack up to any that you've tasted in New York. Small place downtown, he mans the wood-burning oven every night. There is usually a one- to two-hour wait for the tiny res-taurant. His pizza is artisan, and he only uses hand-selected ingredients. He makes his own mozzarella and sausage. (The **Sausage and Caramel-ized Onion pizza** is my favorite.) It truly is the best pizza I've ever had. I just can't get in there enough."

A QUESTION FOR DANNY MEYER

What do you suggest we eat?

"Pizza from Sally's or Frank Pepe's in New Haven. Sausage and mushroom is my favorite, but clams and bacon are a close second."

On the same street in New Haven's Little Italy, the Wooster Square area, are two venerable and renowned pizza restaurants: Pepe's, or, as it says on the pizza box, the Original Frank Pepe Pizzeria Napoletana (1925); and Sally's Apizza (1938). On a good day—a very good day—New Haven is but an hour and a half up I-95 from New York City, and there's plenty for gastro-tourists coming in for the day to occupy themselves with. My family made the trip and we started our day at Louis' Lunch, the prototypical burger place. After more burgers and a couple of hours lolling around the green of the Yale campus, we were ready for some pizza.

We parked the car opposite Sally's and walked along Wooster Street to Pepe's at three thirty on what turned out to be a warm early-fall Saturday afternoon. There was a line out the door, as I expected. I was looking forward eagerly to Pepe's famous pizza with fresh clams. But when I went up front to check on the rate of turnover inside, I saw a sign—NO CLAMS. Clams, clams, there were no clams, and apparently there hadn't been for a couple of days.

When we got inside, Pepe's revealed itself to be a fair-sized establishment with two full rooms of booths. There's also an annex next door called The Spot. The oven up front in the main restaurant is huge, and the pizza peels used to take pies out of the oven need to be fifteen feet long or so to reach all the way in back. At least one has been customized, with two poles bound together to ensure the appropriate reach. There's a hook in the ceiling to hang the peels from when they're not being used. Here the art of the cooking must be in precise timekeeping: following the numerous pies that are cooking at one time and knowing when each is ready. There's a fine line between well done and charred to oblivion.

The pies themselves are enormous. Having already hit two burger places, we asked for one pie for the four of us, **an eighteen-inch pie with pepperoni and sausage on one half.** The pie, served sitting on grease-proof paper atop a tray, was huge and irregular and far larger surely than eighteen inches across in any direction. The crust was thicker than that from a quality New York pizzeria (which is fine; we weren't in New York). It was cheesy, featuring the sharp tang of Pecorino Romano, and notable for the sizable chunks of sausage and islands of pepperoni. Funnily enough, the kids didn't really take to it, and Kara was ambivalent, too. But as soon as I stopped trying to compare it with anything, I got down to it and loved the messy, gloppy pie. Pepe's is a great family restaurant. Opposite us a family of five had ordered four whole pies and a gallon of birch beer and was well on its way to demolishing the lot when we left.

We walked out of Pepe's at 4:45, about fifteen minutes before Sally's opened. Kara went down the street to Libby's Italian Pastry Shop to get a chocolate gelato. I went back to check out Sally's and found a line more than thirty strong. I walked back down to Libby's to pick up the family, and by the time we got back to Sally's, the line was gone and everyone was now inside. I figured perhaps the best time to show up here is 5:05. Even though everyone inside will just have been seated, at least you'll be first in line for the second sitting. Kara waited inside for a **small cheese** to go, and I took the kids to the playground next to the restaurant. While waiting, Kara noticed that the large pizza boxes have vents in the corners to let the steam out. The pizza doesn't get soggy that way.

With our pizza, however, we couldn't do the decent thing and eat the pie hot on the way home, or even later that night. The next night, though, we ate the rest of the Pepe's pie we'd brought home, together with the one from Sally's. This was thin, very charred, and piquant. Just grand. Next time we make this trip, we'll reverse the order, or I'll just head up to New Haven one night myself. I'll try to make sure I arrive on Wooster Street at either 4:30 or 5:05 on the nose.

━━━━━━

Dede Wilson, author of *Wedding Cakes You Can Make* and the *Baker's Field Guide* books, makes a vigorous case for Antonio's Pizza in Amherst, Massachusetts. Dede is from New York, so she knows pizza. Now she lives in Amherst and she says Antonio's blows New York pizza out of the water. Like the best places, Antonio's has its quirks. The way Dede describes it, there can be a crush at the counter, so make your mind up quickly and keep moving to the left. Words to live by. As Dede puts it: "Every slice comes with a very crispy crust—no floppy slices here; these crunch when you bite into them. The toppings are varied but used with a very light hand, and the flavors are just right. Even some of the more outrageous combos are pulled off because restraint is employed.

"The **spinach pie** is amazing. Crisp bottom crust, spinach and mushroom filling with just a bit of feta and mozzarella cheese, and then a top crust that you can actually see through. It is a gossamer top layer that adds to this hearty slice. The **Salad Pizza** features artichokes, olives, tomatoes, fresh spinach, roasted red peppers, balsamic vinaigrette, and extra virgin olive oil. They have BBQ Steak Taco, Avocado Quesadilla, Potato with Provolone, Cheddar and Rosemary . . . none of these are heavy.

"I grew up in New York City, and while that pizza has unique style, which is delicious, I have grown to enjoy Antonio's even more. The coal/wood oven flavor is missing, which the New York slices have, but I find the texture of the crust and flavor of the toppings to be superior here in Amherst."

Lombardi's on Spring Street, in the neighborhood that is now called NoLita in Manhattan, bills itself as "America's first pizzeria"—this legend is written on a mirror in the restaurant's front room. (This distinction can be shaved thin, like a Grammy category. Totonno's says it is "the oldest continuously operating pizzeria in the U.S. run by the same family.") Gennaro Lombardi brought pizza to Spring Street in 1897, we read on the menu, and Lombardi's has operated with a restaurant license since 1905, down the street from the current location.

In the century since then, this neighborhood has turned over many times. This is one of my favorite areas to walk round in the city. I especially love the array of pink shutters on the back of the Puck Building on Jersey Street. Walking down Mulberry Street to the pizzeria on Spring, you pass new, expensive stores hard by the old neighborhood businesses: an acupuncturist and a knife grinder; gourmet food shops, high-priced shoe stores, and a funeral parlor. The street follows the wall of the old St. Patrick's Cathedral, New York's premier Catholic house of worship before the new St. Patrick's on Fifth Avenue was opened in 1879. For restaurants, there are the various delights of Ethiopia, Japan, and Australia along the way and, opposite Lombardi's, Rice to Riches, a new eatery that sells nothing but rice pudding.

Sam and I visited Lombardi's on the fourth of our pizza trips. We sat in the dining room recently added to the narrow existing premises. There's less character in the extension, but the pizza comes out of the same oven where you can read LOMBARDI 1905 spelled out in the tile.

I bucked our regular order by getting two different pies. Sam had a small **Gennaro's Original**—fresh mozzarella and San Marzano tomato sauce topped with Pecorino Romano and fresh basil. (The 14-inch small, six-slice pie is $12.50.) I'd been nurturing a hankering for shellfish on my pizza since I missed out at Pepe's. So at Lombardi's I was happy to see the **Fresh Clam Pie**—hand-shucked clams, oregano, fresh garlic, Pecorino Romano cheese, garlic-infused oil, virgin olive oil, pepper, and parsley. (The small is seventeen dollars.) The two pies inflated our bill, but we took almost a whole one home. We didn't have any toppings, but anchovies and pepperoni would have added five bucks. At Lombardi's, value is to be found in bulk toppings because while you pay three dollars for one, you get five for eight dollars.

Sam expressed satisfaction with his lunch, and I knocked down a slice of his so we could compare notes: the now-familiar combination of crunch and chew of the crust, the crushed tomato rather than tomato sauce base, and the subtle richness of the cheese. The fresh basil gave this pizza a piquant little kick, while the Pecorino Romano was spread with a light hand. It was quite subtle and understated. The fresh clam pie, not so much. I mean this in a good way. Cooked clams will bear a lot of seasoning, and I pounded red pepper flakes on each slice of the pizza to test just how much. The texture was very pleasing, dry and chewy, the clams yielding all their briny flavor to extended mastication. A lot of taste sensations tussled for predominance after I took a few bites. The garlic won out. It lingered, not unpleasantly, long into the afternoon.

At last a window of time presented itself and I could make the long trip into Brooklyn to visit Di Fara for a couple of slices of Domenic De Marco's pizza. No longer any kind of neighborhood secret, Di Fara has found its reputation gaining citywide traction by the day. I wanted to eat there to round out my pizza test, but I was also intensely curious about the pie: Could it possibly be as good as advertised?

I had only a limited period to get to Midwood and back, and I needed the New York City subway to deliver me expeditiously. So when I saw the familiar gaggle of frustrated commuters coming up the stairs at my local stop, hailing cabs or running for the bus, I was disheartened. The next nearest train line was running, and I eventually wound up at Avenue J, looking for the pizza parlor. Di Fara isn't grand by any means, but no one who visits cares a whit. There's only one thing to look at—the pie on the shelf behind the counter.

Everyone who walks up to the modest counter takes a peek over to see what Mr. De Marco's just brought out of the oven. But he works at his own pace, so there may not be anything ready just yet, in which case you're going to have to wait awhile. When I arrived, there were a couple of guys standing at the counter where almost all of a square pie steamed away. Mr. De Marco was holding a sheaf of fresh basil and cutting a few leaves onto the slice he'd taken from the pie. I turned to the fridge to pick out a soda, planning to pick up one of the squares and to ask for a slice, which could come whenever. Big mistake—bam!—a guy swooped in and ordered two squares. A second man called through the open window out from the street for a whole pie with sausage and peppers, and suddenly there was nothing for me.

I was thankful to see there was a plain pizza finishing up in the (non-coal) oven. De Marco took it out, and the cheese was bubbling fiercely on the surface of the slightly irregular pie. He ground up some fresh hard cheese in a mill and sprinkled it over the pie, he cut more basil leaves over it, and it was done. I got my two slices and soda (six dollars) and sat down to eat and watch. Mr. De Marco worked methodically as people passed by, asking through the window how he was doing and what was good today. With great economy of movement, he stretched the dough and ladled on the sauce, sprinkled on the oil and shaved the mozzarella over the pie before placing it in the oven. In a few minutes he checked if it was ready by lifting up a corner and peering at the underside. Soon, out it came. Thus has he made pizza for more than forty years.

And, yes, the pizza tasted wonderful. The crust was perilously thin away from the edge, which was hardened into a good crunchy mouthful. The cheeses and tomato blended into one, a supersavory, salty, sharp, and slightly sweet flavor that threw me back to Totonno's. A postcard lists ingredients: buffalo mozzarella from Caserta, which is Mr. De Marco's hometown in Italy; fior de latte, which is cow's-milk mozzarella; Parmigiana Reggiano; tomatoes from Salerno; and Bertolli olive oil. There are potted herbs growing in the window of the restaurant and sprigs of oregano on the counter you can rub onto your pie. The genius is in the simplicity of the ingredients and the perfection of the execution, and I was thankful I had witnessed it firsthand. Sometimes you should save the best till last.

PIZZA SUMMARY

RUN, DON'T WALK, FOR . . .

- Whatever is just out of the oven at Di Fara, in Brooklyn.
- The thinnest thin crust and sharp bite of Pecorino Romano at Totonno's in Brooklyn.
- Go by land or by sea to Grimaldi's in Brooklyn.

- In New Haven, plan two meals: a family-size pie at Pepe's and another one at Sally's, down the street.

IF YOU'VE NEVER TRIED . . .

- If you eat a lot of pizza and have never tried real thin-crust pizza out of a furnacelike oven and then you do, you'll be hard pressed to go back to the other kind.

23

THE DESSERT TROLLEY AND THE END OF THE MEAL

*At least once in the life of every human, whether he be brute or
trembling daffodil, comes a moment of complete gastronomic satisfaction.*
—M. F. K. Fisher, *Serve It Forth* (1937)

If I had to pick a couple of times I felt such extreme contentment I'd
pick the two times I ate dessert I recall with particular fondness. I
wouldn't want to say they're once- or twice-in-a-lifetime experiences, because I hope I have more of these delights to come. I don't characterize
myself as a devoted dessert eater, which is perhaps why these two items
and the circumstances in which I ate them stick in my mind. That and the
fact that I have four servings of one of them waiting in the fridge right
now. Thus situated, it is removed from its original context, but I'm still
sitting pretty.

These two items notwithstanding, a quick survey of the food I
had written about in the manuscript for this book showed me that I was

otherwise woefully deficient in this whole genre, specifically pies and other desserts that come out of the oven. It's not that I don't like sweet stuff; I just don't eat it that often. Perhaps it's something I inherited from certain of my ancestors who'd eat only boiled chicken and vegetables. There's a slight feeling of guilty excess associated with sweet comestibles: don't need 'em. I don't seem to have passed any of this on because my kids have decided that dessert is mandatory with every meal, sometimes even after the main course. My own prejudice had spilled over onto this book, and I needed to rectify it.

A day or so after my realization, my wife, mind-reading again, e-mailed me a link about an upcoming lecture at the 92nd Street Y: "America's Sweet Tooth: The Delicious History of Our Favorite Desserts," by Francine Segan. Sold!

When the evening of the lecture arrived, I enjoyed telling my son I was going out to attend a meeting on dessert. The lecture was great—enjoyable and informative and pitched just right for the mix of food professionals and amateur enthusiasts like me. I may even have had as much fun as my son imagined I would. We also got to try a number of dishes Francine had made, so not only did I go to a meeting about dessert, I also got to eat dessert for dinner.

Francine Segan is a food historian and the author of *The Philosopher's Kitchen*; *Shakespeare's Kitchen*, in which she re-creates recipes from ancient Greece and Rome and from sixteenth- and seventeenth-century England; and also *Movie Menus*. In a ninety-minute lecture, she covered a tremendous amount of ground. She zipped from the settlers to the time of the first American cookbook, *American Cookery*, by Amelia Simmons, published in 1796, with her **Election Cake**, made in quantities suitable for a political rally. (Start with thirty quarts of flour, ten pounds of butter, and fourteen pounds of sugar . . .)

The first dessert we got to try was a nameless settler dish that would have been cooked in a Dutch oven. It was somewhat like a bread pudding or a *pain perdu*, made with eggs, milk, bread, butter, apples, and raisins, and topped with a marmalade laced with bourbon. The body of the pudding was convincingly old-fashioned (you could imagine that this had been made a couple of hundred years ago), but the bourbon marmalade seemed very modern. They made for a terrific combination.

Moving on, we touched on the famous Boston cream pie, which has been around since the mid-1850s. The Parker House Hotel in Boston opened in 1856, and a French chef made a pie, a chocolate cream pie, for the occasion. The dish found immortality as the Boston cream pie. The

Boston cream pie is more of a cake than a pie, but in the middle of the nineteenth century, you would more likely have baked something like this in a pie tin than a cake tin. By the way, the Parker House Hotel also originated Parker House dinner rolls, and both culinary inventions are still available on-site.

Most of us know that the phrase "as American as apple pie" is based on a fallacy—apple pie isn't American at all. Francine Segan reminds us that the apple itself wasn't indigenous to North America and was imported by the English. The first apple orchard in North America was planted in Boston in the 1600s. The classic apple pie, with cinnamon and nutmeg in the filling and a baked crust, can be traced in England at least as far back as 1510, during the reign of Henry VIII.

A common theme in the lecture was how technological advances through history quickly prompted broad changes in eating habits. When icehouses became more common in the eighteenth century, this allowed French-style ice cream with eggs, as popularized by Thomas Jefferson, to take hold. And when affordable iceboxes were introduced in the 1920s, recipes for dishes that "cooked" in the refrigerator became the rage. Francine showed us cookbooks published by GE and Kelvinator, manufacturers of iceboxes, in which each recipe was prepared using your brand-new icebox. And when someone figured out how to produce marshmallows commercially in the 1930s, they became the centerpiece of every new dessert.

Two old-style dishes came up in conversation at the lecture, **charlotte russe** and Nesselrode pie. The former was mentioned as being difficult, if not impossible, to find these days, and the latter as downright impossible. Individual charlotte russes — sponge and cream in little paper cups — people could remember eating round New York in days gone by. The Nesselrode pie was more mysterious.

Mrs. Beeton includes a Nesselrode pudding in her *Book of Household Management*, first published in England in 1861. The pudding, following a recipe of the original French cooking god Marie-Antoine Carême, is an iced custard that begins with forty chestnuts, a pound of sugar, a pint of cream, and twelve egg yolks. Mrs. Beeton also has a charlotte russe, a decadent pudding of a cream filling in a ladyfinger case. In Mrs. Beeton's book, both puddings are part of the third course of a dinner menu suggested by Mrs. Beeton for twelve in February. The third course comes after the meat and before the real desserts and includes Orange Jelly, Clear Jelly, Gateau de Riz, Sea-kale, and Maids of Honor (a kind of tart).

Count Nesselrode was a foreign minister for the tsarist Russian empire in the nineteenth century who died in 1862, the year after Mrs. Beeton's cookbook was published. It's the chestnuts that put the "Nesselrode" in Nesselrode pudding and pie. As food writer Arthur Schwartz, the "Food Maven," notes, for some reason Count Nesselrode was associated with chestnuts and his name was attached to various recipes that included them. The pie used to be made in New York City by Hortense Spier, who ran a restaurant in the 1940s and then a bakery that supplied a lot of New York restaurants. Schwartz says that Nesselrode pie is now extinct.

As for charlotte russes, my friend Deborah learned to make them during a course at Peter Kump's cooking school, but she never had cause to do so professionally in her work as a pastry chef. It is still possible to find the charlotte russe here and there. Leon's Bakery on Knapp Street in Brooklyn makes one in the form of a small sponge cake with whipped cream and a cherry on top. It comes in a paper cup from which you eat the cake. No spoon allowed.

———

What Shall We Eat? prints a very laissez-faire recipe for charlotte russe: "Line the bottom of a mold with Savoy biscuits, or sponge cakes, and fill it with any kind of cream according to taste." Some of the many creams are included in the book's next chapter.

The cookbook includes a lot of desserts, some of which probably don't get made much anymore. College pudding is an amalgam of breadcrumbs, suet, currants, flour, egg, brandy, and nutmeg. For Montagu pudding, mix a half pound of suet, four tablespoons of flour, four eggs, and four tablespoons of milk. Add half a pound of raisins and sugar and boil for four hours, in a pudding basin presumably. Gloucester pudding combines eggs, butter, flour, sugar, and bitter almonds and is "baked in cups." You're on your own entirely with Queen Cake: one pound sugar, one pound butter, fourteen ounces flour, ten eggs, brandy, wine, lemon essence, cinnamon, cloves, and nut-meg. There are no directions.

Another dessert dish the book suggests is called, oddly, German Puffs. Put a half pound of butter into half a pint of milk and heat. When it boils, add a cup of flour and beat. When cold, add six beaten eggs, a half cup of sugar, and grated lemon. "Bake."

———

Francine Segan talked about a couple of desserts with surprise or mystery ingredients. She made some cupcakes using a **Mystery Cake** recipe. The cupcakes were passed round the room. They tasted like most other cupcakes, though not as rich as many. They were somewhat orange in color, which was a big clue. Alas, some show-off had shouted out the answer immediately—the mystery ingredient was revealed as being a can of Campbell's Tomato Soup, which I may never have guessed. I stuck one of the cupcakes in my bag and showed it to my kids when I got home. They were rightly suspicious when I tried to press a piece on them. They had no clue as to what might be in the cake, and were aghast when they found out.

I was encouraged by Francine's lecture to make a **Mock Apple Pie**. There's no mystery here: the recipe uses crushed Ritz crackers instead of apples. I was curious—could doctored Ritz crackers actually taste like apples in a pie? It seemed unlikely. The recipe calls for two *cups* of sugar that's made into a syrup with grated lemon peel and lemon juice to fill a nine-inch pie pan. Needless to say, the result is extraordinarily sweet. The consistency of the filling is quite smooth, and the taste underlying the sugar, once you've got past the blinding glare of the sugar, is of lemon.

I served the pie to some friends at a New Year's Eve party. One said it was like lemon curd; others recognized it for what it was. I actually

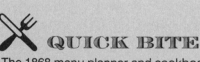

QUICK BITE

The 1868 menu planner and cookbook *What Shall We Eat? A Manual for Housekeepers* includes, as an idea for a dinner in March, something called Winibeg Pudding. "Pound and sift five crackers, and mix with a cup of boiling water, one of sugar, and the juice and peel of a lemon. Bake in a coat." If we can take a coat to be a crust, this sounds very much like a precursor to the classic Mock Apple Pie.

thought it was pretty good, but I had a low level of expectation. I almost made two pies, thinking that one would never be enough for eight adults and nine children, but the one I took along was only half finished. Many of the assembled company had been gracious enough to try a piece, but each had taken just a half-inch sliver. The mock apple pie was created in the tough times of the thirties, so it is perhaps not surprising that a little of it goes a very, very long way.

Francine includes recipes for **Icebox Cake**, Mystery Cake, and Mock Apple Pie in her book *Movie Menus: Recipes for Perfect Meals with Your Favorite Films*. She provides modern versions of old recipes so you can make a meal to accompany your movie. There are stuffed dates for *Gladiator* and Old West Baked Beans, if you have the stomach for them, for *Blazing Saddles*. Mystery Cake and Mock Apple Pie are Depression-era dishes. Francine's recipe for the cake comes from a 1933 issue of *American Cookery Magazine*, and the pie recipe was printed on the side of the Ritz cracker box in the 1930s, when, as Francine says, crackers were practically free but apples cost a penny.

QUICK BITE

Whoopie pies, or gobs, are found in many places throughout Pennsylvania Dutch country. I bought one at Kitchen Kettle Village in Intercourse and took a small nibble before I handed it off to my kids to taste. Needless to say, I never got it back. Firm, rich chocolate cake, creamy white filling. Say no more. There's a Maine recipe for it included in *Eating New England,* by Juliette Rogers and Barbara Radcliffe Rogers. Here's how the pie is described by Juliette Rogers.

A whoopie pie, I learned, is rich chocolate cake packed to travel. The frosting—and it is always a pure white, shortening-based frosting when you buy [whoopie pies] at the market—is conveniently enclosed by cake, so it isn't messy. The cake, in two gigantic, pillowy cookies on either side, should be a moist, dark chocolate brown, and have a good crumb.

The recipe includes **Marshmallow fluff,** which is made in Lynn, Massachusetts.

I had a yen for a piece of real apple pie, so one afternoon in Soho I dropped into Once Upon a Tart, on Sullivan Street. I bought a small **Alsatian Apple Tart** and a cup of coffee and walked out of the store intending to drink the coffee and take the tart home. Alas, the poor tart never made it.

Chef Jerome Audureau, who hails from Avignon, in the south of France, makes beautiful tarts. The store also sells salads, savory tarts, frittatas, and so on. Together with his American partner, Frank Mentesana, Jerome Audureau has written a *Once Upon a Tart* cookbook.

What I ate was a tart, not a pie. The apple was sliced paper thin and lightly glazed. The crust flaked and fell away in my hand (I could have used a plate), and the tart simply bursts with the apple flavor, more so than most pies whose fillings are adulterated in some way. Sheepishly, on my way home, I said to myself that I must remember to buy at least two next time.

One summer treat I look forward to is a piece of **raspberry crumb pie** from Tate's Bakery in Southampton, New York. The crumb is rich and crunchy and soaked in raspberry syrup. If you love raspberries like I do, you cannot fail to appreciate this pie because it tastes as if the very essence of every raspberry you've ever eaten has been captured right here. As I write this, a tremendously strong childhood image flashed into my head, of eating raspberries by the handful straight off the canes on the allotment behind my grandparents' terraced house. When I was five or six, I'd eat raspberries till my hands were red and my belly was packed. Any berry with the slightest tinge of red was fair game. Tate's makes unusual **chocolate chip cookies,** which are thin and very crunchy. Their **strawberry rhubarb pie** is also fabulous. My parents grew rhubarb at the bottom of our garden. (More properly, it grew itself. It was just there.) Stewed and served straight up with sugar—I loved it.

There's no shortage of great pie around the country—what's your favorite? Monisha Primlani also nominates **strawberry rhubarb pie,** this from Arthur Gordon's Irregardless Cafe, in Raleigh, North Carolina. The pie "has been mastered to a bittersweet perfection," she says. The cafe "is a treat in itself . . . the food is creative." The menu changes daily. If you like music with your food, check out the nightly jazz, with dancing on Saturdays.

NANAIMO BARS

Dana Cree says that Nanaimo bars "were often made by my grandmother, as they're one of my father's favorites. They're a chocolate-and-cream layer thing, not a brownie, not even baked. They come from a town in British Columbia called Nanaimo. There they began to surface in ladies' community cookbooks, and in the shops around 1955. I have seen these regional treats as far south as a tiny mountain coffee shop in Mill City, a village on the way to Bend, Oregon. There they sold the original and a peanut butter version, which I had never seen before."

For an account of the Nanaimo bar and the official recipe, as selected by the Canadian city of Nanaimo in 1986, visit the Web site www .nanaimo.ca.

If you look in an old cookbook, there are likely to be large numbers of recipes for pre-freezer desserts: puddings and creams and manges other than blancmange, which no one really eats anymore either. *What Shall We Eat?* is full of these simple, if obsolete, dishes with sweet names:

- Pomme Mange (apples, sugar, water)
- Flemish Cream (cream, brandy, isinglass)
- Rhenish Cream (isinglass, egg yolks, lemons, wine, sugar)
- French Flummery (isinglass, cream, sugar, rose water, orange flower water)
- Bohemian Cream (strawberries, sugar, lemon, isinglass, whipped and molded)
- Snow Cream (cream, egg whites, white wine)

Mrs. Porter's New Southern Cookery Book and Companion for Frugal and Economical Housekeepers, published in Philadelphia in 1871, includes a Jaune (yellow) Mange with egg yolks, lemon juice, and almonds, a blancmange with almonds, and a Jacque Mange made with white wine. *The Settlement Cookbook* features something called a Lalla Rookh Cream, whose characterizing feature is the maraschino cherries you put on top.

Finally, from *Eighteen Colonial Recipes* is "Burnt Cream," from a "Receipt used by the Jefferson Family at Monticello":

Boil two quarts of milk with a large piece of orange peel. To one half a pound of sugar add the yolks of seven eggs and the whites of two. Stir them well together and add two or three handfuls of flour and pour in the boiling milk. Stir all well together and strain it through a sieve and put it on the fire and stir until it thickens. Add one ounce of fresh butter and pour it into a deep dish. Sift powdered sugar over it and glaze it with a hot shovel. Use any flavoring you like.

QUICK BITE

Mrs. Kander also has a recipe for the medicinal-tasting **horehound** candy made with the herb of the same name. Take an ounce of dry horehound and boil it up with a cup and a half of water and a pound and three-quarters of brown sugar. Once it's thickened, pour the mixture into a baking dish, mark off the squares, and let it cool. You can buy horehound candy, but none of the stuff I've tried has been up to much.

CHEESECAKE

Shopping at the uptown Fairway one day, and seduced by an attractive display, I made an impulsive purchase of a **Junior's Cheesecake.** I winced a little at the checkout—the one-and-a-half-pound cheesecake was $18.99, and groaned even more when I got home and saw that I'd purchased a sugar-free low-carb cheesecake, which is made with the sweetener Xylitol. It still packs a dietetic wallop—each serving has 259 calories in it—but this was not "the cheesecake that made Brooklyn great," which is a Junior's slogan, printed, along with pictures of the Brooklyn Bridge, on the box.

Fortunately, a real Junior's cheesecake was served at the New Year's Eve party for which I made my Mock Apple Pie. This pie was much more like it: ultrarich and creamy with just a hint of a crust. It was topped with strawberries, which helped cut the sweetness and cream of the cheesecake. If pressed, I like a good ricotta cheesecake better, but this was good and it redeemed Junior's for me.

Nectarines were named after the nectar consumed by the Olympian gods, and their flavor is widely acknowledged to be, in a word, divine . . . A beautiful ripe

QUICK BITE

While eating a dinner we'd picked up from Joe's Stone Crab in Miami Beach, I kept my eye on the **Key lime pie.** I'd bought a whole pie ($19.95). It came with a can of nondairy whipped product, which I don't think the pie really needs. On inspection, the pie presented as a lovely, smooth yellow disk set in a thick graham cracker crust. Each of the assembled company tucked into a piece, or two. First thing, it smacked tartly of the limes and then the flavor settled toward the general richness of the filling. If you really want to know, the pie box lists the ingredients. In addition to the crackers and limes, there's butter in here, with sugar, egg yolks, and sweetened condensed milk. (Do yourself a favor at least once and get some Key lime pie in you.) The commingling of these fine ingredients helps explain why this is a veritable king—a king among pies.

nectarine makes such pleasurable eating that we serve the best nectarines of midsummer all by themselves with a few raspberries.

—*Alice Waters,* Chez Panisse Fruit *(2002)*

M. F. K. Fisher wrote about eating a slab of chocolate on a frigid Alpine mountainside when she described her eating nirvana. As I read her depiction of the scene, I recalled a far more leisurely meal I had enjoyed a number of years ago and its quite perfect ending—one of my gastronomic moments for sure. I read a page or so more of Fisher, and she quotes Keats describing eating a nectarine—it "melted down my throat like a large beatified Strawberry," he writes—and funnily enough, it was a nectarine I had been thinking of.

Twelve or more years ago, Kara and I drove down Route 1 from San Francisco to Los Angeles with our friends Jean and Paul. An Anglo-Scottish alliance living in London, Jean and Paul are committed food people. I'd sent them all of Waters's Chez Panisse cookbooks, and they made a recipe with quail that I believe involved the purchase of a special de-boning implement. We visited Berkeley on our West Coast trip, and it was natural for us to want to eat at Alice Waters's famous Chez Panisse restaurant.

On a hot day in August we ate lunch at the café. I wish I'd made a note of what we ate first, but I didn't, and that memory is lost. But for dessert, I ordered a **white nectarine,** which was an exotic fruit to me. I remember it came chilled on a plate and tasted like the freshest thing I'd ever eaten. Just a plain white nectarine. It was like I was eating a piece of summer. I savored it as slowly as I could.

Much more recently, I was eating my burger at the Apple Pan in Los Angeles and was thinking ahead to dessert. George Motz told me to be sure to try the Apple Pan banana cream pie. The burgers are good at the Apple Pan, George told me, but don't miss the **banana cream pie.** George knows what he's talking about, so I was primed and ready. I'd been looking forward to my pie all day. I knew the pies were made fresh daily in the restaurant, and as I was eating, I could see through a window to my right fifteen of them sitting on racks, waiting for me.

> ### QUICK BITE
>
> There's one exception to my dessert disinclination in restaurants. I am an absolute sucker for bread pudding. It's on the menu; I'll order it. The most extravagant one I've had recently was the **warm bread pudding with caramelized apples and crème anglaise** at Kate Mantilini in Los Angeles. Layers of sweet, sweet bread, warm apple, and beautiful custard, which is how I think of crème anglaise.

My burger finished, I ordered a piece of pie. The pie is so simple, deriving, the menu says, from a Missouri recipe from 1886. I looked it over when it came. The crust was very thin. The banana custard filling held a deep layer of thickly sliced fruit and the pie was topped with an ungodly amount of whipped cream. I felt tingling physical excitement eating the thing; I can't say why. It is perfect. Sweet but not piercingly so. The thick cream resists the crunch of the crust, and the great big banana flavor bursts right through. That much fresh cream will enhance anything you eat it with, but it takes the other ingredients here to extreme heights.

I took a second piece with me to share with my friend Rick. I'm not blessed with steely self-control as far as snacking is concerned, but the pie somehow made it through a whole night in the fridge without being disturbed. It met its end seconds after Rick picked me up the next morning, polished off by the side of the road in a few joy- and delight-filled seconds. Rick agreed that this was something special.

A few months later I was happy to be able to take my family to the Apple Pan. We ate our burgers at the counter, and then, for just $16.50, I picked up a whole banana cream pie to go. After a couple of ceremonial photos of me and my pie outside the restaurant, we left for home. The ride back to our apartment I could hardly bear. I held the pie on my knees but I was sorely wracked with trepidation the whole journey: Was the pie hot or uncomfortable in any way? Was I holding it level? Was the inside of the box lid pressing down on the cream? We got home fine, and the pie was just as I remembered it. Eating the pie again wasn't quite the same as experiencing it for the first time, but it was close enough.

It was today that we went back to the Apple Pan. So, one more time, this sublime pie, the best thing I've eaten in years, is waiting for me, not ten feet away, in the fridge. Resistance is futile. This time I'm not going to let it stand overnight. So, excuse me, I have to go. I've got some work to do.

THE DESSERT TROLLEY
AND THE END OF THE MEAL SUMMARY

RUN, DON'T WALK, FOR . . .

- **Banana cream pie** from the Apple Pan, in Los Angeles. I don't know why this had such a profound effect on me, but it did.
- **Key lime pie** from Joe's Stone Crab, in Miami Beach.
- Any pie with raspberries.

IF YOU'VE NEVER TRIED . . .

- Make a **mock apple pie**—it's easy (I managed it), it's a surprise, and it's actually edible, in small pieces.
- Finish off your meal with the simplest dessert on the menu—one perfect piece of fresh fruit can be the best exclamation point to the whole meal.

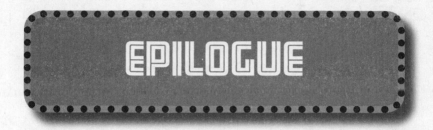

EPILOGUE

I feel like I've only scratched the surface of this enormous subject. Almost every time I mention this book to someone, I hear about something new I want to try or a place I really should have included. Any grievous omissions, please let me know about, so I can refine the 1,001 things with your help. Thank you.

After *Eat This!* had been typeset and proofread and while corrections were being made, my family made a trip to Phoenix, Arizona. Far too late to add new material, but yet. . . . While in Phoenix, it was a blisteringly hot few days (99 degrees in March), we checked out the Roaring Fork restaurant in Scottsdale, so I could try their Big Ass burger. You have to eat at the bar to get one, or have it to go to snack on, as I did. The burger was Big Assed as advertised. On Sam's birthday we celebrated at Cowboy Ciao, also in Scottsdale, and feasted on the unusual and inventive food. My Stuffed Pork Rib Chop was filled with Shropshire blue cheese, served atop a thick slab of ancho bread pudding, smothered in raisin-fig compote, apple jus, and with pan-grilled vegetables on the side to boot. For Sam's birthday desserts, we essayed an assault on the Chocolate–Peanut Butter "Pot Pie" and then the "Cuppa' Red Hot Chocolate (sort of)," but they were too fancy for him. We asked our terrific server what ice cream they had. He'd already scored points by choosing my entrée for me (since I couldn't decide, and he'd offered), and by recommending the Stetson Chopped salad—an odd and surprisingly successful mélange of smoked salmon, arugula, couscous, homemade trail mix, and dried sweet corn—

that you toss yourself. I knew dried sweet corn was discussed in this book, and here was something I'd love to mention and a new trail to follow. Then I heard the ice cream selection: this flavor, that flavor, and *sweet corn*. Sweet corn ice cream! What would that be like? But I had to decline. I'd run out of room.

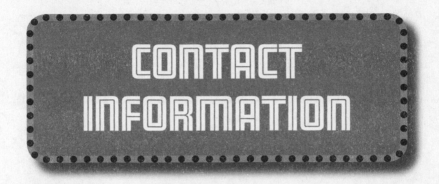

CONTACT INFORMATION

17th Street Bar & Grill, 32 N 17th Street, Murphysboro, IL 62966, 1-618-684-8610

96th Street Steakburgers, 4715 E 96th Street, Indianapolis, IN 46240, 1-317-844-6351 / www.96thstreetsteakburgers.com

AAA South Dakota Pheasant Hunting, 112 S Harmon Drive, Mitchell, SD 57301, 1-605-996-2231 / www.sdpheasanthunting.com

Abalone Farm, PO Box 136, Cayucos, CA 93430, 1-805-995-2495 / www.abalonefarm.com

Absolute Bagels, 2788 Broadway, New York, NY 10025, 1-212-932-2052

Acme Bread, 1 Ferry Building, San Francisco, CA 94105, 1-415-288-2978

Acme Oyster and Seafood House, 724 Iberville Street, New Orleans, LA 70130 and locations, 1-504-525-1160 / www.acmeosyterhouse.com

Ajo Café, 3132 E Ajo Way, Tucson, AZ 85713, 1-520-294-1100

Allie's Donuts Inc., 3661 Quaker Lane, North Kingstown, RI 02852-3006, 1-401-295-8036

Alligator Alley, 1321 E Commercial Boulevard, Oakland Park, FL 33334, 1-954-771-2220 / www.alligatoralleyflorida.com

Allman's, 1299 Jeff Davis Highway, Fredericksburg, VA 22401, 1-540-373-9881

Almar Orchards, 1431 Duffield Road, Flushing, MI 48433, 1-810-659-6568

Al's #1 Italian Beef, 1079 W Taylor Street, Chicago, IL 60607, 1-630-858-9121

Altoona's Original Texas Hot Dogs, 1122 12th Avenue, Altoona, PA 16601, 1-814-942-6381

American Coney Island, 118 W Lafayette, Detroit, MI 48226, 1-313-961-7758 / www.americanconeyisland.com

Anderson Orchard, 369 E Greencastle Road, Mooresville, IN 46158, 1-317-831-4181 / www.andersonorchard.com

Andy's Frozen Custard, 4820 Highway 54, Osage Beach, MO 65065, and locations, 1-573-302-0020 / www.eatandys.com

Andy's Valley Service, 2374 Highway 141, Trout Lake, WA 98650, 1-509-395-2211

Angelo's Coney Island #1, 1816 Davison Road and Franklin Avenue, Flint, MI 48506, 1-810-233-4000 / www.angelosconeyisland.com

Annabelle Candy Co. (Big Hunk), 27211 Industrial Boulevard, Hayward, CA 94545, 1-510-783-2900 / www.annabelle-candy.com

Ann's Chicken Fry House, 4106 NW 39th Street, Oklahoma City, OK 73112, 1-405-943-8915

Anthony-Thomas Factory and Retail Store, 1777 Arlingate Lane, Columbus, OH 43228, and locations, 1-614-272-9221 / www.anthony-thomas.com

Antonio's Pizza, 31 N Pleasant Street, Amherst, MA 01002, 1-413-253-0808

The Apple Pan, 10801 W Pico Boulevard, Los Angeles, CA 90064, 1-310-475-3585 / www.applepan.com

Aquavit, 65 E 55th Street, New York, NY 10022, 1-212-307-7311 / www.aquavit.org

Arctic Circle, 7210 S State Street, Midvale, UT 84047, and branches / www.articcirclerest.com

Arenzville Burgoo Festival (September), Arenzville, IL / www.burgoo.org

Ariccia, The Hotel at Auburn University, 241 S College Street, Auburn, AL 36830, 1-334-844-5140 / www.auhcc.com/ariccia

Arrows Restaurant, Berwick Road, PO Box 803, Ogunquit, ME 03907, 1-207-361-1100 / www.arrowsrestaurant.com

Arthur and Pat's, 239 Ocean Street, Marshfield, MA 02050, 1-781-834-9755

Arthur Bryant's Barbecue, 1727 Brooklyn Avenue, Kansas City, MO 64127, 1-816-231-1123

Artie's Delicatessen, 2290 Broadway, New York, NY 10024, 1-212-579-5959 / www.arties.com

Azalea's Café, 4 Aviles Street, Saint Augustine, FL 32084, 1-904-824-6465

Babbo, 110 Waverley Place, New York, NY 10011, 1-212-777-0303 / www.babbonyc.com

Bar Americain, 152 W 52nd Street, New York, NY 10019, 1-212-265-9700 / www.baramericain.com

Barney Greengrass, 541 Amsterdam Avenue, New York, NY 10024, 1-212-724-4707 / www.barneygreengrass.com

Bartley's Dockside Dining, Western Avenue, Kennebunkport, ME 04046, 1-207-967-5050 / www.bartleys-dockside.com

Bartolino's, 2524 Hampton Avenue, St. Louis, MO 63129, 1-314-644-2266 / www.bartolinosrestaurants.com

Bartolino's South, 5914 S Lindbergh Boulevard, St. Louis, MO 63123, 1-314-487-4545 / www.bartolinosrestaurants.com

Bauder Pharmacy, 3802 Ingersoll Avenue, Des Moines, IA 50312, 1-515-255-1124

Baumgartner's Cheese Store and Tavern, 1023 16th Avenue, Monroe, WI 53566, 1-608-325-6157

Bayona, 430 Dauphine Street, New Orleans, LA 70112, 1-504-525-4455 / www.bayona.com

Bennett's Ice Cream, Farmers Market, 6333 W 3rd Street, Los Angeles, CA 90036, 1-323-939-6786

Ben's Best Deli, 96-40 Queens Boulevard, Rego Park, NY 11374, 1-718-897-1700 / www.bensbest.com

Ben's Chili Bowl, 1213 U Street, NW, Washington, DC 20009, 1-202-667-0909 / www.benschilibowl.com

Berkeley Springs Apple Butter Festival (October), 127 Fairfax Street, Berkeley Springs, WV 25411, 1-800-447-8797 / www.berkeleysprings.com/apple

Big Apple Barbecue Block Party (June), New York City / www.bigapplebbq.org

Big Bob Gibson Bar-B-Q, 1715 6th Avenue SE, Decatur, AL 35601, 1-256-350-6969 / www.bigbobgibsonbbq.com

Big Bob Gibson Bar-B-Q, 2520 Danville Road SW, Decatur, AL 35604, 1-256-360-0404 / www.bigbobgibsonbbq.com

Big Daddy's Rib Shack, 3623 12th Street NE, Washington, DC 20017, 1-202-636-4111

Big Pig Jig (October), Exit 109, Interstate 75, Vienna, GA 31092, 1-229-268-8275 / www.bigpigjig.com

The Bite, 29 Basin Road, Menemsha, MA 02552, 1-508-645-9239 / www.thebitemenemsha.com

Black Bear Restaurant, 10375 Ute Pass Avenue, Green Mountain Falls, CO 80819, 1-719-684-9648 / www.coloradoeats.com/blackbear

Blue Ash Chili Restaurant, 9565 Kenwood Road, Cincinnati, OH 45242, 1-513-984-6107 / www.blueashchili.com

Blue Ribbon, 97 Sullivan Street, New York, NY 10012, 1-212-274-0404 / www.blueribbonrestaurants.com

Blue Smoke, 116 E 27th Street, New York, NY 10016, 1-212-447-7733 / www.bluesmoke.com/blue/index.html

Bobcat Bite, 420 Old Las Vegas Highway, Santa Fe, NM 87505, 1-505-983-5319 / www.bobcatbite.com

Bob's Coffee and Donuts, Farmers Market, 6333 W 3rd Street, #450, Los Angeles, CA 90036, 1-323-933-8929

Bouchon, 6534 Washington Street, Yountville, CA 94599, 1-707-944-8037 / www.frenchlaundry.com

Boudin Bakery, Fisherman's Wharf, 160 Jefferson Street, San Francisco, CA 94133, and locations, 1-415-928-1849 / www.boudinbakery.com

Bragg Farm, Route 14 N, East Montpelier, VT 05651, 1-802-223-5757 / www
.braggfarm.com

Bratfest (Memorial Day), Madison, WI / www.bratfest.com

Briarhurst Manor, 404 Manitou Avenue, Manitou Springs, CO 80829, 1-719-
685-1864 / www.briarhurst.com

Brigantine, 2725 Shelter Island Drive, San Diego, CA 92106, and locations,
1-619-224-2871 / www.brigantine.com

Brooklyn Ice Cream Factory, Fulton Ferry Landing Pier, Brooklyn, NY 11201,
1-718-246-3963

Brother Jimmy's BBQ, 1485 2nd Avenue, New York, NY 10021, 1-212-288-0999
/ www.brotherjimmys.com

The Brown, A Camberley Hotel, 335 West Broadway, Louisville, KY 40202,
1-502-583-1234 / www.brownhotel.com

Brunswick Stew Cook-Off (October), Lawrenceville, VA 23868, 1-434-848-
6773

Buckhorn Exchange, 100 Osage Street, Denver, CO 80204, 1-303-534-9505

The Burger Joint, Le Parker Meridien, 118 W 57th Street, New York, NY
10019, 1-212-245-5000 / www.parkermeridien.com/burger.htm

C & K Barbecue, 4390 Jennings Station Road, St. Louis, MO 63121, 1-314-385-
8100

Café du Monde, 800 Decatur Street, New Orleans, LA 70116-3306, 1-504-581-
2914 / www.cafedumonde.com

Cafe Pasqual's, 121 Don Gaspar Avenue, Santa Fe, NM 87501, 1-505-983-9340 /
www.pasquals.com

Calabria Pork Store, 2338 Arthur Avenue, Bronx, NY 10478, 1-718-367-5145 /
www.arthuravenuebronx.com/latticino.htm

Camellia Grill, 626 S Carrollton Avenue, New Orleans, LA 70118, 1-504-861-
9311

Cape Porpoise Lobster Company, 15 Pier Road, Cape Porpoise, ME 04014,
1-207-967-4268 / www.capeporpoiselobster.com

Caprial's Bistro, 7015 SE Milwaukie Avenue, Portland, OR 97202, 1-503-236-
6457 / www.caprialandjohnskitchen.com

Carl's, 2200 Princess Anne Street, Fredericksburg, VA 22401

Carmine's Seventh Avenue, 1802 E 7th Avenue, Ybor City, FL 33605, 1-813-248-
3834 / www.carminesnyc.com

Carvel, 73 East Montauk Highway, Hampton Bays, NY 11946, and locations,
1-631-728-8145 / www.carvel.com

CASI Terlingua International Chili Championship (November), Terlingua,
TX / www.chili.org

Cato Corner Farm, 178 Cato Corner Road, Colchester, CT 06415, 1-860-537-
3884 / www.catocornerfarm.com

Cattlemen's Steak House, 2458 N Main Street, Fort Worth, TX 76106, 1-817-
624-3945 / www.cattlemenssteakhouse.com

Cattlemen's Steakhouse, 1309 S Agnew, Oklahoma City, OK 73108, 1-405-236-0416 / www.cattlemensrestaurant.com

Cereality Bar and Café, 100 S Wacker, Chicago, IL 60606, 1-312-506-0010 / www.cereality.com

Cereality Bar and Café, 3631 Walnut Street, Philadelphia, PA 19104, 1-215-222-1162 / www.cereality.com

Cereality Bar and Café, Arizona State University, Memorial Union Building, Tempe, AZ 85287, 1-480-242-4743 / www.cereality.com

Cheeseboard Pizza Collective, 1512 Shattuck Avenue, Berkeley, CA 94709, 1-510-549-3055 / www.cheeseboardcollective.coop

Chelo's, 2225 Post Road, Warwick, RI 02886, and locations, 1-401-737-7299 / www.chelos.com

Chelsea Market, 75 9th Avenue, New York, NY 10011 / Individual vendors: www.chelseamarket.com/enter/concourse/contact.html

Cherry Republic, 6026 S Lake Street, Glen Arbor, MI 49636, 1-800-206-6949 / www.cherryrepublic.com

Chez Panisse, 1517 Shattuck Avenue, Berkeley, CA 94709, 1-510-548-5525 / www.chezpanisse.com

Cinnamon Café, 229 N Main Street, Lawrenceville, VA 23868, 1-434-848-2226

City Fish Co., Pike Place Market, 1535 Pike Place, Seattle, WA 98101 / www.cityfish.com/products.htm

Clam Box, 246 High Street, Ipswich, MA 01938, 1-978-356-9707 / www.ipswichma.com/clambox

Clare and Carl's Hot Dog Stand, 8 Tom Miller Road, Plattsburgh, NY 12901, 1-518-562-5378

Claudio's, 111 Main Street, Greenport, NY 11944, 1-631-477-0627 / www.claudios.com

Clayton Farmers Market, Maryland and North Central Avenue, Clayton, MO 63105, 1-636-227-7596

Cokato Corn Carnival, Cokato, MN / www.cokato.mn.us

Cold Hollow Cider Mill, 3600 Waterbury-Stowe Road, Waterbury Center, VT 05677, 1-802-244-8771

The Columbia Restaurant, 2117 E 7th Avenue, Ybor City, FL 33605, and locations, 1-813-248-4961 / www.columbiarestaurant.com

Coney Island Lunch, 515 Lackawanna Avenue, Scranton, PA 18503, 1-570-961-9004 / www.texas-wiener.com

Coney Island Station, 114 S 4th Street, La Crosse, WI 54601, 1-608-782-6314 / www.coneyislandhotdog.com

Cooper's Old Time Pit Bar-B-Q, 505 W Dallas, Llano, TX 78643, 1-325-247-5713 / www.coopersbbq.com

Corky's BBQ and Ribs, 5259 Poplar Avenue, Memphis, TN 38119, and locations, 1-901-685-9744 / www.corkysbbq.com

The Corner Bistro, 331 W 4th Street, New York, NY 10014, 1-212-242-9502

Cotton Bottom Inn, 2820 E 6200 S, Salt Lake City, UT 84121, 1-801-273-9830

Cotton Patch Café, 159 Union, Eutaw, AL 35462, 1-205-372-4235

Country Table Restaurant, 740 E Main Street, Mount Joy, PA 17552, 1-717-653-4745 / www.countrytablerestaurant.com

Court Deli, 96 E 161st Street, Bronx, NY 10451, 1-718-993-1380

Cousin Jenny's Gourmet Cornish Pasties, 129 S Union Street, Traverse City, MI 49684, 1-231-941-7821

Cozy Corner, 745 N Parkway, Memphis, TN 38105, 1-901-527-9158

Crackpot Restaurant, 8102 Loch Raven Boulevard, Towson, MD 21286, 1-410-828-1095 / www.restaurant.com/crackpot.com

Crosstown Bar-B-Q, 202 S Avenue C, Elgin, TX 78621, 1-512-281-5594

Cupcake Café, 545 9th Avenue, New York, NY 10018, and 18 W 18th Street, New York, NY 10011, 1-212-465-1530 / www.cupcakecafe.com

Dahlia Lounge, 2001 4th Avenue, Seattle, WA 98121, 1-206-682-4142 / www.tomdouglas.com/dahlia

Dairy Queen, 1474 Plaza Way, Walla Walla, WA 99362, 1-509-525-6599

Danish Days (July), Viborg, SD / www.danishdays.com

Danish Days Festival (September), Solvang Conference and Visitors Bureau, Solvang, CA 93446, 1-800-468-6765 / www.solvangusa.com

Da Silvano, 260 6th Avenue, New York, NY 10014, 1-212-982-2343 / www.dasilvano.com

DB Bistro, 55 W 44th Street, New York, NY 10036, 1-212-391-2400 / www.danielnyc.com/dbbistro

DeKalb Corn Fest, Inc., 164 E Lincoln Highway, Suite 3, DeKalb, IL 60115, 1-815-748-CORN (2676) / www.cornfest.com

Della Fattoria Downtown, 141 Petaluma Boulevard N, Petaluma, CA 94952, 1-707-763-0173 / www.dellafattoria.com

Del Posto, 85 10th Avenue, New York, NY 10011, 1-212-497-8090 / www.delposto.com

Depot Hotel, 806 4th Street, Napa, CA 94558, 1-707-252-4477 / www.thedepot-napa.com

Di Fara Pizzeria, 1424 Avenue J, Brooklyn, NY 11230, 1-718-258-1367

Dinosaur Bar-B-Que, 646 W 131st Street, New York, NY 10027, and locations, 1-212-694-1777 / www.dinosaurbarbque.com

Dixie Chili, 733 Monmouth Street, Newport, KY 41071, and locations, 1-859-291-5337 / www.dixiechili.com

Domilise's, 5240 Annunciation Street, New Orleans, LA 70115, 1-504-889-9126

Dominguez, 2951 24th Street, San Francisco, CA 94110, 1-415-821-1717

Dooky Chase, 2301 Orleans Avenue, New Orleans, LA 70119, 1-504-821-0600 / www.dookychaserestaurant.com

Down Home Diner, 1039 Reading Terminal Market, Philadelphia, PA 19107, 1-215-627-1955 / www.downhomediner.com

Duran Central Pharmacy, 1815 Central Avenue, Northwest, Albuquerque, NM 87104, 1-505-247-4141

Durgin-Park, 340 Faneuil Hall Market Place, Boston, MA 02109, 1-617-227-2038 / www.durgin-park.com

Duryea's Lobster Deck, 65 Tuthill Road, Montauk, NY 11954, 1-631-668-2410

Dutch Oven Pro, 366 E Brown Farm Lane, Draper, UT 84020, 1-801-319-0778 / www.dutchovenpro.com

Earl's Rib Palace, 4414 W Reno, Oklahoma City, OK 73107, and locations, 1-405-949-1220 / www.earlsribpalace.com

Early Girl Eatery, 8 Wall Street, Asheville, NC 28801, 1-828-259-9292 / www.earlygirleatery.com

East Manor, 4645 Kissena Boulevard, Flushing, NY 11355, 1-718-888-8998

Edelweiss Chocolates, 444 N Canon Drive, Beverly Hills, CA 90210, 1-310-275-0341 / www.edelweisschocolates.com

El Charro, 311 N Court, Tucson, AZ 85701, 1-520-622-1922 / www.elcharrocafe.com

El Guero Canelo, 5201 S 12th Avenue, Tucson, AZ 85706, 1-520-295-9005 / www.elguerocanelo.com

Eli's Vinegar Factory, 431 E 91st Street, New York, NY 10128, 1-212-987-0885 / www.elizabar.com

El Nuevo Frutilandia, 3077 24th Street, San Francisco, CA 94110, 1-415-648-2958

El Pescador Fish Market, 627 Pearl Street, La Jolla, CA 92037, 1-858-456-2526

El Rey de Las Fritas 9343 SW 40th Street, Miami, FL 33165, and locations, 1-305-223-9944

Empress Chili, 8340 Vine Street, Cincinnati, OH 45216, and locations, 1-513-761-5599

Equal Exchange, 50 United Drive, West Bridgewater, MA 02379, 1-774-776-7400 / www.equalexchange.com

Ess-a-Bagel, 359 1st Avenue, New York, NY 10010, 1-212-260-2252 / www.ess-a-bagel.com

Ess-a-Bagel, 831 3rd Avenue, New York, NY 10022, 212-980-1010 / www.ess-a-bagel.com

Eva Restaurant and Wine Bar, 2227 N 56th Street, Seattle, WA 98103, 1-206-633-3538 / www.evarestaurant.com

Exotic Meats, 2245 148th Avenue NE, Bellevue, WA 98007, 1-800-680-4375 / www.exoticmeats.com

Ezell's Fish Camp, 166 Lott's Ferry Road, Butler, AL 36904, 1-205-654-2205

Fairway Market, 2328 12th Avenue, New York, NY 10027, and locations, 1-212-234-3883 / www.fairwaymarket.com

Ferguson's Pub, 2925 Mount Pleasant Street, St. Louis, MO 63111, 1-314-351-1466

Fisherman's Catch Restaurant, 134 Harbor Road, Wells, ME 04090, 1-207-646-8780

Florent, 69 Gansevoort Street, New York, NY 10014, 1-212-989-5779 / www.restaurantflorent.com

Florida Avenue Grill, 1100 Florida Avenue NW, Washington, DC 20009, 1-202-265-1586

Forest Park (Popcorn Festival headquarters), 1018 S John Steele Drive, Brazil, IN 47834, 1-812-448-2307 / www.popcornfest.net

Fore Street, 288 Fore Street, Portland, ME 04101, 1-207-775-2717

The Fort Restaurant, 19192 Highway 8, Morrison, CO 80465, 1-303-697-4771 / www.thefort.com

Four Seas Restaurant, 731 Grant Avenue, San Francisco, CA 94108, 1-415-989-8188 / www.fourseasr.com

Franco's Place, 233 Haddon Avenue, Westmont, NJ 08108, 1-856-854-0771

Frank Pepe Pizzeria Napoletana, 157 Wooster Street, New Haven, CT 06511, 1-203-865-5762

Froelich's Gator Farms, 26256 E Highway 50, Christmas, FL 32709, 1-407-568-5104

The Fry Bread House, 4140 N 7th Avenue, Phoenix, AZ 85013, 1-602-351-2345

Fuller's Old Fashion BBQ, 3201 Roberts Avenue, Lumberton, NC 28306, 1-910-738-8694 / www.fullersbbq.com

Gahm Mi Oak, 43 W 32nd Street, New York, NY 10001, 1-212-695-4113

Gallagher's, 114 W Mill Street, Waterloo, IL 62298-1205, 1-618-939-9933

Garrett's Popcorn Shop, 670 N Michigan Avenue, Chicago, IL 60611, 1-312-944-2630

Gennaro, 665 Amsterdam Avenue, New York, NY 10025, 1-212-665-5348

Geno's Steaks, 1219 S 9th Street, Philadelphia, PA 19147, 1-215-389-0659 / www.genosteaks.com

George's of Galilee, 250 Sand Hill Road, Narragansett, RI 02882, 1-401-783-2306 / www.georgesofgalilee.com

Gethsemani Farms, 3642 Monks Road, Trappist, KY 40051, 1-502-549-3117 / www.gethsemanifarms.org

Ghirardelli Soda Fountain and Chocolate Shop, 801 Lincoln Road, Miami Beach, FL 33139, and branches, 1-305-532-2538 / www.ghirardelli.com

Glier's Goettafest (August), Riverfront Levee, Newport, KY / www.goettafest.com

Gold City Supermarket, 46-31 Kissena Boulevard, Flushing, NY 11355, 1-718-762-6188

Gold Star Chili, 1802 Race Street, Cincinnati, OH 45210, 1-513-241-5461 / www.goldstarchili.com

Graeter's Ice Cream, 41 E 4th Street, Cincinnati, OH 45202, and locations, 1-513-381-0653 / www.graeters.com

Gramercy Tavern, 42 E 20th Street, New York, NY 10003, 1-212-477-0777 / www.gramercytavern.com

Granny's Chocolate Creations, 1035 N McQueen Road, Suite 116, Gilbert, AZ 85233, 1-866-362-CHOC (2642) / www.grannyschocolate.com

Gran-Val Scoop, 233 Granby Road (Route 189), Granville, MA 01034, 1-413-357-6632 / www.gran-valscoop.com

Gray's Grist Mill, Adamsville Road, Adamsville, RI 02801, 1-508-636-6075

The Gun Barrel Steak & Game House, 862 W Broadway, Jackson Hole, WY 83002, 1-307-733-3287 / www.gunbarrel.com

Guss' Pickles, 504 A Central Avenue, Cedarhurst, NY 11516, 800-620 GUSS (4877) / www.gusspickle.com

Guss' Pickles, 85 Orchard Street, New York, NY 10002, 1-516-569-0909

H & H Bagels, 2239 Broadway, New York, NY 10024, 1-212-595-8003 / www.handhbagel.com

H & H Bagels, 639 W 46th Street, New York, NY 10036, 1-212-595-8000 / www.handhbagel.com

H and J McNally's Tavern, 8634 Germantown Avenue, Philadelphia, PA 19118, 1-215-247-9736 / www.mcnallystavern.com

Hadley, Inc., 83-555 Airport Boulevard, Thermal, CA, 1-760-399-5191 (wholesale) / www.hadley.com

Hallo Berlin Juicy Fruit Stand, 54th Street and 5th Avenue, New York, NY, 1-212-947-9008 / www.halloberlinrestaurant.com

Halo Burger, 800 S Saginaw Street, Flint, MI 48502, and locations, 1-810-238-1839 / www.haloburger.com

Hammons Products Company, 105 Hammons Drive, Stockton, MO 85785, 1-888-4BW-NUTS (29-6887) / www.black-walnuts.com

Hamptons Wine and Food Festival (August), 29 Prospect Avenue, Sea Cliff, NY 11579, 1-631-613-3110 / www.hamptonswineandfood.com

Han Bat Restaurant, 53 W 35th Street, New York, NY 10001, 1-212-629-5588

Happy Joe's Pizza and Ice Cream, 2430 Spruce Hills Drive, Bettendorf, IA 52722, and locations, 1-563-359-5457

Harbourside Lobstermania, Water Street, East Greenwich, RI 02818, 1-401-884-6363 / www.harboursideri.com

Hard Times Café, 314 Jefferson Davis Highway, Fredericksburg, VA 22401, and locations, 1-540-899-6555 / www.hardtimes.com

Hatch Chile Festival (Labor Day), 1-505-267-5050 / www.nmchili.com

Haute Chocolate, 9823 Montgomery Road, Cincinnati, OH 45242-6401, 1-513-793-9999

Hershey's Chocolate World, 100 W Hersheypark Drive, Hershey, PA 17033, 1-717-534-4900 / www.hersheys.com/chocolateworld

Higgins Restaurant and Bar, 1239 SW Broadway, Portland, OR 97205, 1-503-222-9070 / www.higgins.citysearch.com

Highland County Maple Festival (March), Highland County Chamber of

Commerce, PO Box 223, Monterey, VA 24465, 1-540-468-2550 / www.high landcounty.org

Hires Big H, 425 S 700 E, Salt Lake City, UT 84102, 1-801-364-4582 / www.hiresbigh.com

Hob Nob Hill, 2271 1st Avenue, San Diego, CA 92101, 1-619-239-8176 / www.hobnobhill.com

Holmquist Hazelnut Orchards, 9821 Holmquist Road, Lynden, WA 98264, 1-360-988-9240 / www.holmquisthazelnuts.com

Hot Dog Johnny's, US Highway 46, Buttzville, NJ 07829, 1-908-453-2882 / www.hotdogjohnny.com

Hot Doug's, 3324 N California, Chicago, IL 60618, 1-773-279-9550

Hot Grill, 669 Lexington Avenue, Clifton, NJ 07011, 1-973-772-6000

The Hungarian Pastry Shop, 1030 Amsterdam Avenue, New York, NY 10025, 1-212-866-4230

ICS World's Championship (October), Omaha, NE / www.chilicookoff.com

Idaho Candy Company (Idaho Spud), PO Box 1217, Boise, ID 83701, 1-800-8-YUMYUM (986986) / www.idahospud.com

Imo's Pizza, 742 S 4th Street, St. Louis, MO 63102, and locations, 1-314-421-4667 / www.imospizza.com

In-N-Out Burger, 3640 Cahuenga Boulevard, Studio City, CA 90068, and locations, 1-800-786-1000 / www.in-and-out.com

International Bar-B-Q Festival (May), PO Box 434, Owensboro, KY 42302, 1-270-926-6938 / www.bbqfest.com

International Burgoo Cook-Off (October), Webster Springs, WV, 1-304-847-7291 / www.websterwv.com

International Dutch Oven Society World Championship Cook-Off, Logan, UT / www.idos.org

International Mustard Day (August), Mount Horeb Mustard Museum, 100 W Main Street, Mount Horeb, WI 53572, 1-800-438-6878 / www.mustardweb.com

International Pickle Day (September), Orchard Street, New York, NY 10002, 1-212-226-9010 / www.LowerEastSideNY.com

International Ramp Cook-Off and Festival (April), Elkins, WV, 1-304-636-2717 / www.randolphcountywv.com

Irregardless Cafe, 901 W Morgan Street, Raleigh, NC 27603, 1-919-833-8898 / www.irregardlesscafe.com

Island Burgers and Shakes, 799 9th Avenue, New York, NY 10019, 1-212-307-7934

Jacques Torres Chocolate, 66 Water Street, Brooklyn, NY 11201, 1-718-875-9772 / www.mrchocolate.com

Jacques Torres Chocolate Haven, 350 Hudson Street, New York, NY 10014, 1-212-414-2462 / www.mrchocolate.com

James Coney Island, 701 Town & Country Boulevard, Houston, TX 77024, 1-713-973-9143 / www.jamesconeyisland.com

Janos and J Bar, 3770 E Sunrise Drive, Tucson, AZ 85718, 1-520-615-6100 / www.janos.com

Jim's Original Hot Dog, 700 W O'Brien Street, Chicago, IL 60607, 1-312-733-7820

Jim's Steaks, 400 South Street, Philadelphia, PA 19147, 1-215-928-1911 / www.jimssteaks.com

Joe's Stone Crab, 11 Washington Avenue, Miami Beach, FL 33139, 1-305-673-4611 / www.joesstonecrab.com

John Cope's Food Products, 156 W Harrisburg Avenue, Rheems, PA 17570, 1-800-745-8211 / www.copefoods.com

Johnsonville Brat Days, Sheboygan, WI (August), 1-920-803-8980 / www.sheboyganjaycees.com

Junior's, 386 Flatbush Avenue Extension, Dekalb Avenue, Brooklyn, NY 11201, 1-718-852-5257 / www.juniorscheesecake.com

Justtomatoes.com, Westley, CA 95387, 1-209-894-5371

Kai, Sheraton Wild Horse Pass Resort, 5594 W Wild Horse Pass Boulevard, Chandler, AZ 85226, 1-602-225-0100 / www.wildhorsepassresort.com

Kate Mantilini, 9101 Wilshire Boulevard, Beverly Hills, CA 90210, 1-310-278-3699

Katz's Delicatessen, 205 E Houston Street, New York, NY 10002, 1-212-254-2246

Kellogg's Cereal City USA, 171 W Michigan Avenue, Battle Creek, MI 49017, 1-800-970-7020 / www.kelloggscerealcity.com

Kelly's, 410 Revere Beach Boulevard, Revere, MA 02151-4705, 1-781-284-9129

Kimball Farm, Route 124, Jaffrey, NH 03452, 1-603-532-5765

Kim Van Restaurant, 2649 Gravois Avenue, St. Louis, MO 63118, 1-314-865-1321

Kirsten Dixon, 2463 Cottonwood Street, Anchorage, AK 99508, 907-274-2710 / www.kirstendixon.com

Kitchen Kettle Village, Route 340, Intercourse, PA 15392, 1-800-732-3538 / www.kitchenkettlevillage.com

Kitchen Kettle Village Rhubarb Festival (May), Route 340, Intercourse, PA 15392, 1-800-732 3538 / www.kitchenkettlevillage.com

Klicker's Strawberry Acres, 106 Strawberry Lane, Walla Walla, WA 99362, 1-509-525-2494

Koegel's Meats (Corporate), 3400 W Bristol Road, Flint, MI 48507 / www.koegelmeats.com

Kohr Bros., Wonderland Pier, Ocean City Boardwalk, North End, Ocean City, NJ 08226, and locations / www.kohrbros.com

Kokkari Estiatorio, 200 Jackson Street, San Francisco, CA 94111, 1-415-981-0983 / www.kokkari.com

Kokomo Cafe, 6333 W 3rd Street, Suite 120, Los Angeles, CA 90036, 1-323-933-0773 / www.kokomocafe.com

Kolache Festival (September), Burleson County Chamber of Commerce, 301 N Main Street, Caldwell, TX 77836, 1-979-567-000 / www.bc/chamber.com

Kolache Shoppe, 113 Burnet Road, Suite 112, Austin, Texas 78757, 1-512-458-5542 / www.kolacheshop.com

Kopp's Frozen Custard Stand, 5373 N Port Washington Road, Milwaukee, WI 53217, and locations, 414-961-2006 / www.kopps.com

K-Paul's Louisiana Kitchen, 416 Chartres Street, New Orleans, LA 70130, 1-504-524-7394 / www.kpauls.com

Kreuz Market, 619 N Colorado Street, Lockhart, TX 78644, 1-512-398-2361

Lafayette Coney Island, 114 W Lafayette, Detroit, MI 48226, 1-313-964-8198

Lake Champlain Chocolates, 750 Pine Street, Burlington, VT 05401, 1-802-864-1808 / www.lakechamplainchocolates.com

Lamb's Grill Café, 169 S Main Street, Salt Lake City, UT 84111, 1-801-364-7166

La Mexicana, 2804 24th Street, San Francisco, CA 94110, 1-415-648-2633

Lancaster Central Market (Tuesday, Friday, Saturday), 23 N Market Street, Lancaster, PA 17603, 1-717-291-4723

La Superica Taco, 622 Milpas Street, Santa Barbara, CA 93103, 1-805-963-4940

La Taqueria, 2889 Mission Street, San Francisco, CA 94110, 1-415-285-7117

Laurey's Catering, 67 Biltmore Avenue, Asheville, NC 28801, 1-828-252-1500 / www.laureysyum.com

La Victoria, 2937 24th Street, San Francisco, CA 94110, 1-415-642-7120

Legal Seafoods, 26 Park Plaza, Boston, MA 02116, 1-617-426-4444 / www.legalseafoods.com

Legal Seafoods, Logan Airport, East Boston, MA 02128, Terminal C Food Court, 1-617-568-2800 / www.legalseafoods.com; Terminal B Food Court, 1-617-568-2811

Leona's Restaurante de Chimayo, Chimayo, NM 87522, 1-505-351-4569

Leonard's Hawaii, 933 Kapahulu Avenue, Honolulu, HI 98616, 1-808-737-5591 / www.leonardshawaii.com

Leon's Pastry Shop, 2137 Knapp Street, Brooklyn, NY 11229, 718-646-9012

Leo's Live Seafood, 4098 Legoe Bay Road, Lummi Island, WA 98262, 1-360-758-7318 / www.leoslive.com

Le Tub, 1100 N Ocean Drive, Hollywood, FL 33019, 1-954-921-9425

Levana Restaurant, 141 W 69th Street, New York, NY 10023, 212-877-8457 / www.levana.com

Lexington Market, 400 W Lexington Street, Baltimore, MD 21201, 1-410-685-6169

Libby's, 98 McBride Avenue, Paterson, NJ 07501, 1-973-278-8718

Libby's Italian Pastry Shop, 139 Wooster Street, New Haven, CT 06511, 1-203-772-0380

Light My Fire, Farmers Market, 6333 W 3rd Street, Los Angeles, CA 90036

Lilly's, 1147 Bardstown Road, Louisville, KY 40204, 1-502-451-0447 / www.lillyslapeche.com

Lobster Roll (Lunch), 1980 Montauk Highway, Napeague, NY 11954, 1-631-267-3740

Locke-Ober, 3 Winterplace, Boston, MA 02108, 1-617-542-1340 / www.lockeober.com

Lombardi's, 32 Spring Street, New York, NY 10012, 1-212-941-7994 / www.lombardispizza.com

Los Panchos Taco Shop, 1595 Pacific Highway, San Diego, CA 92101, and locations, 1-619-232-9233

Louis' Lunch, 261-263 Crown Street, New Haven, CT 06510, 1-203-562-5507 / www.louislunch.com

Lou Malnati's, 6649 N Lincoln Avenue, Lincolnwood, IL 60712, and locations, 1-847-673-0800 / www.loumalnatis.com

LSVN Vegetarian Chili Cook-Off (November), Austin, TX / www.lsvn.org

Lucy's Sweet Surrender, 12516 Buckeye Road, Shaker Heights, OH 44120, 1-216-752-0828 / www.lucyssweetsurrender.com

McClard's Bar-B-Q, 505 Albert Pike, Hot Springs, AR 71901, 1-501-623-9665 / www.mcclards.com

MacFarlane Pheasants Inc., 2821 S US Highway 51, Janesville, WI 53546, 1-608-757-7881 / www.pheasant.com

Magic Fountain, 9825 Main Road, Mattituck, NY 11952, 1-631-298-5225

Magnolia Bakery, 401 Bleecker Street, New York, NY 10014, 1-888-280-1910

Margie's Candies, 1960 N Western Avenue, Chicago, IL 60647, 1-773-384-1035 / www.margiescandies.nv.switchboard.com

Mario's Italian Lemonade, 1068 W Taylor Street, Chicago, IL 60686

Mars' Cheese Castle, 2800 120th Avenue, Kenosha, WI 53144, 1-800-655-6147 / www.marscheese.com

Mary Mac's Tea Room, 224 Ponce de Leon Avenue NE, Atlanta, GA 30308, 1-404-876-1800 / www.marymacs.com

Melissa's/World Variety Produce, PO Box 21127, Los Angeles, CA 90021, 1-800-588-0151 / www.melissas.com

Memphis Championship Barbecue, 1401 S Rainbow Boulevard, Las Vegas, NV 89146, 1-702-254-0520 / www.memphis-bbq.com/locations.html for locations

Memphis in May International Festival (May), 88 Union Avenue, Suite 301, Memphis, TN 38103, 1-901-525-4611 / www.memphisinmay.org

Michigans Plus, 331 Cornelia Street, Plattsburgh, NY 12901, 1-518-561-0537

Mike's Famous Roastbeef and Seafood, 237 Hamilton Street, Saugus, MA 01906, 1-781-233-8260

Milk Pail Farm, 757 Mecox Road, Water Mill, NY 11976, 1-631-537-2565 / www.milkpail.com

Millersport Sweet Corn Festival, Millersport, OH 43046 / www.sweetcornfest.com

Minnestalgia, 41640 State Highway 65, McGregor, MN 55760, 1-218-768-4917 / www.minnestalgia.com

Mondel's Homemade Chocolates, 2913 Broadway, New York, NY 10025, 1-212-864-2111 / www.mondelchocolates.com

Montana Avenue, 6390 E Grant Road, Tucson, AZ 85715, 1-520-298-2020 / www.foxrestaurantconcepts.com

Monterey Fish Market, 1582 Hopkins, Berkeley, CA 94707, 1-510-525-5600 / www.montereyfishmarket.com

Moonlite Bar-B-Q Inn, 2840 W Parrish Avenue, Owensboro, KY 42301, 1-800-322-8989 / www.moonlite.com

Morgan Valley Lamb, PO Box 517, Delta, UT 84624, 1-435-864-4997 / www.morganvalleylamb.com

Morningside Park Farmers Market (Saturdays), 110th Street and Manhattan Avenue, NY, Community Markets, 1-914-923-4837 / www.communitymarkets.biz

Morse Farm, 1168 County Road, Montpelier, VT 05602, 1-800-242-2740 / www.morsefarm.com

Mount Horeb Mustard Museum, 100 W Main Street, Mount Horeb, WI 53572, 1-800-438-6878 / www.mustardweb.com

Mountain Brauhaus, Route 299/Route 44/55, Gardiner, NY 12525, 1-845-255-9766 / www.mountainbrauhaus.com

Mountain Creamery, 33 Central Street, Woodstock, VT 05091, 1-802-457-1715

Mozzicato DePasquale Bakery and Pastry Shop, 329 Franklin Avenue, Hartford, CT 06114, 1-860-296-0426 / www.mozzicatobakery.com

Mr. Broadway Glatt Kosher, 1372 Broadway, New York, NY 10018, 1-212-921-2152 / www.mrbroadwaykosher.com

Murray's Cheese, 254 Bleecker Street, New York, NY 10014, 1-212-243-3289 / www.murrayscheese.com

Myanmar Restaurant, 7810 Lee Highway C, Falls Church, VA 22042, 1-703-289-0013

Myers of Keswick, 634 Hudson Street, New York, NY 10014, 1-212-691-4194 / www.myersofkeswick.com

Myron & Phil's, 3900 W Devon Avenue, Lincolnwood, IL 60712, 1-847-677-6663 / www.myronandphils.com

Namaste Indian Cuisine, 1671 Willow Pass Road, Concord, CA 94520, 1-925-687-7874

Napa Valley Mustard Festival (January–March), Contact: Napa Valley Mustard

Festival, PO Box 3603, Yountville, CA 94599, 1-707-944-1133 / www
.mustardfestival.org

Nathan's Famous, 1310 Surf Avenue, Brooklyn, NY 11224, and locations, 1-718-
946-2202 / www.nathansfamous.com

National Cherry Festival, 109 6th Street, Traverse City, MI 49684, 1-231-947-
4230 / www.cherryfestival.org

Nebraska Czech Festivals, Omaha, Lincoln, Wilber, and Prague / www
.nebraskaczechs.org

Ninfa's, 2704 Navigation Boulevard, Houston, TX 77003, 1-713-228-1175 / www
.mamaninfas.com

Nolechek's Meats, Inc., 104 N Washington Street, Thorp, WI 54771, 1-800-
454-5580 / www.nolechekmeats.com

Norsk Høstfest (October), North Dakota State Fairgrounds, 2005 Burdick
Expressway E, Minot, ND 58702, Contact: Box 1347, Minot, ND 58702,
1-701-852-2368 / www.hostfest.com

Norwill Scandinavian Food, 1400 E Hillsboro Boulevard, #200, Deerfield
Beach, FL 33441, 1-866-598-4506 / www.norwill.com

Oklahoma Czech Festival (October), Yukon, OK 73099, 1-405-206-8142

Olathe Sweet Corn Festival, Olathe, CO 81425, 1-866-363-CORN (2676) or
1-970-323-6006 / www.olathesweetcornfest.com

Old Homestead, 56 9th Avenue, New York, NY 10011, and locations, 1-212-
242-9040 / www.theoldhomesteadsteakhouse.com

Old Town Bar and Restaurant, 45 E 18th Street, New York, NY 10003, 1-212-
529-6732 / www.oldtownbar.com

Olmstead Orchards, 360 Frazer Road, Grandview, WA 98930, 1-877-882-1946 /
www.olmsteadorchards.com

Olvera Street, Olvera Street and Cesar Chavez Avenue, Los Angeles, CA
90012, 1-213-628-1274

Omni Parker House Hotel, 60 School Street, Boston, MA 02108, 1-617-227-
8600 / www.omnihotels.com

Once Upon a Tart, 135 Sullivan Street, New York, NY 10012, 1-212-387-8869 /
www.onceuponatart.com

Opie's Barbecue, 125 Spur 191, Spicewood, TX 78669, 1-830-693-8660

The Original Pantry, 877 S Figueroa Street, Los Angeles, CA 90017, 1-213-972-
9279 / www.pantrycafe.com

Original Rainbow Cone, 9233 S Western Avenue, Chicago, IL 60620, 1-773-
238-7075

Original Terlingua International Championship Chili Cookoff (November),
Terlingua, TX / www.abowlofred.com

Owl Bar & Cafe, 77 US Highway 380, San Antonio, NM 87832, 1-505-835-9946

The Oystercatcher, 901 Grace Street, Coupeville, WA 98239, 1-360-678-0683

Packo's Front Street Restaurant, 1902 Front Street, Toledo, OH 43605, 1-419-
691-6054 / www.tonypackos.com

Pan Lido, 3147 22nd Street, San Francisco, CA 94110, 1-415-282-3350

Parker's Barbecue, 2514 US Highway 301 S, Wilson, NC 27893, 1-252-237-0972

Parker's Maple Barn, 1316 Brookline Road, Mason, NH 03048, 1-603-878-2308 / www.parkersmaplebarn.com

Pat's King of Steaks, 1237 E Passyunk Avenue, Philadelphia, PA 19147, 1-215-468-1546 / www.patskingofsteaks.com

Patsy Grimaldi's Pizzeria, 133 Clinton Street, Hoboken, NJ 07030, 1-201-792-0800

Patsy Grimaldi's Pizzeria, 19 Old Fulton Street, Brooklyn, NY 11201, 1-718-858-4300

Patsy's Pizza, 2287 1st Avenue, New York, NY 10035, 1-212-534-9783 / www.patsyspizzeriany.com

Penn Cove Mussel Festival (March), PO Box 1345, Coupeville, WA, 98239 / www.musselfest.com

Penn Cove Shellfish, PO Box 148, Coupeville, WA 98239, 1-360-678-4803 / www.penncoveshellfish.com

Peter's Sushi Spot, 3337 Fairbanks Road, Anchorage, AK 99503, 1-907-276-5188 / www.peterssushispot.com

Pete's Famous Hot Dogs, 1925 2nd Avenue N, Birmingham, AL 35203, 1-205-252-2905

Pete's Place, 120 SW 8th, Krebs, OK 74554, 1-918-423-2042 / www.petes.org

Philippe, The Original, 1001 North Alameda Street, Los Angeles, CA 90012, 1-213-628-3781 / www.philippes.com

Picco Pizzeria, 316 Magnolia Avenue, Larkspur, CA 94939, 1-415-945-8900

The Pickle Guys, 49 Essex Street, New York, NY 10002, 1-212-656-9739; 1-888-4 PICKLE (742553)

Pike Place Market PDA, 85 Pike Street, Room 500, Seattle, WA 98101, 1-206-682-7453

Pink's Famous Chili Dogs, 709 N La Brea, Los Angeles, CA 90038, 1-323-931-4223 / www.pinkshollywood.com

Pittsburgh Rare, Sheraton Station Square Hotel, 300 W Station Square Drive, Pittsburgh, PA 15219, 1-412-803-3824 / www.pittsburghrare.com

Pizzeria Bianco, 623 E Adams Street, Phoenix, AZ 85004, 1-602-258-8300 / www.pizzeriabianco.com

Pizzeria Due, 619 N Wabash Avenue, Chicago, IL 60611, 1-312-943-2400

Pizzeria Uno, 29 E Ohio Street, Chicago, IL 60611, 1-312-321-1000 / www.unos.com

The Place, 891 Boston Post Road, Guilford, CT 06437, 1-203-453-9276

Pleasant Ridge Chili, 6032 Montgomery Road, Cincinnati, OH 45213, 1-513-531-2365

Prejean's, 3480 I-49, North Lafayette, LA 70507, 1-337-896-3247 / www.prejeans.com

Price Hill Chili, 4920 Glenway Avenue, Cincinnati, OH 45238, 1-513-471-9507

Primanti Brothers Restaurant, 46 18th Street, Pittsburgh, PA 15222, and locations, 1-412-263-2142 / www.primantibros.com

Prime Select Seafoods, PO Box 846, Cordova, AK 99574, 1-907-424-7750 / www.pssifish.com

Primo Hoagies, 6105 New Jersey Avenue, Wildwood Crest, NJ 08260, 1-609-523-6590 / www.primohoagies.com

Punch Neapolitan Pizza, 704 Cleveland Avenue S, St. Paul, MN 55116, 1-651-696-1066

The Purity Ice Cream Company, 700 Cascadilla Street, Ithaca, NY 14850, 1-607-272 1545 / www.purityicecream.com

Quivey's Grove, 6261 Nesbitt Road, Madison, WI 53719, 1-608-273-4900 / www.quiveysgrove.com

Rack & Soul, 2818 Broadway, New York, NY 10025, 1-212-222-4800 / www.rackandsoul.com

Raffetto's, 144 W Houston Street, New York, NY 10012, 1-212-777-1261

The Red Bird, 120 W Front Street 105, Missoula, MT 59801, 1-406-549-2906 / www.redbirdrestaurant.com

Red's Eats, 41 Water Street, Wiscasset, ME 04578, 1-207-882-6128

Restaurant Villegas, 1735 W Grand River Avenue, Okemos, MI 48864, 1-517-347-2080 /www.restaurantvillegas.com

Righteous Urban Barbecue, 208 W 23rd Street, New York, NY 10011, 1-212-524-4300 / www.rubbbq.net

Riverside County Fair and National Date Festival (February), Riverside County, Fairgrounds, 46-350 Arabia Street, Indio, CA 92201, 1-800-811-FAIR (3247) / www.datefest.org

Roaring Fork, 4800 N Scottsdale Road, Scottsdale, AZ 85251, 1-480-947-0795 / www.roaringfork.com

Roast to Go, Grand Central Market, 317 S Broadway, Los Angeles, CA 90013, 1-213-625-1385

Roberts Mayfair Hotel, 806 Saint Charles Street, St. Louis, MO 63101, 1-314-421-2500 / www.wyndham.com/hotels/STLMF/main.wnt

The Rogue Creamery, PO Box 3606, Central Point, OR 97502, 1-541-664-1537 / www.roguegoldcheese.com

Runza Drive-In, 141 S Chestnut Street, Wahoo, NE 68066, and locations, 1-402-443-3560 / www.runza.com

Rutt's Hut, 417 River Road, Clifton, NJ 07014, 1-973-779-8615

Sahara Restaurant, 511 E Edgemont Avenue, Montgomery, AL 36111, 1-334-264-9178

Sally's Apizza, 237 Wooster Street, New Haven, CT 06511, 1-203-624-5271

Salt Lick Barbecue Restaurant, 18300 FM Road 1826, Driftwood, TX 78619, 1-512-858-4959 / www.saltlickbbq.com

Salumi, 309 3rd Avenue S, Seattle, WA 98104, 1-206-621-8772 / www.salumicuredmeats.com

Sam's No. 3, 1500 Curtis Street, Denver, CO 80202, 1-303-534-1927 / www.sams no3.com

Sam's No. 3, 2580 S Havana Street, Aurora, CO 80014, 1-303-751-0347 / www. samsno3.com

Scandinavian Festival in Junction City, Oregon (August) / www.scandinavian festival.com

Scharffen Berger Chocolate Maker, 1 Ferry Building, San Francisco, CA 94105, 1-415-981-9150

Schiller's Liquor Bar, 31 Rivington Street, New York, NY 10002, 1-212-260-4555

The Schmitter, Citizens Bank Park, One Citizens Bank Way, Philadelphia, PA 19148, 1-215-463-6000

Schwabl's Restaurant, 789 Center Road, West Seneca, NY 14224, 1-716-674-9821

Semifreddi, 3084 Claremont Avenue, Berkeley, CA 94705, 1-510-596-9942

Servatii Pastry Shop & Deli, 3888 Virginia Avenue, Cincinnati, OH 45227, 1-513-271-5040

Shadeau Breads, 1336 Main Street, Cincinnati, OH 45202, 1-513-665-9270

Shake Shack, Madison Square Park, New York, NY 10010, 1-212-889-6600 / www.shakeshacknyc.com

The Shed, 113½ E Palace Avenue, Santa Fe, NM 87501, 1-505-982-9030 / www. sfshed.com

Shelton Oyster Fest (October), Contact: Shelton Skookum Rotary Club Foundation, PO Box 849, Shelton, WA 98584, 1-800-576-2021

Shooting Star Saloon, 7350 E 200 S, Huntsville, UT 84317, 1-801-745-2002 / www.ogdencvb.org/shootstar.html

ShopNatural, 350 S Toole Avenue, Tucson, AZ 85701, 1-520-884-0745 / www .shopnatural.com

Shorty's Saloon, 576 9th Avenue, NY 10036, 1-212-967-3055

Showcase of Citrus, 5010 US Highway 27, Clermont, FL 34711, 1-352-394-4377 / www.showcaseofcitrus.com

Sifers Candy Company, 5112 Merriam Drive, Merriam, KS 66203 / www.valo milk.com

Skyline Chili, 1007 Vine Street, Cincinnati, OH 45202, and locations, 1-513-721-4715 / www.skylinechili.com

Slightly North of Broad, 192 E Bay Street, Charleston, SC 29401, 1-843-723-3424 / www.slightlynorthofbroad.net

Smoki O's, 1545 N Broadway, St. Louis, MO 63102, 1-314-621-8180

Snake Creek Grill, 650 W 100 S, Heber City, UT 84032, 1-435-654-2133 / www .snakecreekgrill.com

Solly's Grille, 4629 N Port Washington Road, Milwaukee, WI 53212, 1-414-332-8808

Solvang Restaurant, 1672 Copenhagen Drive, Solvang, CA, 93463, 1-805-688-4645 / www.solvangrestaurant.com

Sonny Bryan's Smokehouse, 2202 Inwood Road, Dallas, TX 75235, and locations, 1-214-357-7120 / www.sonnybryans.com

South Kingstown Farmers Market, University of Rhode Island, Route 138, Kingstown, RI 02881, 1-401-789-1388

Southside Market & BBQ, 1212 Highway 290 E, Elgin, TX 78621, 1-512-285-3407 / www.southsidemarket.com

Spiedie Fest and Balloon Rally (August), PO Box 275, Westview Station, Binghamton, NY 13905, 1 607 765 6604 / www.spiediefest.com

Squire House Restaurant, 632 S Main Street, Emporia, VA 23847, 1-434-634-0046

Standard Candy Company, 715 Massman Drive, Nashville, TN 37210, 1-615-889-6360

Stone Haus Farm Bed and Breakfast/Hodecker's Celery Farm, 360 S Esbenshade Road, Manheim, PA 17545, 1-717-653-8444 / www.stonehausfarm bnb.com

Sundae School, 210 Main Street, East Orleans, MA 026436, 1-508-255-5473

Sun Prairie Sweet Corn Festival, Angell Park, Sun Prairie, WI 53590, 1-608-837-4547 / www.sunprairiechamber.com

Suomi Restaurant, 54 Huron Street, Houghton, MI 49931, 1-906-482-3220

Sushi Nozawa, 11288 Ventura Boulevard, Studio City, CA 91604, 1-818-508-7017

Sweatman's BBQ, 2113 Highway 15 N, St. George, SC 29477, 1-843-563-7574

Sweet Energy, 195 Acorn Lane, Colchester, VT 05446, 1-800-979-3380 / www.sweetenergy.com

Tarantini Panzarotti, 349 Marlton Avenue, Camden, NJ 08105, 1-856-966-5725

Tate's Bake Shop, 43 N Sea Road, Southampton, NY 11968, 1-631-283-9830 / www.tatesbakeshop.com

Taylor Café, 101 N Main Street, Taylor, TX 76574, 1-512-352-2828

Taylor's Automatic Refresher, 1 Ferry Plaza, San Francisco, CA 94105, 1-866-328-3663 / www.taylorsrefresher.com

Taylor's Automatic Refresher, 933 Main Street, St. Helena, CA 94574, 1-707-963-3486 / www.taylorsrefresher.com

Taylor Shellfish Farms, Inc., Headquarters and Store, 130 SE Lynch Road, Shelton, WA 98584, 1-360-426-6178 / www.taylorshellfishfarms.com

Tears of Joy Hot Sauce Shop, 618 E 6th Street, Austin, TX 78701, 1-512-499-0766 / www.tearsofjoysauces.com

Ted Drewe's Frozen Custard, 4224 S Grand Boulevard, St. Louis, MO 63111, 1-314-352-7376 / www.teddrewes.com

Ted Drewe's Frozen Custard, 6726 Chippewa, St. Louis, MO 63109, 1-314-481-2652 / www.teddrewes.com

Ted's Restaurant, 1044 Broad Street, Meriden, CT 06450, 1-203-237-6660 / www.steamedcheeseburger.com

Testicle Festival (August), Rock Creek Lodge, 7 Rock Creek Road, Clinton, MT 59825, 1-406-825-4868 / www.testyfesty.com

Texas Hot Wieners, 101 58th Street, Altoona, TX 16602, 1-814-942-9992

Todoroff's, 1200 W Parnall Road, Jackson, MI 49201, and locations, 1-517-841-1000 / www.todoroffs.com

Tolbert's Restaurant, 423 Main Street, Grapevine, TX 76051, 1-817-421-4888

Tomasita's Santa Fe Station, 500 S Guadalupe, Santa Fe, NM 87501, 1-505-983-5721

Tommy DiNic's, Reading Terminal Market, 12th and Arch streets, Philadelphia, PA, 19107, 1-215-923-6175

Tony Jr.'s, 118 S 18th Street, Philadelphia, PA 19103, 1-215-568-4630 / www .tonylukes.com

Tony Luke's Beef and Beer Sports Bar, 26 E Oregon Avenue, Philadelphia, PA 19148, 1-215-465-1901 / www.tonylukes.com

Totonno's, 1544 2nd Avenue, New York, NY 10028, 1-212-327-2800 / www .totonnos.com

Totonno's Pizzeria Napolitano, 1524 Neptune Avenue, Brooklyn, NY 11224, 1-718-372-8606 / www.totonnos.com

Tristan, 55 N Market Street, Charleston, SC 29401, 1-843-534-2155 / www.tri standining.com

Ubon's Restaurant, 1029 Highway 51, Madison, MS 39110, 1-601-607-3322

Ubon's Restaurant, 801 N Jerry Clower Boulevard, Yazoo City, MS 39194, 1-662-716-7100

Ukrop's Super Markets, 2001 Maywill Street, Suite 100, Richmond, VA 23230, 1-804-340-3004 / www.ukrops.com for store locator

Union Grill, 413 S Craig Street, Pittsburgh, PA 15213, 1-412-681-8620

University of Missouri Chestnut Roast (October), New Franklin, MO / www .centerforagroforestry.org

Urban Organic, 240 6th Street, Brooklyn, NY 11215, 1-718-499-4321 / www .urbanorganic.net

Vaccaro's Italian Pastry Shop, 222 Albemarle Street, Baltimore, MD 21202, 1-410-685-4905 / www.vaccarospastry.com

Valentino's Pizza, 3457 Holdrege Street, Lincoln, NE 68503, and locations, 1-402-467-3611 / www.valentinos.com

Varsity Drive-In, 61 North Avenue NW, Atlanta, GA 30308, 1-404-881-1706 / www.thevarsity.com

Veniero's Pasticceria & Caffé, 342 E 11th Street, New York, NY 10003, 1-212-674-7070 / www.venierospastry.com

Versailles Restaurant and Bakery, 3555 SW 8th Street, Miami, FL 33135, 1-305-444-0240; 1-305-445-7614

Veselka, 144 2nd Avenue, New York, NY 10003, 1-212-228-9682 / www
.veselka.com

Walters Hot Dogs, 937 Palmer Avenue, Mamaroneck, NY 10543 / www.walters
hotdogs.com

Watershed, 406 W Ponce De Leon Avenue, Decatur, GA 30030, 1-404-378-
4900 / www.watershedrestaurant.com

Wayside Restaurant & Bakery, Route 302, Montpelier, VT 05602, 1-802-223-
6611

Weaver D's, 1016 E Broad Street, Athens, GA 30601, 1-706-353-7797

West Point Sweet Corn Festival, West Point, IA 52656, 1-319-837-6313 / www
.westpointcornfestival.com

West Side Market (Monday, Wednesday, Friday, Saturday), 1925 W 25th Street,
Cleveland, OH 44113, 1-216-579-0634 / www.westsidemarket.com

White House Sub Shop, 2301 Arctic Avenue, Atlantic City, NJ 08401, 1-609-
345-1564

Whole Foods Market, 6350 W 3rd Street, Los Angeles, CA 90036, and locations, 1-323-964-6800 / www.wholefoodsmarket.com

Whole Hog Café, 2516 Cantrell Road, Little Rock, AR 72202, and locations,
1-501-664-5025 / www.wholehogcafe.com

Wickham's Fruit Farm, Main Road, Cutchogue, NY 11935, 1-631-734-6441 /
www.wickhamsfruitfarm.com

Wiener's Circle, 2622 N Clark Street, Chicago, IL 60614, 1-773-477-7444

Wild Edibles, Grand Central Market, Grand Central Terminal, New York, NY
10017, 1-212-687-4255 / www.wildedibles.com

Wildwood Restaurant and Bar, 1221 NW 21st Avenue, Portland, OR 97209,
1-503-248-9663 / www.wildwoodrestaurant.com

Willows Inn, 2579 W Shore Drive, Lummi Island, WA 98262, 1-360-758-2620 /
www.willows-inn.com

Wilmington Banana Split Festival (June), Wilmington, OH / www.bananasplit
festival.com

Wilson's Holy Smoke BBQ, 1851 Post Road, Fairfield, CT 06824, 1-203-319-
7427

Winstead's, 1200 Main Street, Kansas City, MO 64105-2122, and locations,
1-816-221-3339 / www.winsteadskc.com

Wolfy's, 2734 W Peterson Avenue, Chicago, IL 60659, 1-773-743-0207

Woodman's, 121 Main Street, Essex, MA 01929, 1-978-768-6057 / www.wood
mans.com

Yankee Doodle Coffee and Sandwich Shop, 258 Elm Street, New Haven, CT
06511, 1-203-865-1074 / www.thedoodle.com/index.html

Yankee Pier, 286 Magnolia Avenue, Larkspur, CA 94939, 1-415-924-7676 / www
.yankeepier.com

Yeh's Bakery, 5725 Main Street, Flushing, NY 11355, 1-718-939-1688

Yonah Schimmel Knish Bakery, 137 E Houston Street, New York, NY 10003, 1-212-477-2858 / www.knishery.com

Zachary's Chicago Pizza, 5801 College Avenue, Oakland, CA 94618, 1-510-655-6385 / www.zacharys.com

Zanzibar's Coffee Adventure, 2723 Ingersoll Avenue, Des Moines, IA 50312, 1-515-244-7694 / www.zanzibarscoffee.com

Zellwood Sweet Corn Festival, 4253 W Ponkan Road, Zellwood, FL 32798, 1-407-886-0014 / www.zellwoodcornfestival.com

Zia's, 5256 Wilson Avenue, St. Louis, MO 63110, 1-314-776-0020 / www.zias.com

Zippy's Restaurant, 1450 Ala Moana Boulevard, Honolulu, HI 96814, and locations, 1-808-973-0870 / www.zippys.com

Zip's Café, 1036 Delta Avenue, Cincinnati, OH 45208, 1-513-871-9876 / www.zipscafe.com

AMERICA'S STATE FAIRS

Note that not every fair is a state fair as such. Alabama has not had a state fair since 2001, but there is the "North Alabama State Fair" in Muscle Shoals. Also, fairs have a greater or lesser connection to the state administration. Web sites are usually (but not universally) informative. Some contact addresses for fairs are different from the physical address of the fairgrounds. Most fairs provide a way of getting in touch by e-mail. The month cited is generally the month in which the fair is held.

Alabama: September, North Alabama State Fair, 65 Sports Plex Drive, Muscle Shoals, AL 35662, 1-256-383-3247 / www.northalabamastatefair.org

Alaska: August/September, Alaska State Fair, 2075 Glenn Highway, Palmer, AK 99645, 1-907-745-4827 / www.alaskastatefair.org

Arizona: October–November, 1826 W McDowell Road, Phoenix, AZ 85007, 1-602-252-6771 / www.azstatefair.com

Arkansas: October, Arkansas State Fairgrounds, 2401 W Roosevelt Road, Little Rock, AR 72206; Contact: 2600 Howard Street, Little Rock, AR 72206, 1-501-372-8341 / www.arkansasstatefair.com

California: August–September, Cal Expo, 1600 Exposition Boulevard, Sacramento, CA 95815, 1-916-263-FAIR (3247); 1-877-CAL-EXPO (225-3976) / www.bigfun.org

Colorado: August–September, 1001 Beulah Avenue, Pueblo, CO 81004; Contact: 1-800-876-4567; 1-719-561-8484 / www.coloradostatefair.com

Connecticut: July, Connecticut Agricultural Fair, Fairgrounds, Route 63, Goshen, CT 06756, 1-860-491-3628 / www.ctagriculturalfair.org

Delaware: July, Delaware State Fair, Routes 316 and 13, Harrington, DE 19952;

Contact: Delaware State Fair, Inc., Dupont Highway, PO Box 28, Harrington, DE 19952-0028, 1-302-398-3269 / www.delawarestatefair.com

Florida: February, Florida State Fairgrounds, 4800 Highway 301 N, Tampa, FL 33610, 1-813-621-7821; 1-800-345-FAIR (3247); Contact: Florida State Fairgrounds, PO Box 11766, Tampa, FL 33680, 1-813-621-7821; 1-800-345-FAIR (3247)

Georgia: September–October, Macon City Park, Macon, GA 31201; Contact: PO Box 4105, Macon, GA 31208, 1-478-746-7184 / www.georgiastatefair.com

Hawaii: May–June, 50th State Fair, Aloha Stadium, 99-500 Salt Lake Boulevard, Honolulu, HI 96818, 1-808-682-5767 / www.ekfernandez.com/fair_carnival01.html

Idaho: September, Eastern Idaho State Fair, PO Box 250, Blackfoot, ID 83221, 1-208-785-2480 / www.idaho-state-fair.com

Illinois: August, Illinois State Fairgrounds, 801 Sangamon Avenue, Springfield, IL 62706; Contact: Emmerson Building, 801 Sangamon Avenue, State Fairgrounds, PO Box 19427, Springfield, Illinois 62794, 1-217-782-6661 / www.agr.state.il.us/isf

Indiana: August, State Fairgrounds, 1202 E 38th Street, Indianapolis, IN 46205, 1-317-927-7535 / www.in.gov/statefair

Iowa: August, E 30th Street and E University Avenue, Des Moines, IA 50317; Contact: Iowa State Fair, PO Box 57130, Des Moines, IA 50317-0003, 1-515-262-3111 / www.iowastatefair.com

Kansas: September, Kansas State Fair, 2000 N Poplar Street, Hutchinson, KS 67502, 1-620-669-3600 / www.kansasstatefair.com

Kentucky: August, Kentucky Exposition Center, 937 Philips Lane, Louisville, KY 40209; Contact: PO Box 37130, Louisville, KY 40233, 1-502-367-5002 / www.kystatefair.org

Louisiana: October–November, State Fair of Louisiana, 3701 Hudson Avenue, Shreveport, LA 71109, 1-318-635-1361 / www.statefairoflouisiana.com

Maine: July–August, Bangor State Fair, 100 Dutton Street, Bangor, ME 04401, 1-207-947-5555 / www.bangorstatefair.com

Maryland: August–September, 2200 York Road, Timonium, MD 21093; Contact: Maryland State Fair and Agriculture Society, Inc., PO Box 188, Timonium, MD 21094-0188, 1-410-252-0200 / www.bcpl.net/-mdstfair

Massachusetts: September, Eastern States Exposition ("The Big E"), 1305 Memorial Avenue, West Springfield, MA 01089, 1-413-737-2443 / www.thebige.com

Michigan: August, Michigan State Fairgrounds and Exposition Center, 1120 W State Fair Avenue, Detroit, MI 48203, 1-313-369-8250/54 / www.michigan.gov/mistatefair

Minnesota: August–September, 1265 N Snelling Avenue, St. Paul, MN 55108, 1-651-288-4400 / www.mnstatefair.org

Mississippi: October, Mississippi Coliseum, and Fair Grounds, 1207 Mississippi Street, Jackson, MS 39202; Contact: Mississippi State Fair Commission, PO Box 892, Jackson, MS 39205, 1-601-961-4000 / www.msfair.net

Missouri: August, Missouri State Fair, 2503 W 16th Street, Sedalia, MO 65301; Contact: 1-800-422-FAIR (3247); 1-660-827-8150 / www.mostatefair.com

Montana: July–August, Montana ExpoPark, 400 3rd Street NW, Great Falls, MT 59404; Contact: Montana State Fair, 400 3rd Street NW, Great Falls, MT 59404, 1-406-727-8900 / www.montanastatefair.com

Nebraska: August–September, 1800 State Fair Park Drive, Lincoln, NE 68508; Contact: PO Box 81223, Lincoln, NE 68501, 1-402-474-5371 / www.statefair .org

Nevada: August, Reno Livestock Event Center, 1350 N Wells Avenue, Reno, NV 89512, 1-775-688-5767 / www.nvstatefair.com

New Hampshire: Hopkinton State Fair, 392 Kearsarge Avenue, Contoocook, NH 03229, 1-603-746-4191 / www.hsfair.org

New Jersey: August, Sussex County Fairgrounds, 37 Plains Road, Augusta, NJ 07822; Contact: New Jersey State Fair, PO Box 2456, Branchville, NJ 07826, 1-973-948-5500 / www.newjerseystatefair.org

New Mexico: September, New Mexico State Fair, Expo New Mexico, 300 San Pedro Boulevard NE, Albuquerque, NM 87108; Contact: PO Box 8546, Albuquerque, NM 87198, 1-505-265-1791 / www.exponm.com

New York: August/September, 581 State Fair Boulevard, Syracuse, NY 13209, 1-800-475-FAIR (3247); 1-315-487-7711 / www.nysfair.org

North Carolina: October, 1025 Blue Ridge Boulevard, Raleigh, NC 27607, 1-919-821-7400 / www.ncfair.org

North Dakota: July, North Dakota State Fair, 2005 Burdick Expressway E, Minot, ND 58702; Contact: North Dakota State Fair, PO Box 1796, Minot, ND 58702, 1-701-857-7620 / www.ndstatefair.com

Ohio: August, The Ohio Expo Center and State Fair, 717 E 17th Avenue, Columbus, Ohio 43211, 1-888-OHO-EXPO (646-3976) / www.ohioexpo center.com

Oklahoma: September, Oklahoma State Fair Arena, 333 Gordon Cooper Boulevard, Oklahoma City, OK 73107; Contact: Oklahoma State Fair Office, 500 Land Rush Street, Oklahoma City, OK 73107, 1-405-948-6700 / www .okstatefair.com

Oregon: July–August, Oregon State Fair and Expo Center, 2330 17th Street NE, Salem, OR 97303-3201, 1-503-947-3247 / www.oregonstatefair.org

Pennsylvania: May–June, Philadelphia Park Racetrack, Street Road, Bensalem, PA 19020, 1-215-525-1789 / www.pennsylvaniafair.com

Rhode Island: August, Washington County Fair, Richmond Townhouse Road, Richmond, RI 02891 / www.washingtoncountyfair-ri.com

South Carolina: October, 1200 Rosewood Drive, Columbia, SC 29201; Contact: South Carolina State Fair, PO Box 393, Columbia, SC 29202, 1-803-799-3387 / www.scstatefair.org

South Dakota: August–September, South Dakota State Fair, 890 3rd Street SW, Huron, SD 57350, 1-800-529-0900 / www.sdstatefair.com

Tennessee: September, Tennessee State Fairgrounds, 625 Smith Avenue, Nashville, TN 37203; Contact: Tennessee State Fair, PO Box 40208, Nashville, TN 37204, 1-615-862-8980 / www.tennesseestatefair.org

Texas: September–October, Fair Park, 1200 S 2nd Avenue, Dallas, TX 75210-1012; Contact: PO Box 159090, Dallas, TX 75315, 1-214-670-8400 / www.bigtex.com; www.fairpark.org

Utah: September, 155 North 1000 West, Salt Lake City, UT 84116, 1-801-538-8400 / www.utah-state-fair.com

Vermont: August–September, The Vermont State Fair, 175 S Main Street, Rutland, VT 05701, 1-802-775-5200 / www.vermontstatefair.net

Virginia: September–October, State Fair of Virginia, Richmond Raceway Complex, 600 E Laburnum Avenue, Richmond, VA 23222; Contact: PO Box 26805, Richmond, VA 23261, 1-804-569-3200 / www.statefair.com/site.asp

Washington: Evergreen State Fair in Monroe (including Puyallup Fair) / www.wastatefairs.com/fairdates.htm

West Virginia: August, State Fair of West Virginia, 107 W Fair Street, Lewisburg, WV 24901 / www.wvstatefair.com

Wisconsin: August, Wisconsin State Fair Park, 640 S 84th Street, West Allis, WI 53214; Contact: 640 S 84th Street, West Allis, WI 53214, 1-414-266-7000 / www.wsfp.state.wi.us

Wyoming: August, Wyoming State Fair and Rodeo, 400 W Center, Douglas, WY 82633; Contact: 400 W Center, PO Drawer 10, Douglas, WY 82633, 1-307-358-23398 / www.wystatefair.com

SUGGESTIONS FOR FURTHER READING

These are some of the tasty books referred to in this book:

Aidells, Bruce. *Bruce Aidells's Complete Book of Pork*. New York: Morrow Cookbooks, 2004.

———. *Bruce Aidell's Complete Sausage Book*. Berkeley, Calif.: Ten Speed Press, 2000.

Allegra, Antonia. *Napa Valley: The Ultimate Winery Guide*, 4th ed. San Francisco: Chronicle Books, 2004.

Almond, Steve. *Candyfreak*. New York: Harcourt, 2004.

Arnold, Sam. *Eating Up the Santa Fe Trail*. Golden, Colo.: Fulcrum Publishing, 2001.

Beard, James. *James Beard's American Cookery*. Boston: Little, Brown, 1972.

Beeton, Mrs. *Mrs. Beeton's Book of Household Management*. New York: Oxford World's Classics, 2000.

Calta, Marialisa. *Barbarians at the Plate: Taming and Feeding the Modern Family*. New York: Perigee, 2005.

Carville, James. *Stickin'*. New York: Simon & Schuster, 2000.

Cather, Willa. *O Pioneers!* New York: Signet Classics, 2004.

Child, Julia, and Jacques Pépin. *Jacques and Julia Cooking at Home*. New York: Knopf, 1988.

Colwin, Laurie. *Home Cooking*. New York: Knopf, 1988.

Connelly, Michael. *The Black Ice*. New York: Warner Books, 2003.

Coolidge, Dane. *Arizona Cowboys*. New York: Dutton, 1938.

Corr, Anne Quinn. *The Seasons of Central Pennsylvania*. University Park: Pennsylvania State University Press, 2000.

Dekura, Hideo, Brigid Treloar, and Ryuichi Yoshii. *The Complete Book of Sushi*. North Clarendon, Vt.: Tuttle Publishing, 2004.

Dent, Huntley. *The Feast of Santa Fe*. New York: Simon & Schuster, 1985.

Dixon, Kirsten. *Riversong Lodge Cookbook*. Portland, Ore.: Alaska Northwest Books, 2002.

———. *The Winterlake Lodge Cookbook*. Portland, Ore.: Alaska Northwest Books, 1993.

Duggan, Tara. *The Working Cook: Fast and Fresh Meals for Busy People*. San Francisco: San Francisco Chronicle Books, 2006.

Dupree, Nathalie. *Nathalie Dupree's Southern Memories*. Athens: University of Georgia Press, 2004.

———. *New Southern Cooking*. Athens: University of Georgia Press, 2004.

Duyff, Roberta Lawson. *365 Days of Healthy Eating from the American Dietetic Association*. Hoboken, N.J.: John Wiley & Sons, 2003.

———. *The American Dietetic Association Complete Food and Nutrition Guide*. Hoboken, N.J.: John Wiley & Sons, 2002.

Edge, John T. *Hamburgers and Fries*. New York: G. P. Putnam's Sons, 2005.

Engel, Alison, and Margaret Engel. *Food Finds*. 3rd ed. New York: Morrow, 2000.

Eugenides, Jeffrey. *Middlesex*. New York: Farrar, Straus & Giroux, 2002.

Farmer, Fannie. *The Boston Cooking-School Cook Book*. 100th anniversary edition. New York: Knopf, 1996.

Fernández-Armesto, Felipe. *Near a Thousand Tables*. New York: The Free Press, 2002.

Fisher, M. F. K. *Consider the Oyster*. New York: North Point Press, 1988.

———. *How to Cook a Wolf*. New York: North Point Press, 1988.

———. *Serve It Forth*. New York: North Point Press, 2002.

Fitzgibbon, Theodora. *A Taste of Ireland*. North Pomfret, Vt.: Trafalgar Books, 1995.

Garvin, Alexander. *The American City: What Works, What Doesn't*. New York: McGraw-Hill, 2002.

Hearn, Lafcadio. *La Cuisine Creole*. New Orleans: F. F. Hausell, 1903.

Heller, Joseph. *Catch-22*. New York: Simon & Schuster, 1961.

Hesser, Amanda. *Cooking for Mr. Latte*. New York: W. W. Norton, 2004.

How We Cook in Tennessee. Jackson, Tenn.: Silver Thimble Society of the First Baptist Church, 1906.

Jenkins, Steven. *The Cheese Primer*. New York: Workman, 1996.

Jewett, Sarah Orne. *The Country of the Pointed Firs*. New York: Library of America, 1994.

Joachim, David. *A Man, a Can, a Plan*. Emmaus, Pa.: Rodale Press, 2002.

———. *The Tailgater's Cookbook*. New York: Broadway, 2005.

Johnson, Ronald. *The American Table*. New York: Fireside Books, 1991.

Joyce, James. *Ulysses*. New York: Modern Library, 1992.

Kagel, Katherine. *Cafe Pasqual's Cookbook*. San Francisco: Chronicle Books, 1993.

Kander, Lizzie. *The Settlement Cookbook*. Milwaukee, Wisc.: The Settlement Cook Book Co., 1921.

Kaminsky, Peter. *Pig Perfect*. New York: Hyperion, 2005.

Kirschenbaum, Lévana. *Levana's Table: Kosher Cooking for Everyone*. New York: Stewart, Tabori & Chang, 2002.

Kuralt, Charles. *Charles Kuralt's America*. New York: Putnam, 1995.

Kurlansky, Mark. *The Big Oyster: History on the Half-Shell*. New York: Ballantine Books, 2006.

———. *Salt*. New York: Penguin, 2003.

Langer, Adam. *Crossing California*. New York: Riverhead Books, 2004.

———. *The Washington Story*. New York: Riverhead Books, 2006.

———. *Larousse Gastronomique*. New York: Crown, 1988.

Lewis, Alfred Henry. *The Sunset Trail*. Whitefish, Mont.: Kessinger Publishing, 2005.

Liebling, A. J. *Between Meals*. New York: Modern Library, 1995.

McCullough, David. *Truman*. New York: Simon & Schuster, 1992.

Melville, Herman. *Moby-Dick*. New York: Penguin Classics, 2002.

Mentesana, Frank, and Jerome Audureau. *Once Upon a Tart*. New York: Knopf, 2003.

Morton, Julia. *Fruits of Warm Climates*. Boynton Beach, Fla.: Florida Flair Books, 1987.

Norris, Frank. *McTeague*. New York: Modern Library, 1996.

Oliver, Jamie. *Jamie's Dinners*. New York: Hyperion, 2004.

Orcutt, Georgia, and John Margolies. *Cooking USA*. San Francisco, Calif.: Chronicle Books, 2004.

Parker, Robert B. *Cold Service*. New York: Berkley, 2006.

Pellegrino, Frank. *Rao's Cookbook*. New York: Random House, 1998.

Pinner, Patty. *Sweets: A Collection of Soul Food Desserts and Memories*. Berkeley, Calif.: Ten Speed Press, 2006.

Pollack, Penny, and Jeff Ruby. *Everybody Loves Pizza*. Cincinnati, Ohio: Emmis Books, 2005.

Porter, Mrs. M. E. *Mrs. Porter's New Southern Cookery Book and Companion for Frugal and Economical Housekeepers*. Philadelphia: John E. Potter & Co., 1871.

Rhett, Blanche S. *200 Years of Charleston Cooking*. New York: Harrison Smith and Robert Haas, 1930.

Rodgers, Rick. *The Baker's Dozen Cookbook*. New York: William Morrow, 2001.

Rogers, Juliette, and Barbara Radcliffe Rogers. *Eating New England*. Woodstock, Vt.: The Countryman Press, 2002.

Rommelmann, Nancy. *Everything You Pretend to Know About Food*. New York: Penguin Books, 1998.

Roosevelt, Theodore. *Hunting Trips of a Ranchman and the Wilderness Hunter.* New York: Modern Library, 1996.

Root, Waverly, and Richard de Rochemont. *Eating in America.* New York: The Ecco Press, 1981.

Rosengarten, David. *It's All American Food.* New York: Little, Brown, 2005.

Schlosser, Eric. *Fast Food Nation.* New York: Houghton Mifflin, 2001.

Scott, Natalie, and Caroline Merrick Jones. *Gourmet's Guide to New Orleans.* New Orleans: Scott and Jones, 1933.

Scottoline, Lisa. *Killer Smile.* New York: HarperCollins, 2004.

Segan, Francine. *Movie Menus.* New York: Villard Books, 2004.

———. *The Philosopher's Kitchen.* New York: Random House, 2004.

———. *Shakespeare's Kitchen.* New York: Random House, 2003.

Shapiro, Laura. *Perfection Salad.* New York: Farrar, Straus & Giroux, 1986.

Siegelman, Stephen. *The Marshall Field's Cookbook.* Book Kitchen, 2006.

Sokolov, Raymond. *Fading Feast.* Jaffrey, N.H.: Nonpareil Books, 1998.

———. *Why We Eat What We Eat.* New York: Touchstone, 2002.

Steinbeck, John. *Cannery Row.* New York: Penguin Books, 1983.

Steingarten, Jeffrey. *It Must Have Been Something I Ate.* New York: Knopf, 2002.

———. *The Man Who Ate Everything.* New York: Knopf, 1987.

Tolbert, Francis X. *A Bowl of Red.* Garden City, N.Y.: Doubleday & Co., 1966.

Trillin, Calvin. *American Fried.* New York: Doubleday, 1974.

Twain, Mark. *Life on the Mississippi.* New York: Penguin Classics, 1985.

Volland, Susan. *Cooking for Mr. Right.* New York: New American Library, 2005.

———. *Love and Meatballs.* New York: New American Library, 2004.

Warren, Ann, and Joan Lilly. *Cupcake Café Cookbook.* New York: Doubleday, 1998.

Waters, Alice. *Chez Panisse Fruit.* New York: HarperCollins, 2002.

———. *Chez Panisse Menu Cookbook.* New York: Random House, 1982.

Weaver, Dexter. *Automatic Y'all.* Athens, Ga.: Hill Street Press, 1999.

Weir, Joanne. *From Tapas to Meze.* Berkeley, Calif.: Ten Speed Press, 2004.

———. *Weir Cooking in the City.* New York: Simon & Schuster, 2004.

What Shall We Eat?: A Manual for Housekeepers. New York: G. P. Putnam's Sons, 1868.

Wheeler, Clementine, ed. *Greenwich Village Gourmet.* New York: The Bryan Publications, 1949.

Wilcox, Estelle Wood. *Buckeye Cookery.* Minneapolis, Minn.: Buckeye Publishing Company, 1880.

Wister, Owen. *Lady Baltimore.* Nashville: J. S. Sanders, 1992.

———. *The Virginian.* New York: Signet Classics, 2002.

Wolfert, Paula. *The Cooking of Southwest France.* Hoboken, N.J.: John Wiley & Sons, 2003.

———. *The Slow Mediterranean Kitchen.* Hoboken, N.J.: John Wiley & Sons, 2003.

ACKNOWLEDGMENTS

Reading long and fulsome acknowledgments is a little like looking at some-one else's mail. I got a lot of help with this book, and I'll try to be brief and save the longer expressions of gratitude for another place. But I must thank my wife, Kara Welsh, for the idea and the constant encouragement. And thanks to my pizza buddy Sam and to Lindsay, who were always happy to try new things. At HarperCollins, my editor, David Roth-Ey, was always thoughtful and on the money. Thanks also to Jeanette Perez, Gregory Kulik, Jenna Dolan, Jamie Kerner-Scott, Kolt Beringer, Carrie Kania, and Michael Morrison. My agent, Laura Dail, was wonderful throughout, thank you. And Lisa Ekus, thank you for going so far out of your way to help.

Thank you so much to all my friends for eating with me. Bud Kliment matched gastronomic nouse with textual acuity. Many thanks also to Rick Mandler, Bob Magee, and Paula Wong, Ivan Held, Will Frears, Jason Pugatch, Buzz Welsh, Craig and Heather Welsh, Doug Welsh, Jessica Jonap, and Michael Levinson, Jean McNicol, and Paul Taylor.

The first food expert I called, Hsiao-Ching Chou, was extremely kind. She said food people tend to be effusive and so it proved. Thanks to Steve Almond for his substantial contribution. And thanks to Molly Abraham, Bruce Aidells, Antonia Allegra, Kathy Allen, Diane Arne, Sam Arnold, Clen Atchley, Allison Beadle, Pam Becker, John Birdsall, Ron Blasingame, Joe Bonwich, Joe Broom, Linda Carucci, James Carville, Chef Bobo, Bryan Bracewell, Cathy Burch, Anne Burke, Shannon Byrne, Julia Caldwell, Kenny Callaghan, Rick Callendar, Marialisa Calta, Mark Calvino, Pam Campbell, Linda Carucci, Dale Carson, Nicole Starr Castillo, Kristen Cook, David Corey, Erik Cosselmon, Anne Quinn Corr, Dana Cree, Thomas Crone, Delores Custer, Jerilyn DeBoer, Paul Dentrone, Peter and

Florence DeRose, Carole DeSanti, Mike Davis, Kirsten Dixon, Brandi Dobbins, Brooke Dojny, Sean Dougherty, Katelyn Doyle, Marjorie Drucker, Tara Duggan, Nathalie Dupree, Roberta Duyff, Bonnie Eckre, Jonathan Eig, George Emerich, Carol Fenster, Barbara Fenzl, Michael Feigenbaum, Michael Flamini, Gary Flinn, Marlo Fogelman, Bethany Fong, William Ford, Jennifer Fragleasso, Cynthia Frank, Sam Frears, Edwin Froelich, Nina Froes, Jamie Gillmor, Joline Glenn, Kari Greenfield, Kurt Groetsch, Ann and Peter Haigh, Kate Hanzalik, Teresa Nielsen Hayden, Meredith Halpern, and David Must, Barb Hill, Jason Homa, Maria Hunt, Sheila Jackman, Steven Jenkins, David Joachim, Lawrence Johnson, Cassie Jones, Terri Kalish, David Kamen, Paula Katz, Robert Kennedy, John Kessler, Siritrang Khalsa, Lévana Kirschenbaum, Lisa Kovitz, Sandy Krebs, Deborah Kwan, Beverly Lancaster-Hyde, Kristen Laney, Adam Langer, Jeff Lassen, C. Lindquist, Gordie and Kaye Little, Chris Lyons, Carolyn McLemore, Robin McMillan, Kat Macaraeg, Sean Maguire, Ellen Malloy, Laurey Masterton, Victor Matthews, Danny Meyer, Nancy Meyer, Mike Mills, Ed Mitchell, T. C. Mitchell, Doug Moe, Merle Moore, Kelly Moss, George Motz, Linda Murray, Megan Newman, Deirdre O'Hearn and Richard Eckerstrom, Lynne Olver, Georgia Orcutt, Louise Owens, Iggy Palacios, Juanita Panlener, Rick Pascocello, Bob Pastorio, Valerie Phillips, Patty Pinner, Heidi Posnien, Caprial Prence, Joe Prichard, Monisha Primlani, Kathleen Purvis, David Remillard, Karen Rivara, Gary Roark, Paula Rocco, Maria Rodriguez, Kathryn Ross, David Roth, Gary Schatsky, Jake Scherrer, James Scherzi, Holly Schmidt, Denise Schwartz, Rick Sebak, Francine Segan, Merv and Angie Shenk, Sara Silvia, Riley Starks, Sheryl Stebbins, Evan Stein, Kathy Stephenson, Chuck Stokes, Dick Stubbs, Joe Surak, Nadya Swedan, Ellen Sweets, Bryant Tenorio, Ruth Thomas, Jane Tobler, Jacques Torres, Amy Traverso, Amy Treadwell, Andy Van Laar, Eric Villegas, Susan Volland, Diana von Glahn, Otis Walker, Gwen Walters, Joanne Weir, Kelly Welsh, Dan Weissman, Prudence Wickham, Janos Wilder, Dede Wilson, Paula Wolfert, Seana Wood, and Madlen Zahir.

To everyone I mention here, and to anyone who helped in any way, goes the credit for the ideas and the information. Any faults in executing their leads are down to me.

SUBJECT INDEX

REGIONAL INDEX